ORAL PATHOLOGY

THIRD EDITION

ORAL PATHOLOGY

THIRD EDITION

JOHN L. GIUNTA, B.S., D.M.D., M.S., F.A.C.D.

Professor of Oral Pathology
Tufts University School of Dental Medicine
Staff Associate in Oral Pathology
Forsyth School of Dental Hygiene
Lecturer on Oral Pathology
Harvard School of Dental Medicine
Boston, Massachusetts
Diplomate, American Board of Oral Pathology
Diplomate, American Board of Oral Medicine

1989
B.C. Decker Inc • Toronto • Philadelphia

Publisher

B.C. Decker Inc
3228 South Service Road
Burlington, Ontario L7N 3H8

B.C. Decker Inc
320 Walnut Street
Suite 400
Philadelphia, Pennsylvania 19106

Sales and Distribution

United States and Puerto Rico
The C.V. Mosby Company
11830 Westline Industrial Drive
Saint Louis, Missouri 63146

Canada
McAinsh & Co. Ltd.
2760 Old Leslie Street
Willowdale, Ontario M2K 2X5

Australia
McGraw-Hill Book Company Australia Pty. Ltd.
4 Barcoo Street
Roseville East 2069
New South Wales, Australia

Brazil
Editora McGraw-Hill do Brasil, Ltda.
rua Tabapua, 1.105, Itaim-Bibi
Sao Paulo, S.P. Brasil

Colombia
Interamericana/McGraw-Hill de Colombia, S.A.
Apartado Aereo 81078
Bogota, D.E. Colombia

Europe
McGraw-Hill Book Company GmbH
Lademannbogen 136
D-2000 Hamburg 63
West Germany

France
MEDSI/McGraw-Hill
6, avenue Daniel Lesueur
75007 Paris, France

Hong Kong and China
McGraw-Hill Book Company
Suite 618, Ocean Centre
5 Canton Road
Tsimshatsui, Kowloon
Hong Kong

India
Tata McGraw-Hill Publishing Company, Ltd.
12/4 Asaf Ali Road, 3rd Floor
New Delhi 110002, India

Indonesia
P.O. Box 122/JAT
Jakarta, 1300 Indonesia

Italy
McGraw-Hill Libri Italia, s.r.l.
Piazza Emilia, 5
I-20129 Milano MI
Italy

Japan
Igaku-Shoin Ltd.
Tokyo International P.O. Box 5063
1-28-36 Hongo, Bunkyo-ku,
Tokyo 113, Japan

Korea
C.P.O. Box 10583
Seoul, Korea

Malaysia
No. 8 Jalan SS 7/6B
Kelana Jaya
47301 Petaling Jaya
Selangor, Malaysia

Mexico
Interamericana/McGraw-Hill de Mexico, S.A. de C.V.
Cedro 512, Colonia Atlampa
(Apartado Postal 26370)
06450 Mexico, D.F., Mexico

New Zealand
McGraw-Hill Book Co. New Zealand Ltd.
5 Joval Place, Wiri
Manukau City, New Zealand

Panama
Editorial McGraw-Hill Latinoamericana, S.A.
Apartado Postal 2036
Zona Libre de Colon
Colon, Republica de Panama

Portugal
Editora McGraw-Hill de Portugal, Ltda.
Rua Rosa Damasceno 11A–B
1900 Lisboa, Portugal

South Africa
Libriger Book Distributors
Warehouse Number 8
"Die Ou Looiery"
Tannery Road
Hamilton, Bloemfontein 9300

Southeast Asia
McGraw-Hill Book Co.
348 Jalan Boon Lay
Jurong, Singapore 2261

Spain
McGraw-Hill/Interamericana de Espana, S.A.
Manuel Ferrero, 13
28020 Madrid, Spain

Taiwan
P.O. Box 87–601
Taipei, Taiwan

Thailand
632/5 Phaholyothin Road
Sapan Kwai
Bangkok 10400
Thailand

United Kingdom, Middle East and Africa
McGraw-Hill Book Company (U.K.) Ltd.
Shoppenhangers Road
Maidenhead, Berkshire
SL6 2QL England

Venezuela
McGraw-Hill/Interamericana, C.A.
2da. calle Bello Monte
(entre avenida Casanova y Sabana Grande)
Apartado Aereo 50785
Caracas 1050, Venezuela

NOTICE

The authors and publisher have made every effort to ensure that the patient care recommended herein, including choice of drugs and drug dosages, is in accord with the accepted standards and practice at the time of publication. However, since research and regulation constantly change clinical standards, the reader is urged to check the product information sheet included in the package of each drug, which includes recommended doses, warnings, and contraindications. This is particularly important with new or infrequently used drugs.

Oral Pathology
Third Edition

ISBN 1–55664–184–2

Library of Congress catalog card number: 84–2258

10 9 8 7 6 5 4

To my brother,
Paul David,
an astute dental hygienist
and caring soul
and to my cherished wife,
Jocelyn,
and children, Nonna and Weston

Preface to the Second Edition

The first edition of *Oral Pathology* was part of a multimodule series of textbooks, *Dental Auxiliary Practice: Biological Basis and Clinical Application.* The original module was written according to the outline and contents of the course on pathology (oral pathology) given at the Forsyth School of Dental Hygiene. Augmented by numerous illustrations, it attempted to give factual, concise information on clinical examination, some principles of pathology, inflammation and healing, developmental entities, microbial diseases, white and pigmented lesions, benign and malignant oral diseases, and some of the oral manifestations of systemic diseases.

This second edition has been updated and corrected in all chapters. (Embarrassing errors in the first edition were noted and corrected.) Several new entities have been included. Intentionally, the common conditions and diseases along with normal findings have been emphasized. Utilizing oral diseases, principles of pathology have been introduced. Purposely this is not a complete text on oral pathology. Numerous excellent textbooks cover the subject in greater depth and emphasis. Consequently, there is limited coverage of areas such as developmental syndromes, bone diseases, and many other systemic diseases. There is no coverage of periodontal disease since it demands a separate course and text. Nonetheless, it is hoped that this textbook will again be serviceable as an aid in understanding some basic pathology and oral pathology and as a review for those wanting a short, well-illustrated, and practical book.

I would like to acknowledge my teachers, Dr. Gerald Shklar and Dr. Edmund Cataldo, for their education and the opportunity to do this work and for some of the photographs; Dr. Esther Wilkins-Gallagher for her encouragement and her persuasion for me to add my own artwork; Dr. Gayanne DeVry for the original artwork; and Mary Hayward for her conscientious secretarial help. In addition, I thank Drs. Kabani and Plourde for the photographs on amelogenesis imperfecta.

Preface to the Third Edition

In response to many requests, this third edition has been greatly expanded. Consequently, it is an enlarged and completely updated book with many new features. In particular, there is more on general pathology, although the book is not intended to supplant a general pathology textbook.

In Chapter 1 there is updating on the examination sequence, with the wearing of gloves to emphasize infection control, and there is more on normal structures and structures that can be mistaken for disease. In Chapter 2 more coverage of general pathology has been added to reinforce the principles of pathology with emphasis on the common entities and those with direct bearing on dentistry, such as hepatitis and endocarditis. New illustrations aid the understanding of the principles. In Chapter 3 there is considerable updating and expansion. There is more on inflammation, mediators of inflammation, wound healing, and repair. A completely new section on immunity and immune disease encompasses AIDS, autoimmunity, diabetes, hypersensitivity, and some infectious diseases like hepatitis, with the basics on gingivitis and periodontitis being introduced. In Chapter 4 there is some updating and an addition of some syndromes. In Chapter 5 there is new information on demineralization and remineralization of the teeth. In Chapter 6 the section on viral disease was reworked, with updating on the herpesviruses and aphthous stomatitis. Factitial trauma and hairy leukoplakia were added, along with several new illustrations. Chapter 7 has updating and a new table on stains and discolorations of the teeth. Chapter 8 was greatly expanded in an attempt to include more examples of oral manifestations of systemic diseases and to discuss those diseases to further expand the pathology part of the text. There is a new section on oral manifestations of allergy. AIDS is covered here as well as throughout the text. Numerous new illustrations help to reinforce this section. Chapter 9 on differential diagnosis is new and attempts only to introduce this otherwise complex and comprehensive subject. Several new appendices provide some basic information. One is a listing by differential diagnosis of common oral lesions, which can be used as a guide in studying for regional boards. Overall, there has been an attempt to cover those subjects and areas suggested by the American Association of Dental Schools in their guidelines for teaching pathology and oral pathology.

I would like to acknowledge Dr. Cameron Lowe for his suggestions and help on the basic immunology section.

Contents

ORAL PATHOLOGY

THIRD EDITION

Chapter 1
CLINICAL EXAMINATION

The dental auxiliary, as a member of the health team, is responsible for understanding and recognizing diseases of the teeth and adjacent tissues and disorders of the oral cavity and paraoral area. This knowledge is based on principles of pathology as they relate to the head, neck, and oral structures.

The auxiliary can readily observe the patient at each appointment. By a carefully planned routine examination, the auxiliary will be able to recognize several disease states. Many conditions can be diagnosed readily when they are first observed; others will present as characteristic lesions that may suggest several disease entities. In these cases further information will be required for a definite diagnosis. The dental auxiliary should note and record the observations and should refer those cases that require further diagnosis and treatment to other members of the oral health team.

Observation is the key in maintaining oral health. The head, neck, and oral cavity are areas that can be easily viewed. Both normal and abnormal states of the soft tissue can be inspected by eye alone. Thus, with an understanding of disease states and changes that can occur, the dental auxiliary can detect disease entities that may be present. It is the purpose of this book to acquaint auxiliary personnel with several aspects of disease states with emphasis on those appearing in the oral regions.

Examination Procedure

With knowledge of what is normal and of what one expects to see, the auxiliary can routinely perform a systematic examination of the patient. This simple procedure will take no longer than a few minutes and may yield fruitful information regarding the health status of this area of the body. To be effective, the examination must be *routine, preplanned*, and *orderly*. It should be done at every visit. By using the same sequence of steps at each examination, the examiner will not inadvertently avoid any area. The specific order to be used is a matter of individual choice for each examiner. However, regardless of the order chosen, it is of utmost importance to start in the same site every time and to move in a predetermined pattern.

Utilizing primarily inspection and palpation, the following method of examination is offered as a basis for establishing a logical order and sequence.

Extraoral examination

1. Generalized appraisal of the patient
2. Face
3. Submental and submandibular lymph node areas
4. Parotid glands
5. Temporomandibular joint area
6. Ears
7. Neck and cervical lymph node areas
8. Thyroid gland area

Oral examination

1. Lips and corners of mouth
2. Mucous membrane of lips, labial and buccal vestibulae, gingivae, buccal mucosa, and papillae of parotid ducts
3. Hard palate and palatal gingivae
4. Soft palate
5. Tonsillar areas and posterior pharynx
6. Tongue—dorsum, lateral borders
7. Tongue—ventrum
8. Floor of mouth and lingual gingivae
9. Teeth (occlusion, caries)

The materials required for this examination are a good light, a dental mirror, 2×2 gauze, and an explorer. The patient should be asked to remove eyeglasses, earrings, and any other removable items such as dental prostheses.

Examination Technique

The clinical examination of the patient should begin with a general overall evaluation of the individual. The patient should be observed while walking to the dental chair. This may yield information on the attitude of the patient and of obvious physical problems which may be discussed with the patient. This casual examination takes place prior to seating the patient and before obtaining any history. For example, swollen ankles may indicate edema due to a kidney or a heart problem. After reviewing the medical and dental history, the examination should proceed.

On viewing and palpating the face, the examiner should observe if there is normal symmetry (Fig. 1.1). An asymmetry of the face could be due to a swelling related to an abscessed tooth (Fig. 1.2). Excluding trauma, the most common cause of facial swelling is a dentoalveolar or periodontal abscess. Pigmented lesions such as moles and age spots and ulcers such as skin cancers are readily observable and should be questioned (Figs. 1.3 and 1.4). A rash on the skin of the face may be due to allergy. That a patient has allergies is most important in gathering further historical data that could have a direct bearing on treatment. Some asymmetries can be due to swollen lymph nodes. Whether or not they are swollen, lymph node areas should be palpated.

Lymph nodes are concentrations of lymphatic tissue with various types of lymphocytes and macrophages. Important in draining protein from tissue spaces and fats from the gastrointestinal tract to the blood, as well as in immune surveillance and defense, they react to inflammation, infection, and malignant tumors and enlarge as

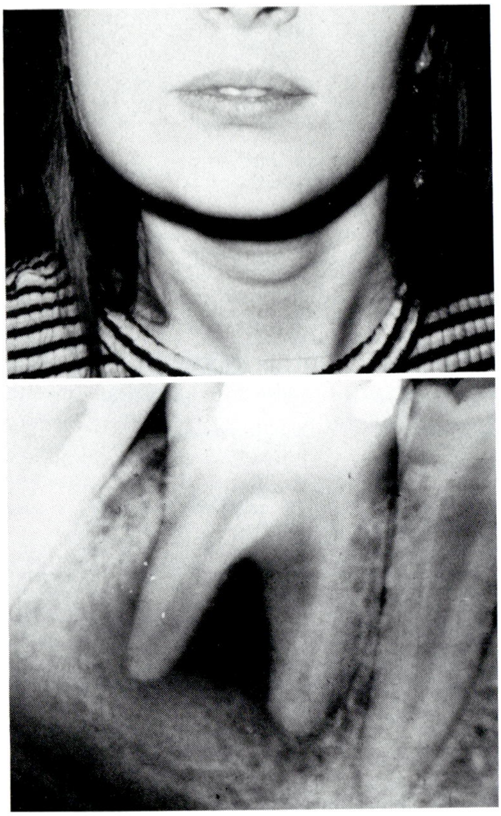

Figure 1.2. Asymmetry of face. Swelling of right cheek (*top*) is due to a dental infection (radiolucency, *bottom*) that has spread (cellulitis).

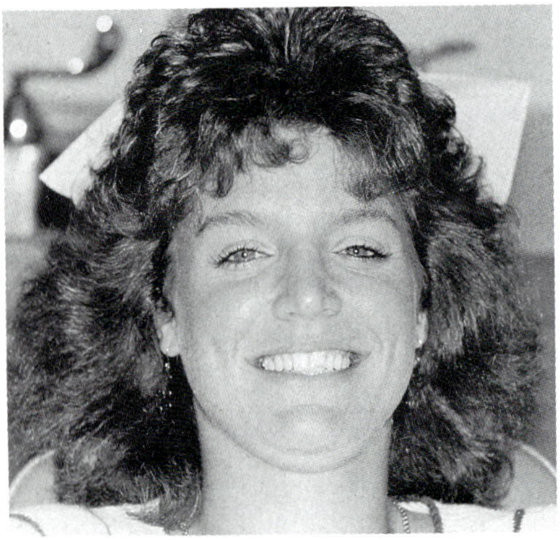

Figure 1.1. Facial view of patient showing normal symmetry.

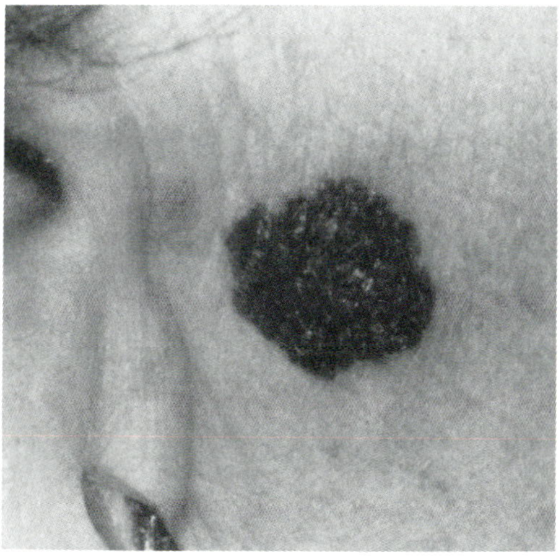

Figure 1.3. Malignant melanoma anterior to right ear. Note dark color and irregular border. Also note paler, even-bordered lesion posterior to melanoma, a common "age spot."

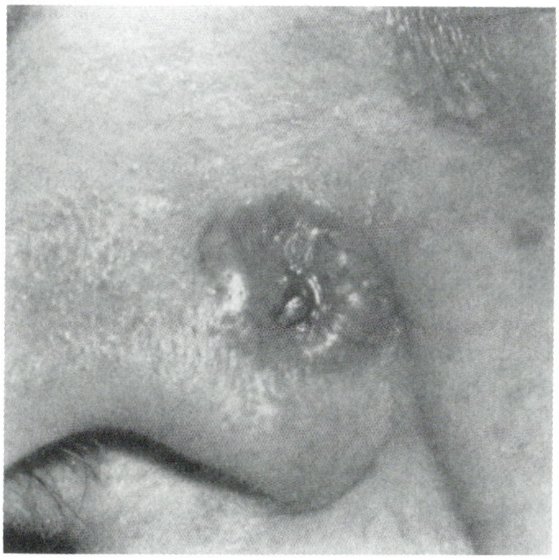

Figure 1.4. Basal cell tumor on left side of nose. A nonhealing craterlike ulcer with shiny, rolled margins.

part of the reaction. They may return to their original size or may remain enlarged if there is scar tissue or calcification. With a malignant tumor they remain enlarged and grow with the tumor. For example, in an infection such as primary herpetic gingivostomatitis, several nodes in many sites in the neck enlarge and are tender. After the disease passes, the nodes gradually regress in size and become asymptomatic. Multiple inflammatory episodes may cause the node to develop sufficient scar tissue or growth so that the node remains enlarged even though there is no stimulus for reaction. Thus, the significance of palpating a node (positive lymphadenopathy) may not always be readily apparent until coupled with other physical findings. If palpable, the nodes may be tender or nontender, mobile or fixed to the adjacent tissues. Malignant tumors can spread to lymph nodes and grow in them, causing permanent enlargement and fixation of the node.

Lymph nodes are oval or bean-shaped structures located along the length of lymphatic vessels. Normally, they are nontender, soft, and cannot be felt unless there is residual enlargement. Therefore, the examiner proceeds to feel beneath the skin for them in their prescribed anatomical areas (Fig. 1.5). Starting from the submental area (Fig. 1.6), one then moves posteriorly to the submandibular area (Figs. 1.7 and 1.8), the parotid region, the ears, and then to the neck. Bimanual palpation is recommended, and for the submandibular area this can be done both intra- and extraorally.

The parotid glands can be palpated for swellings. If the patient clenches the teeth together, any swellings of the parotid area can be felt over the firm masseter muscle. Sometimes the masseter muscles are so large that they resemble swellings of the parotid area (see Fig. 2.5). Next, the temporomandibular joint area can be palpated in front of the ear opening while the patient opens and closes the jaw. Any cracking or history of pain should be noted. Following this, the area behind the ears should be examined. Frequently a tumor or sore may be located there.

Then the cervical and neck nodes should be palpated. By tracing the extent of the sternocleidomastoid muscle both superfi-

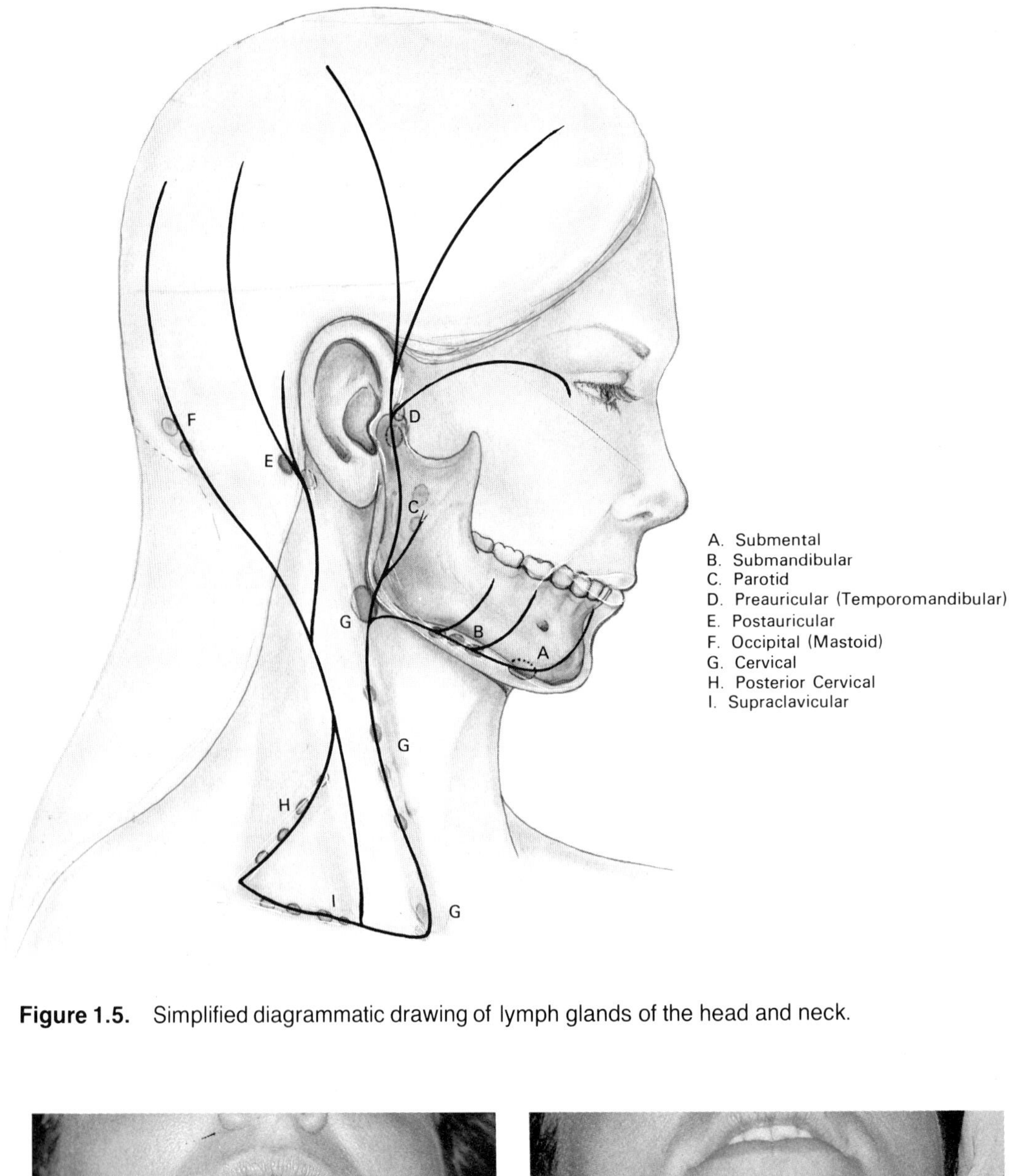

Figure 1.5. Simplified diagrammatic drawing of lymph glands of the head and neck.

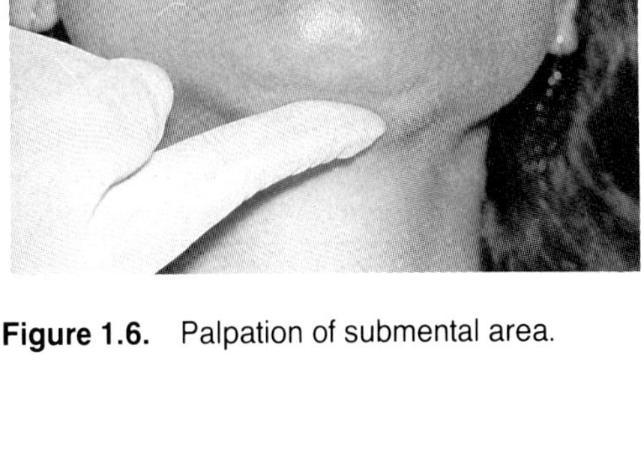

Figure 1.6. Palpation of submental area.

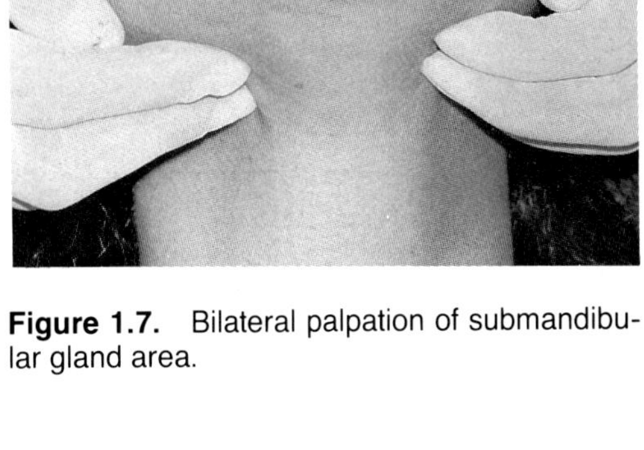

Figure 1.7. Bilateral palpation of submandibular gland area.

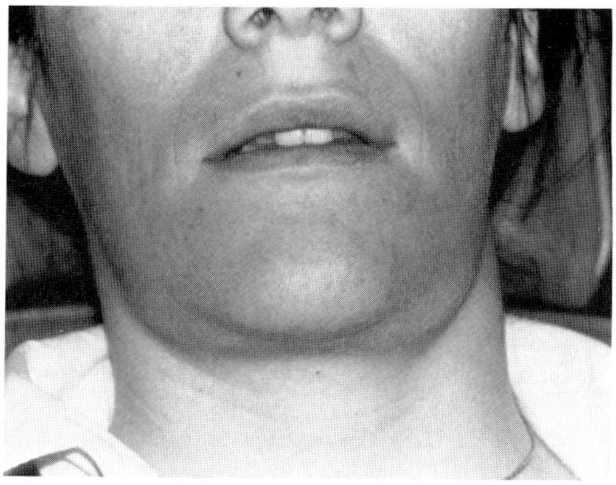

Figure 1.8. Bilateral swellings of reactive submandibular lymph nodes in 24-year-old with primary herpetic gingivostomatitis.

cially and deeply, these nodes may be felt (Fig. 1.9). Positive posterior auricular and occipital lymphadenopathy combined with swollen, sore palatine tonsils is strongly suggestive of infectious mononucleosis (Fig. 1.10). Positive supraclavicular lymphadenopathy can mean that there is a malignant disease from the mediastinum or from the thyroid gland. The thyroid gland itself and abnormalities can be palpated with the hand over the midline of the neck; when the patient swallows, the gland passes under the hand.

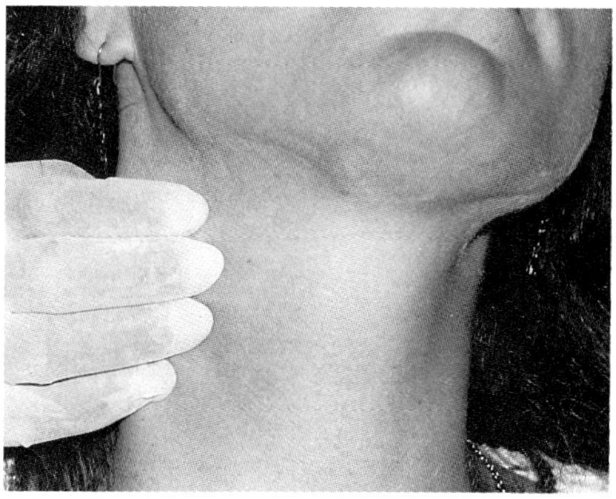

Figure 1.9. Palpation of cervical node area along the sternocleidomastoid muscle.

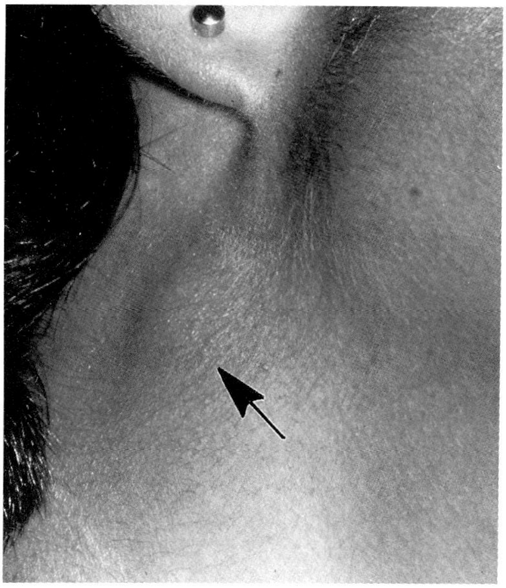

Figure 1.10. Swollen postauricular or postcervical lymph node (*arrow*) in 18-year-old with infectious mononucleosis. The palatine tonsils (see Fig. 6.47) were also swollen and tender and became necrotic.

In beginning the oral examination, first note the lips. A scar on the skin surface may represent the closure of a cleft lip or repair from an accident. Frequently yellow glands show through the vermilion border (Fig. 1.11). Next, after having the patient bring the teeth together (this relaxes the lip muscle), grasp the lips and reflect them to visualize the whole mucosal surface (Fig. 1.12). The maxillary frenum is a normal landmark at the base of the upper lip. Frequently, there is a small tab of extranormal tissue attached to the frenum (Fig. 1.13). In a similar manner, the lower lip is pulled down and inspected (Fig. 1.14). If this surface is dried, the tiny openings of mucous ducts are seen and they express drops of mucus. Then proceed first on one side and then the other to view the labial and buccal vestibules along with the unattached and attached gingivae (Fig. 1.15). Next, reflect the corner of the mouth to expose the buccal mucosa (inner cheeks). Here there are two

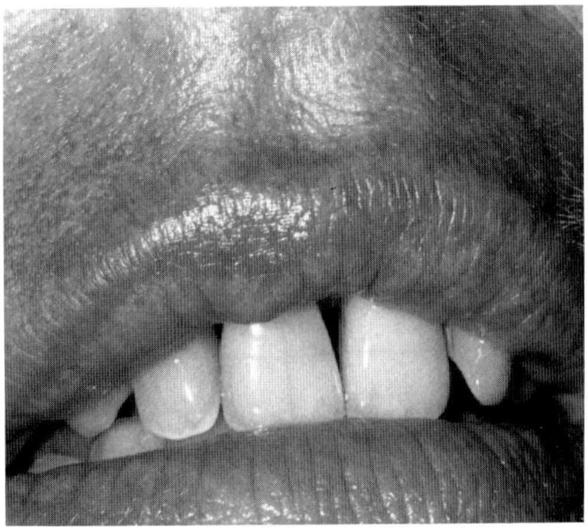

Figure 1.11. Fordyce's glands, ectopic, sebaceous glands, on inner aspect of upper lip.

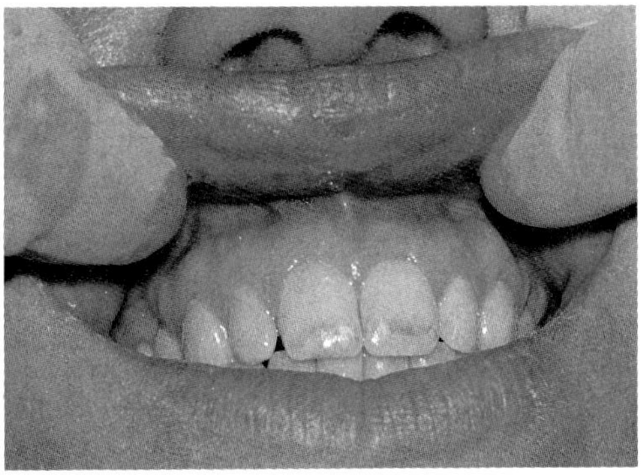

Figure 1.12. Retraction of upper lip.

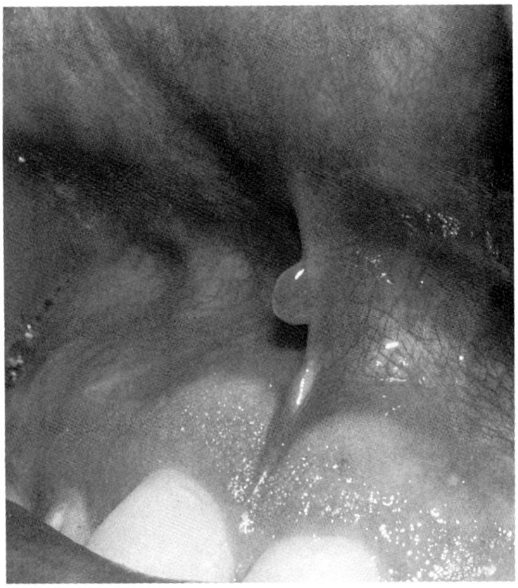

Figure 1.13. A normal mucosal tag projecting from the maxillary labial frenum. Also note normal mucogingival line and stippled gingivae.

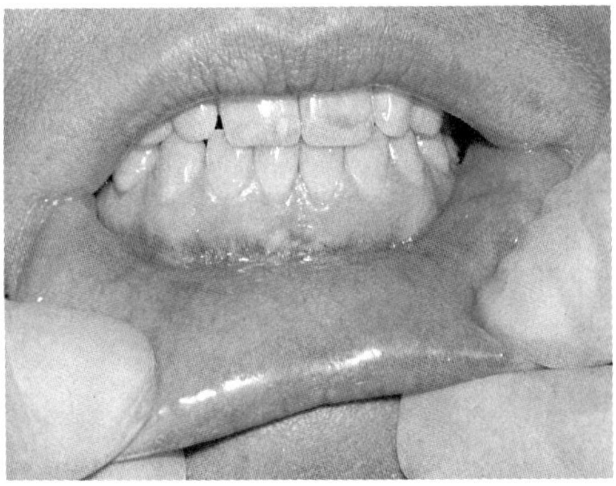

Figure 1.14. Retraction of lower lip.

landmarks. One is the papilla and opening of the parotid (Stensen's) duct of the parotid gland. A clear saliva usually can be seen flowing from the opening (Fig. 1.16). The flow can be tested by squeezing the area of the parotid gland over the posterior lateral border of the ramus of the mandible. No flow may indicate a dry mouth (xerostomia), which may be secondary to medications or radiotherapy, among other reasons. A yellowish, thick flow means there is an infection, usually bacterial, in the parotid gland. The other landmark is not anatomical but is found consistently. This is the white line corresponding to the occlusal or bite line of the teeth and is seen in the middle of the cheek running from the back to the front of the mouth.

Next the hard palate can be viewed, either directly or with the dental mirror (Fig. 1.17). The anterior portion contains the folds of tissue called rugae. Posteriorly, it is whitened due to the keratinized surface. Laterally, where there are numerous

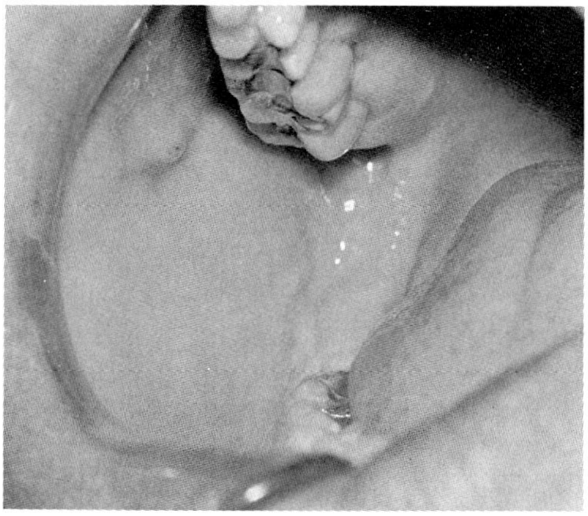

Figure 1.15. Examination of buccal mucosa. Note the papilla of Stensen's duct above the occlusal line and the retromolar area.

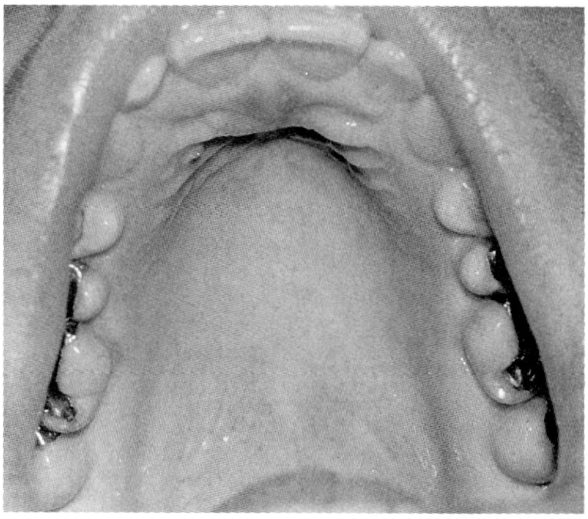

Figure 1.17. Examination of hard palate. Note the incisive papilla, rugae, and blanched color of hard palate.

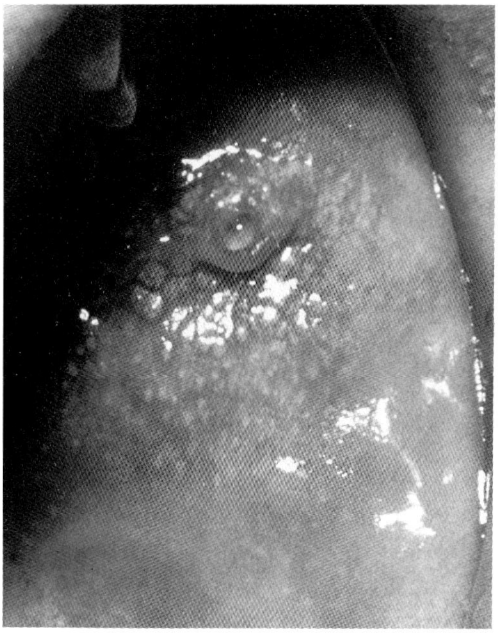

Figure 1.16. A prominent papilla of Stensen's duct with clear, watery saliva coming from the parotid gland. Also note the ectopic sebaceous glands within the buccal mucosa.

minor salivary glands and a prominent vascularity, there is an underlying blueness. The ductal openings are pin-sized and pink. In smokers, they may be reddened and more prominent. A white line can be seen in the midline because there are no glands or fat there, and the connective tissue is bound tightly to the firm bone beneath this area. Frequently, there can be excess bone in this area of the hard palate (torus) (Fig. 1.18).

Moving toward the posterior, the examiner should see the soft palate in its entirety (Fig. 1.19). This includes visualizing the full extent of the pendulous uvula. In this

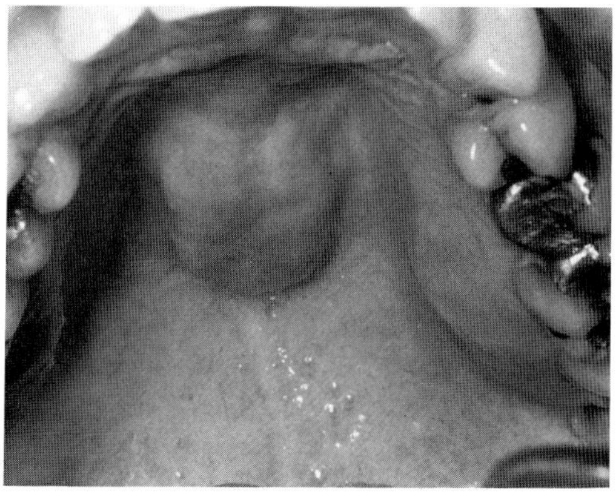

Figure 1.18. Maxillary torus in midline and exostosis on the left lingual alveolar ridge. Both are bony projections and are painless and solid to touch.

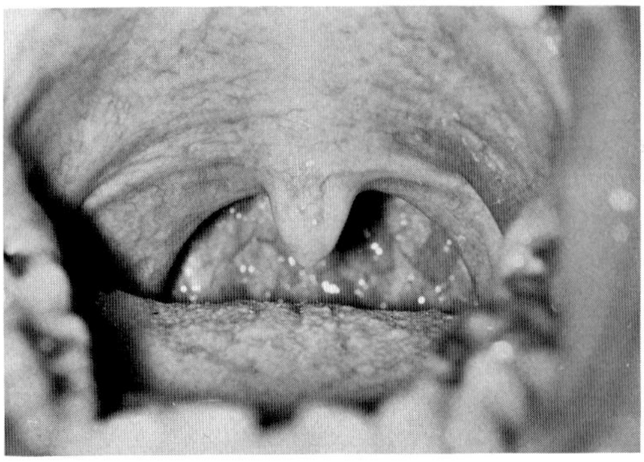

Figure 1.19. Soft palate, uvula, tonsillar fauces, and posterior pharynx, including enlarged pharyngeal tonsils (*right*).

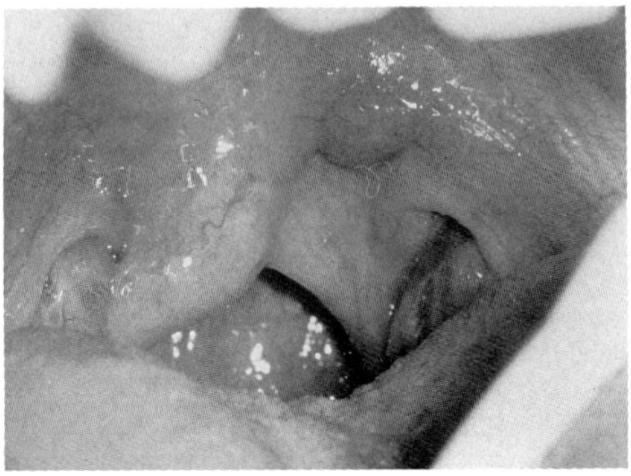

Figure 1.21. Left palatine tonsil in fauces and accessory tonsil at the base of the uvula.

region are many of the oral tonsillar tissues. The major tonsillar tissues are clearly identifiable, multiple aggregates of lymphoid tissue in specific anatomical sites. The minor oral tonsils are not readily identifiable in every patient but may occur randomly in other areas of the mouth, the floor being the most common site (Fig. 1.20). The most prominent are the palatine tonsils on each side situated between the palatoglossal and the palatopharyngeal folds (Fig. 1.21). They may be very large in children but in adults they should be receded between the folds unless they are enlarged by reactivity or tumor. The tonsillar crypts are indentations that can become filled with bacteria. A bacterial plug is a yellow accumulation of bacteria filling the crypt and may cause a tickle in the throat. Another yellow lesion frequently seen is the pseudocyst. If the epithelium at the opening of the crypt fuses, then the normally desquamating cells lining the crypt pile up and expand forming a cystlike, yellow lesion (Fig. 1.22).

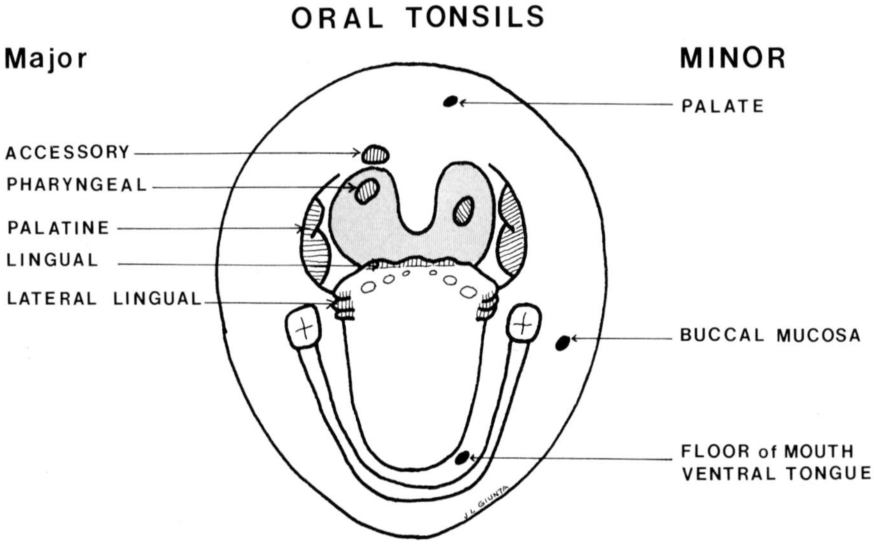

Figure 1.20. Diagram of locations of major and minor oral tonsils.

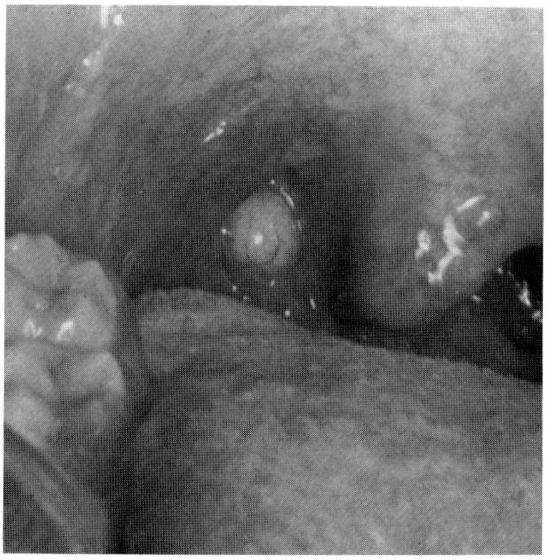

Figure 1.22. Pseudocyst of the right palatine tonsil. Bright yellow, it resembled a fatty tumor, a lipoma.

Pseudocysts can occur in any oral tonsillar tissue and usually spontaneously regress so they do not have to be removed.

Also seen in this area, but not consistently, are the accessory tonsils. They usually are near the base of the uvula and resemble a tumor such as a fibroma (see Fig. 1.21). However, that they decrease in size after being reactive is a clue to their tonsillar nature. If the palatine tonsils have been surgically removed, there may be broad white bands of scar tissue or even fenestrations in the tissue. Frequently, there are "residual" nodules of reactive tonsil that remain and enlarge after the palatine tonsils are "removed."

By reflecting the tongue down and forward with the dental mirror and by asking the patient to say "ah," with good light, the uvular tonsillar area and pharyngeal wall can be noted. Patients with colds may have red streaks in the mucosa in this area.

The tongue should be viewed next. The dorsal surface can be seen easily by asking the patient to extend the tongue. Several aspects of anatomy should be noted. The white "coating," which may be accentuated in some diseases, represents the individual filiform papillae of the tongue. These may be stained brown in heavy smokers or tea drinkers. Interspersed among these are small pink dome-shaped fungiform papillae (Fig. 1.23). These may be quite prominent in some individuals, particularly in disease states in which the filiform papillae are absent. The circumvallate papillae usually are not seen. When they are seen, they appear as large swellings on the posterior surface of the tongue (Fig. 1.24). Because they occur symmetrically and bilaterally in the form of a "V" with the point toward the pharynx, they can usually be distinguished from a pathologic swelling which is usually unilateral.

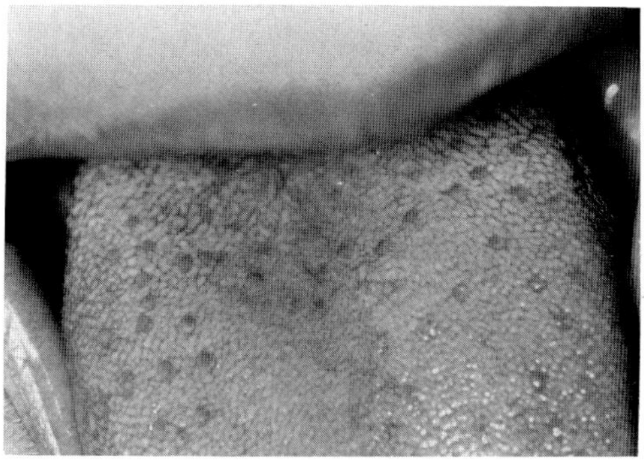

Figure 1.23. Dorsal view of tongue. Note small dome-shaped fungiform papillae among white filiform papillae.

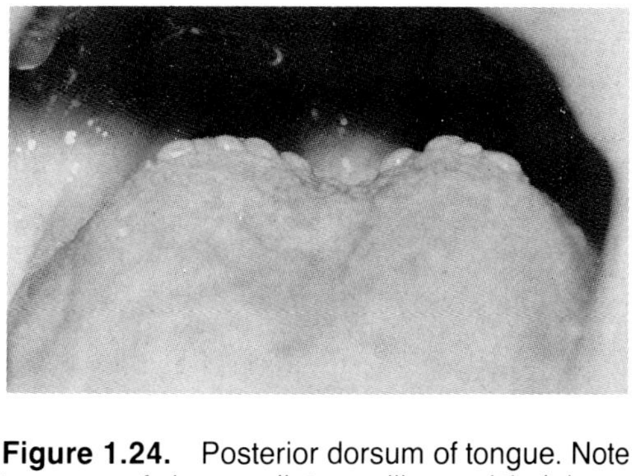

Figure 1.24. Posterior dorsum of tongue. Note two rows of circumvallate papillae and their large size.

The tongue can be viewed easily and controlled well by holding it with 2×2 gauze wrapped around the tip of the tongue (Figs. 1.25 and 1.26). In this manner, the examiner can draw the tongue to each side and view the lateral aspects. The lateral lingual tonsil area, just forward of the extreme posterolateral border, should be noted. Bilaterally they are nodular with vertical crypts and may be swollen and reddened, particularly in smokers and they may develop pseudocysts (Fig. 1.27). In a small number of patients, it may be possible to observe the base of the tongue (Fig. 1.28), which would reveal the true lingual tonsils behind or posterior to the circumvallate papillae. This whole area appears very blue because it is richly vascularized. An enlarged lingual tonsil may mimic a tumor (Fig. 1.29) and must be distinguished from

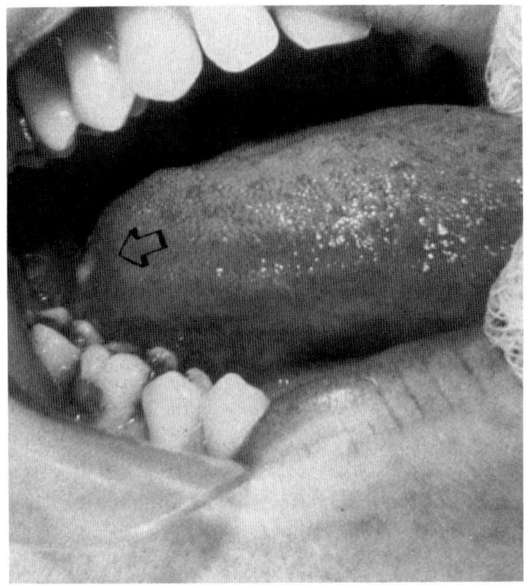

Figure 1.27. Pseudocyst (*arrow*) of the right lateral lingual tonsil. It was yellow, painless, nonremovable, and regressed in 2 months.

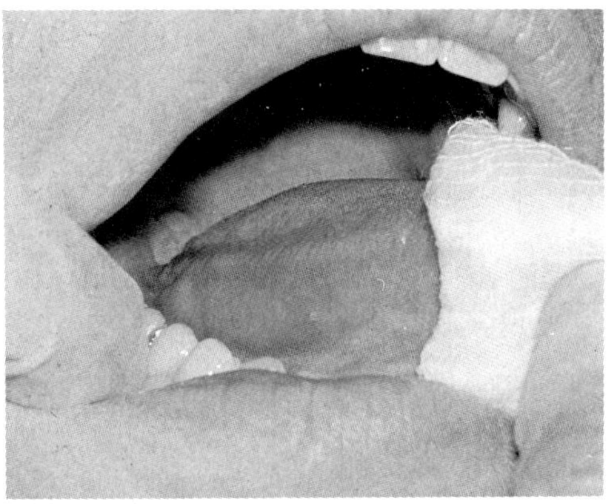

Figure 1.25. Examination of right side of tongue. Note lateral lingual tonsils at the most posterior lateral border.

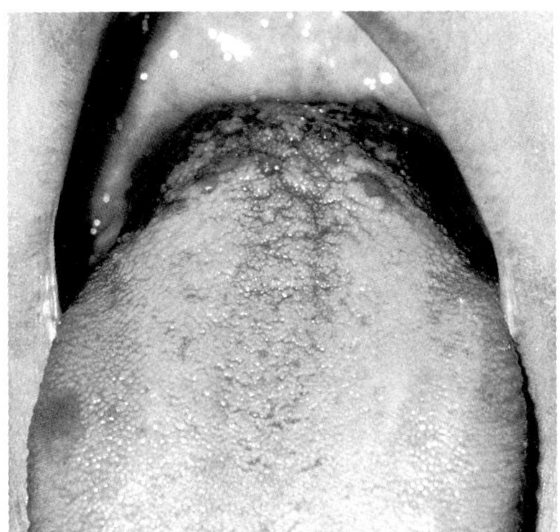

Figure 1.28. Lingual tonsils at the base of tongue behind several circumvallate papillae.

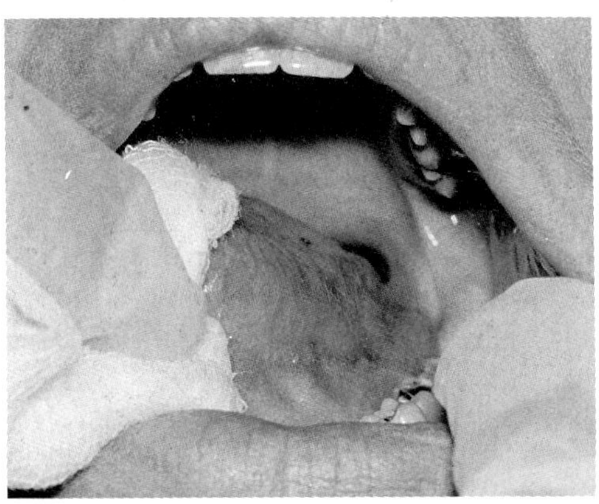

Figure 1.26. Examination of left side of tongue. Note lateral lingual tonsils.

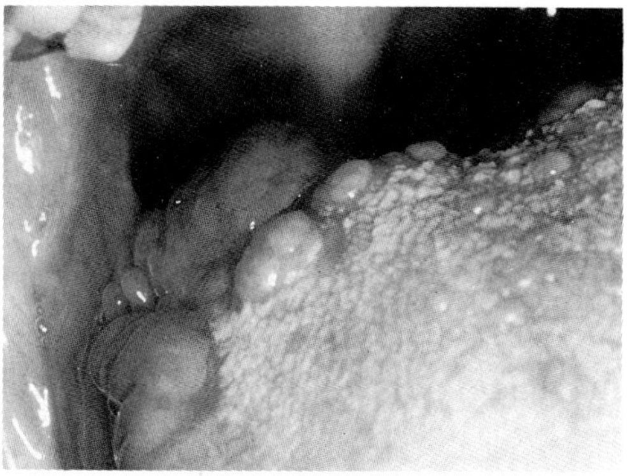

Figure 1.29. Enlarged lingual tonsil behind two circumvallate papillae on the right; lateral lingual tonsil to the left.

one. All of the normal structures of the tongue may be mistaken at times for disease.

The patient should then be asked to touch the palate with the tongue. By doing this, the ventral surface of the tongue and the floor of the mouth can be visualized (Fig. 1.30). Some patients cannot touch the roof of the mouth because of the manner in which the lingual frenum attaches to the tongue (tongue-tie). Not only does the examiner see the lingual frenum, but he or she also notes the large veins running laterally on each side. These become more prominent in elderly patients. Analogous to varicose veins of the lower legs, they are called lingual varicosities or varices, caused by loss of elastic tissue in the vein causing a distention (Fig. 1.31). Then the floor of the mouth is examined. In the anterior portion on each side are the sublingual plicae, or carunculae, which are slightly raised horizontal cylinders of tissue with openings of lingual glands at the surface. Shaped like a "V" pointing toward the anterior teeth, these folds end at a slightly larger swelling with a large ductal opening (submandibular [Wharton's] duct [Fig. 1.32]). Saliva can be readily expressed from these openings by pressing the submandibular glands against the lower borders of the mandible. Sometimes a stone may form in one of the ducts and the flow is impeded or stopped. If there is an edentulous alveolar ridge with substantial resorption, the floor of the mouth may resemble a swelling (Fig. 1.33).

With a dental mirror and direct viewings, the unattached and attached gingivae should be noted (Fig. 1.34). In some patients, particularly in the first several decades of life, a retrocuspid papilla may be noted on the attached gingivae just below

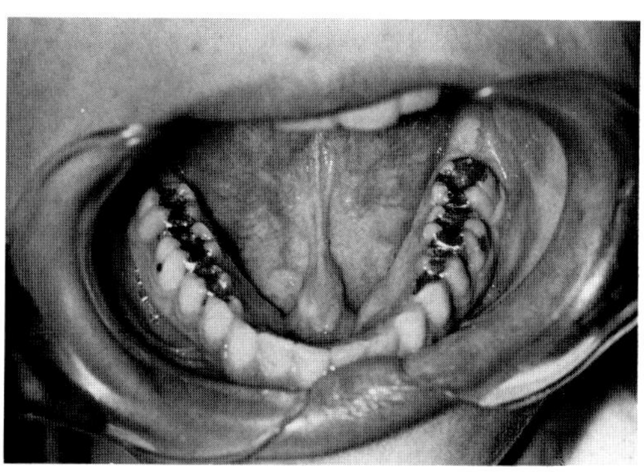

Figure 1.30. Floor of mouth, lingual frenum, and gingivae.

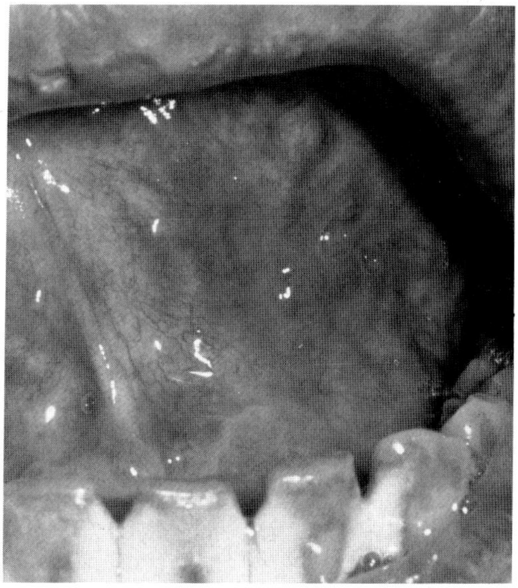

Figure 1.31. Varicosities of veins in ventral surface of tongue. They resemble a tumor of blood vessels, a hemangioma.

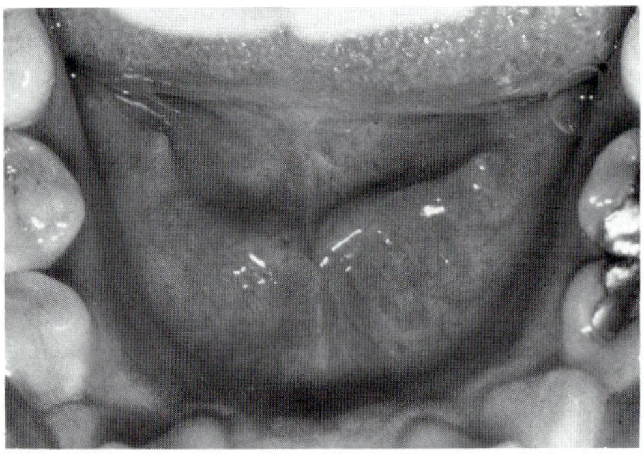

Figure 1.32. Normal floor of mouth showing sublingual carunculae. Note the opening of Wharton's duct near the midline.

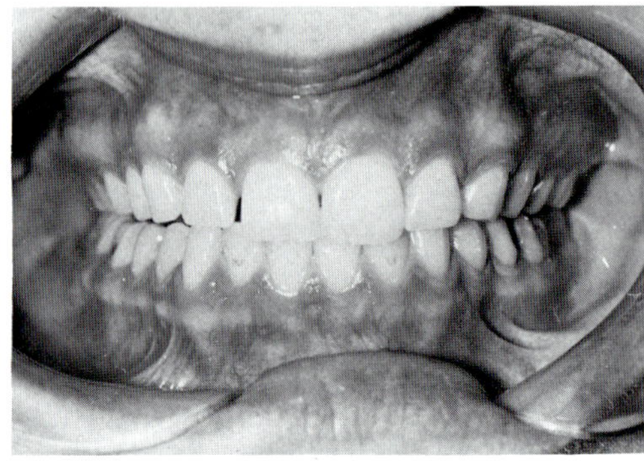

Figure 1.34. Labial and buccal vestibule, gingivae, and teeth.

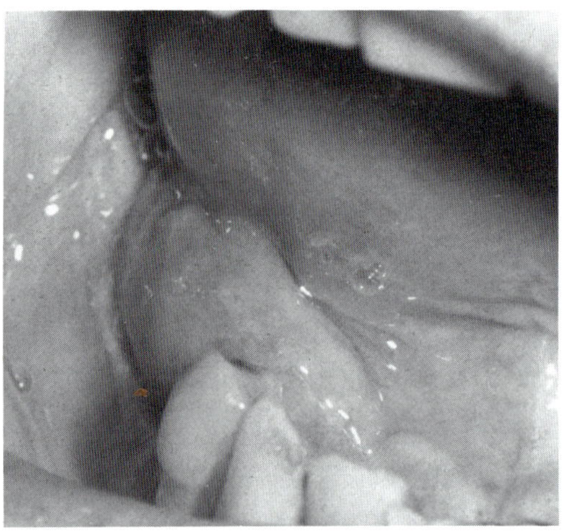

Figure 1.33. Floor of mouth resembling a tumor. The edentulous ridge is so resorbed that normal tissue projects above it.

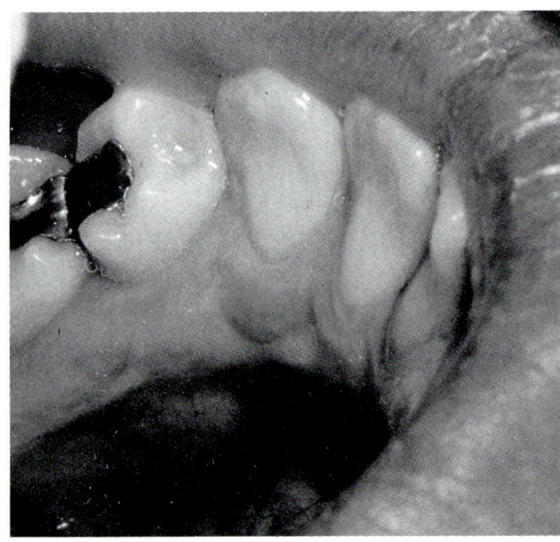

Figure 1.35. Retrocuspid papilla; reddish, slightly raised.

and lingual to the cuspid (Fig. 1.35). A developmental, essentially normal condition, the retrocuspid papilla may be mistaken for disease. These papillae may be bilateral, raised, small nodules, usually 0.5 mm, and have a broad base (sessile) or may be pedunculated (emanating from a thin stalk). There is no treatment, and they may regress with age. Next, the teeth should be checked. After asking the patient to close the teeth together, observe for possible malocclusion. With an explorer, the examiner can check for caries and other defects.

Through routine examination such as this (i.e., methodically and consistently performed), any deviations from normal can be observed. These may range from simple and innocuous defects to very serious and lethal diseases. What is important is that these deviations be observed. The welfare of the patient is enhanced because of astute observation and referral.

Chapter 2
PRINCIPLES OF PATHOLOGY

Pathology is the study of the nature of disease, its causes (etiology), development (pathogenesis), and consequences (prognosis). Disease is defined as any abnormal condition of an organism or one of its parts, especially as a consequence of inherent weakness, physical stimuli, infection, emotional stress, or other factor that may impair normal physiologic functioning. Oral pathology is that branch of pathology that deals specifically with diseases affecting the oral areas—the teeth, adjacent tissues, oral mucosa, and contiguous parts. However, the underlying tissue and cellular reactions that produce the morphologic (concerning structure and form) and physiologic (functional) changes in the oral region are the same basic responses that occur in any other area of the body. Therefore a study of oral disease covers principles of pathology that apply to disease anywhere in the body.

Historically, the nature of disease was a mystery until the advent of the microscope and its application to the study of diseased tissue. Through the microscope it was discovered that organs and tissues are composed of cells and that changes in the cells are responsible for changes in the organs. The altered functional state of cells led to cellular structural changes in many disease states, which the early pathologists began to categorize and classify.

Classification of a disease is a valuable means of identifying a particular disease or type of disease. However, it should be remembered that classification is arbitrary. Many diseases can be classified in many ways. For example, mumps, because it is caused by a virus, can be classed as a viral disease. On the other hand, mumps affects glandular tissue and can be classed as a salivary gland disease. The point is that a classification is a man-made convenience so that disease can be thought of and discussed with some order. The approach in this book is mainly morphologic with particular emphasis on the gross manifestations of various abnormal states. In some instances reference is made to microscopic features, because certain disease states can be appreciated only in microscopic terms. One should keep in mind that we are in an era of biochemistry, cellular biology, and genetics, and many diseases cannot be recognized simply on a morphologic basis but require sophisticated means to determine their presence, especially the metabolic disease states. With the increase in technologic applications, more and more abnormal conditions will be discovered. Regardless of the approach to the study of disease, certain principles emerge.

Organs and tissues are composed of cells in a fluid environment. Physiologically the cell is a small machine that is capable of specific work but requires nutrients and oxygen to perform its function. The nutrients are derived from the alimentary canal, and the oxygen comes from the lungs. The blood vessels carry the nutrients and oxygen to the cells via the surrounding fluid medium. The cell utilizes the nutrients and through metabolism burns the oxygen to produce energy for its work. Waste products including carbon dioxide are excreted by the cell and enter the venous drainage. The carbon dioxide travels to the lungs where it is exchanged for oxygen. The other waste products are broken down in the liver and kidney and are excreted in the urine.

Etiology refers to the cause of disease.

There are many etiologic agents that can injure the host and, ultimately, the reaction of the host to the injury produces signs and symptoms of what is recognized as disease. There is a long list of factors that produce injury, but the reaction of the host in response to these factors is limited. Usually, many injurious agents act on the host by producing a similar or common response.

The etiologic agents are many but can be essentially categorized as endogenous and exogenous. Endogenous refers to those injuries occurring within the cell. These are primarily genetic and constitute hereditary disease. However, there are spontaneous changes that can take place inside the cell, and these changes are not passed on to further generations.

Exogenous refers to those factors originating outside the cell itself. These agents are the most common ones producing disease. They include such stimuli as trauma, drugs, temperature, radiation, parasites (viruses, bacteria, fungi), nutrition, and emotion.

Once one of these agents affects the host, the host's cells are stimulated to react. The response usually takes one of a limited number of patterns that have been categorized utilizing the light microscope. In cellular and tissue injury the stresses act at the molecular and biochemical level and are rarely detected. Eventually, they induce morphologic changes that may be noted as changes in organelles by the electron microscope and as gross changes by light microscopy.

As the cells adjust to the injury, alterations can be seen in the cells. Certain cell types become more prominent than other cell types. Cells may take a specific direction of growth and maturation. With the variation in the external environment, cells adjust and the cellular adjustments assume certain patterns that can be recognized and labeled in a consistent manner. This labeling has led to the categorization of diseases, which serves as a useful diagnostic tool. The responses of the host to injurious agents are outlined in Table 2.1.

Malformations occur primarily from

Table 2.1
Pathologic stimulating factors and responses in host

Factors	Possible responses in host (major categories of disease)
Injury Chemicals Irradiation Genes Nutrition Bacteria Emotions Others	A. *Malformations* Inborn errors (metabolic) hereditary (genetic), congenital (birth defect, developmental anomaly)
	B. *Degenerations* (deposits) → necrosis (death) → scar; necrosis (death) → resolution water, fat, pigments, atrophy (decrease size) necrosis (death) → lysis → infection → abscess
	C. *Circulatory disturbances* Hyperemia (stasis), ischemia, infarct, hemorrhage
	D. *Inflammation* Vascular, cellular proliferation (growth); repair
	E. *Growths* (tumorlike) Hypertrophy (increase in cell size), hyperplasia (increase in cell number), metaplasia (change in cell type)
	F. *Tumors* Benign (hamartoma), malignant

agents injuring the inside of the cell and include both hereditary and developmental disturbances. They also include the inborn errors that result in metabolic disorders, such as the inability of a cell to utilize a specific enzyme properly. In phenylketonuria there is a deficient enzyme that causes an amino acid not to be metabolized and, consequently, to build up in the bloodstream. The PKU laboratory test in newborns can check for this inborn defect, which if undetected can lead to mental retardation early in life. Agenesis and aplasia are terms used to describe the absence of part or all of an organ. For example, a person may be born without a kidney and still live. Dentally, many people have congenitally missing mandibular third molars. Malformations constitute an important part of oral pathology and are discussed further in Chapter 4.

Degenerative change refers to a metabolic disturbance and deterioration of cells or the area immediately surrounding the cells. It is a state that may revert to normal or lead to the death of the cell, noted by the loss of nuclear material (Fig. 2.1). Microscopically within the cytoplasm of the cell one may see accumulation of water, fat, mucin, or pigments. Lipid accumulation within hepatocytes is usually a manifestation of liver cell injury. It is associated with a lack of oxygen, hypoxia, nutritional deficiencies, chemical toxins, and alcohol abuse. For example, in alcoholic ingestion, cells of the liver swell with fat droplets that impair the function of the cell. This may be reversed by stopping the alcoholic intake, thereby returning the function of the cell to normal. However, if the injury is severe and the cell is overwhelmed, necrosis results. Liver failure may lead to jaundice, a yellow discoloration of the skin, sclera, and so on, resulting from an accumulation of bilirubin in the tissues. Necrosis refers to the death of tissue and, microscopically, is noted by changes in the nucleus such as the splitting apart of the nucleus. Without a nucleus to

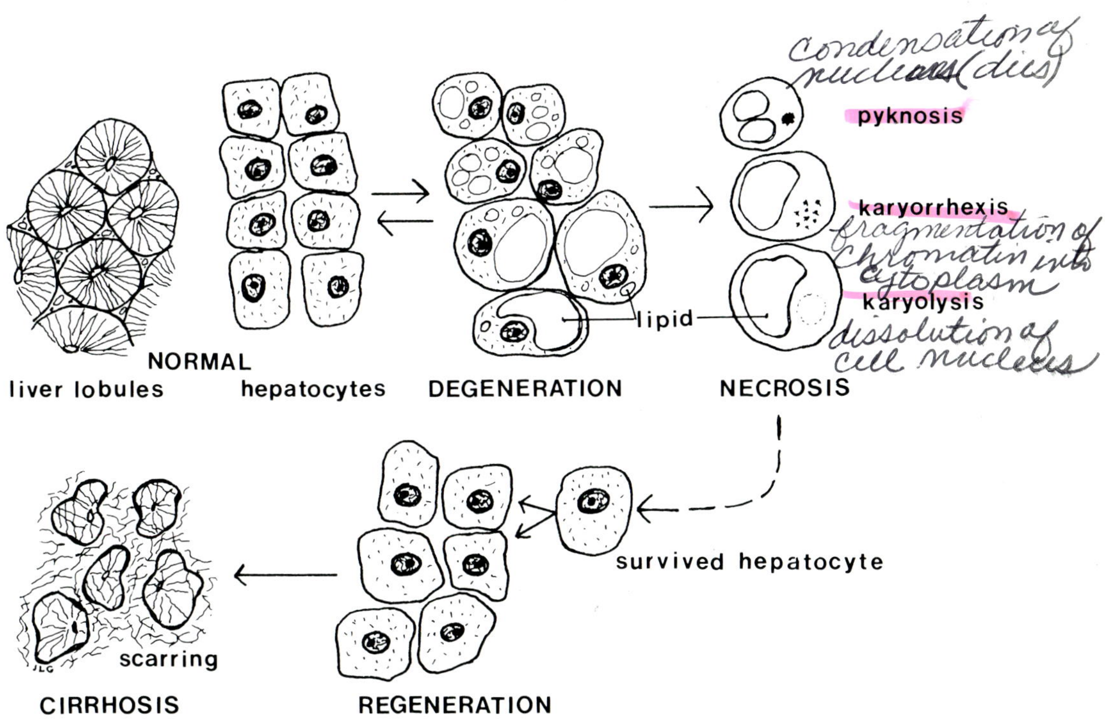

Figure 2.1. Diagram on degeneration, necrosis, and regeneration using the liver with fatty change, cleared droplets in cells, as the example. Three light microscopic changes denoting necrosis are shown at right.

direct activities, the cell dies. The body resolves necrosis in many ways. Most commonly, the necrotic cells are localized and resorbed by other cells, with a scar replacing the area of necrosis. However, other possibilities exist. The necrotic cells may dissolve (lysis) and become liquefied. If the liquid is surrounded by epithelial cells, a cyst remains. If the necrotic cells become infected secondarily, an abscess or collection of pus results. Rather than being resorbed, the necrotic cells may become a focus for calcification and leave a hardened mass. In bone, the necrotic cells may become separated (sequestrated) from the bone cells.

Inactive cells or cells inflicted with a chronic metabolic deficiency may undergo atrophy. Atrophy refers to a decrease in the size of the cell compared to a normal cell. This wasting away of cells may ultimately be reflected in a decrease in the number of cells (numerical atrophy) as the degenerative process proceeds to necrosis of many of the atrophic cells (Fig. 2.2).

On a clinical level, the category of degeneration is not used frequently, but the processes described here are seen often. For instance, an ulcer of the mouth has a necrotic surface. A tooth with deep decay may eventually have an abscess or cyst at the root end of the tooth. These are specific results of degenerative processes. But degenerative changes may be apparent in a more general manner. For example, the ill feeling or malaise that we have with a common cold is caused by degeneration in many cells throughout the body, particularly of the head, neck, and chest if it is an upper respiratory infection.

Circulatory disturbance is an important category of disease. Even under normal conditions there is a constant interplay of hyperemia (activity) and anemia (rest). Hyperemia refers to an increase in the blood supply; anemia, to a decrease in the number of red blood cells. For example, at rest there are capillaries in the lung that are without blood cells. Only a portion of the alveoli are at work. By contrast, during a brisk run, many more alveoli are used and more capillaries are filled with blood cells causing hyperemia.

In pathologic circumstances, there is also hyperemia. In active hyperemia there is an increased inflow of blood to an area. Passive hyperemia refers to a decreased outflow of blood with a stagnation of venous current. This stasis may lead to necrosis of tissues because of lack of oxygen to the site.

Ischemia refers to a reduced oxygen supply to the cells such that they are weakened but not actually killed. In the heart, ischemia of the myocardium is called angina pectoris, meaning chest pain referred from the damaged heart muscle. There are many causes of angina, among which are stress, strenuous exertion, hypertension, anemia, aortic stenosis, and coronary artery spasm or disease. Nitroglycerine is utilized to dilate the blood vessels during a severe attack.

If the tissue continues to lose its oxygen supply eventually it dies. An infarction is the death or necrosis of tissue due to an interrupted blood supply. The common example is myocardial infarction, a lead-

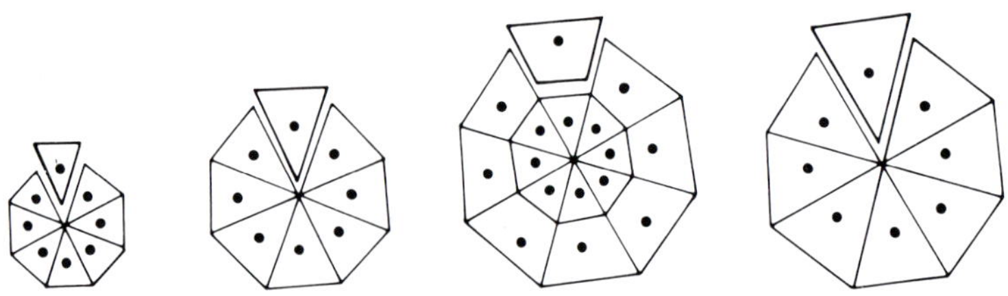

Figure 2.2. Schematic diagram of tissue and cellular changes. The dots represent nuclei within the cell.

ing cause of death in the United States. If the coronary arteries are partly or essentially narrowed to the point that insufficient blood flows to the myocardium, then an infarct develops (Fig. 2.3). Depending on the artery involved and its end-distribution, the patient may die or can recover. The myocardium undergoes degeneration followed by necrosis, with release of enzymes that can be measured to monitor the damage. This is followed by inflammation, a clearing of the damaged cells, and healing by nonfunctional scar tissue. Predisposing factors are hypertension, hyperlipidemia, smoking, diabetes, obesity, being an older male, being a female beyond menopause, and race (blacks are more prone to high blood pressure and strokes). The underlying pathology is usually arteriosclerosis, hardening or the arteries, in the form of atherosclerosis. Atherosclerosis refers to the thickening of the intima and sometimes the media of medium and large blood vessels by the accumulation of a cholesterol-laden plaque. The plaque pushes into the lumen and diminishes its size, impeding the blood flow. Damage to the endothelial lining of the vessel results in the growth of the plaque by blood monocytes (macrophages) embedding into the intima. The macrophages ingest and hold cholesterol and triglycerides and induce fibroblasts to form scar tissue. Atherosclerosis may also cause the most common brain disorder, a stroke or cerebrovascular accident (CVA).

Hemorrhage or bleeding is a circulatory disturbance caused by injury to capillaries, decrease in blood platelets, decrease in fibrinogen, and many other factors. The mechanism to prevent hemorrhage is clot-

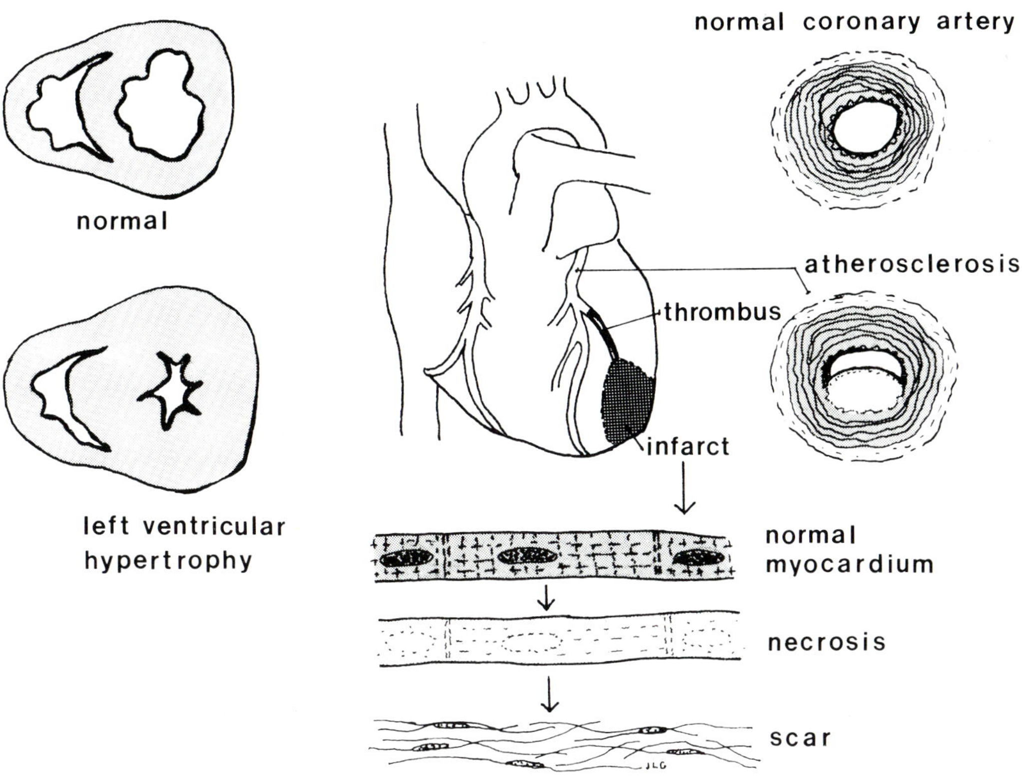

Figure 2.3. Diagram of myocardial ischemia due to atherosclerosis of the coronary vessels leading to a myocardial infarct or necrosis. It contrasts normal ventricular thickness with that in ventricular hypertrophy; normal coronary lumen with smaller lumen due to intimal, fatty plaque. It demonstrates death of the myocardial cells, which heal by scar tissue.

ting. If the inner lining of a blood vessel is damaged, a thrombus may form at the site of damage. Thrombosis is the formation of a plug within a blood vessel. The thrombus or clot is composed of red blood cells, platelets, and fibrin.

The formation of fibrin clots or thrombi is a normal homeostatic mechanism for stopping bleeding (hemostasis) of a damaged or weakened blood vessel. It is balanced by the removal or dissolution of the clot by the plasmin system (Fig. 2.4).

When a blood vessel is damaged, several activities take place to help correct the situation. First, vascular spasm reduces blood flow. Then, because the break in endothelium exposes collagen, the platelets in the blood adhere to the site and release enzymes that attract more platelets to accumulate. This forms a platelet plug that can prevent further blood loss in a small vessel. Following the formation of the plug, fibrin threads are formed during a process called coagulation or clotting.

Through a complex process of chemical chain reactions, the clotting mechanism takes place in three essential phases. In stage 1, prothrombin activator is formed quickly through an extrinsic tissue-activated pathway or more slowly through an intrinsic pathway via coagulation factors within the blood. In stage 2, the prothrombin activator converts prothrombin (a plasma protein formed by the liver) into the enzyme thrombin. In stage 3, thrombin converts fibrinogen (another plasma protein formed by the liver) into fibrin, which eventually becomes stabilized as the threads of the clot.

Following clot formation is clot retraction and clot dissolution. During retraction, with the help of adequate platelets, the damaged edges bind closer together and hold the blood elements within the vessel,

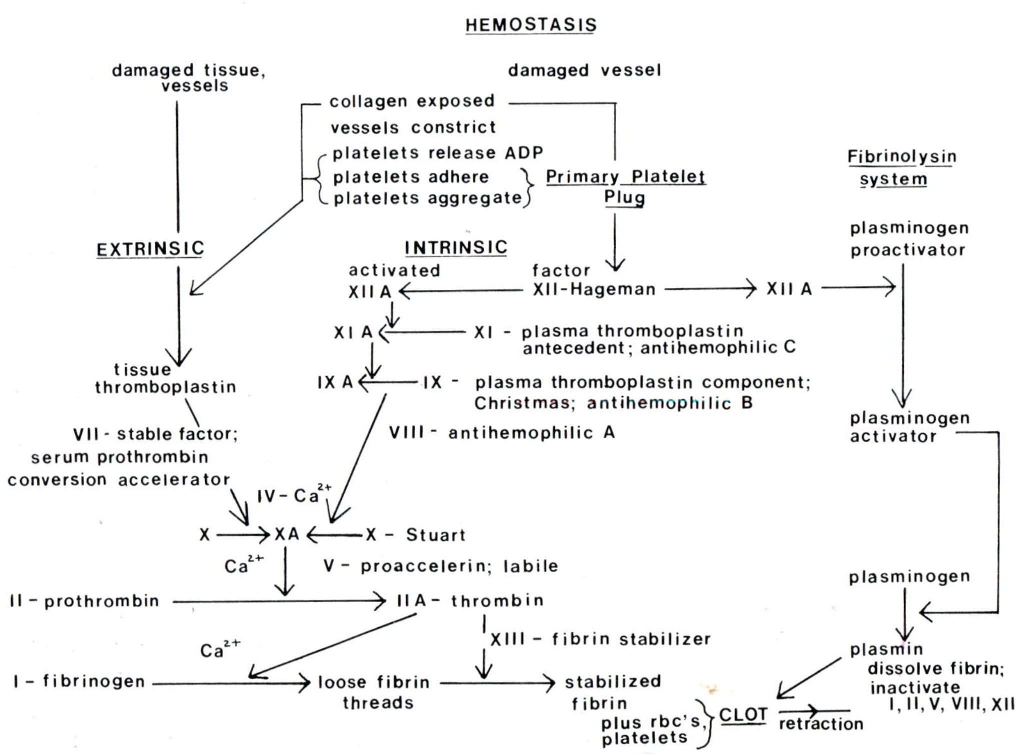

Figure 2.4. Diagram of hemostasis with formation of platelet plug and fibrin clot and the plasmin fibrinolysin system.

except for some serum. Fibrinolysis involves clot dissolution through the formation of plasmin. Plasminogen is an inactive enzyme from the plasma that is incorporated into the formed clot. Several tissue and blood substances (thrombin, factor XII) can help form plasminogen activator, which activates plasminogen to plasmin. The plasmin can digest the fibrin threads and can inactivate other clotting factors.

Blood clots are most common in veins, particularly those of the lower legs, where the superficial veins of the legs often become tortuous and bulge. The blood stagnates within them, and injury is common. This may lead to the formation of a thrombus. Once formed, a thrombus is treated like foreign material, and the body reacts to it in several ways. Certain cells may dissolve it, and the lumen of the vessel becomes patent again. Or, other cells grow into the clot and bind it down to the wall so that it does not become free. Eventually new channels or capillaries are formed, and in time blood can flow through the vessel again. However, sometimes the clot or a portion of it may dislodge from the site of its formation and be transported to a distant site where it can lodge in a smaller vessel. The detached clot is then termed an embolus or more specifically a thromboembolus. The detached and floating clot is the most common threat in patients following major surgery, because clots may form readily in legs that are immobile. However, there are other types of emboli, namely, air, bacteria, cells, fat, or foreign materials. Both the thrombus and emboli are significant, because they can partly or completely occlude vessels and cause ischemia to a vital area. For instance, a clot in a vessel to the brain could lead to apoplexy (a stroke). Besides a clot, a CVA may be caused by hemorrhage into the brain tissue, as by an aneurysm.

An aneurysm is a sac or bulge in the wall of an artery caused by a weakening of the artery wall. It may be caused by atherosclerosis, in which case it is found in the abdominal aorta. If congenital, it is usually found in the circle of Willis at the base of the brain and is called a berry aneurysm. It can be associated with hypertension and can burst, causing hemorrhage and a cerebrovascular accident, or it may be fatal. Other causes of aneurysms are syphilis and septic emboli causing damage. Blood can dissect through the layers of the damaged vessels, may perforate, and can cause death. The risk factors for a CVA are the same as those listed for heart disease plus a weakened blood vessel.

Hypertension is a common disease of the heart and blood vessels. A persistent blood pressure reading of 140/90 or above is considered high blood pressure. The most common variety has no known cause and is called primary or essential hypertension. In secondary hypertension (15 percent) there is atherosclerosis, kidney disease, or an adrenal disorder. Hypertension can cause damage to the heart, kidneys, and brain if it is uncontrolled. With increased pressure, the heart pumps harder and the myocardium thickens (hypertrophy). Hypertension is controlled with diet, decreased sodium, and medications to dilate or relax vessels and to decrease retention of water and sodium (diuretics).

Hypertension, congenital or acquired damage to the cardiac tissues, and pulmonary disease can be causes of congestive heart failure. In heart failure the ventricular muscle cannot contract enough to sustain an adequate circulation. This leads to secondary effects on other organs. If the left ventricle fails, there is a backup of fluid in the pulmonary circulation causing edema and difficulty in breathing. In addition, the right ventricle dilates causing dilatation and congestion in the vena cava and resulting in edema and congestion in the liver with eventual swelling of the ankles. If the left ventricle fails to supply sufficient output of blood forward, the kidney, normally getting 25 percent of the cardiac output, receives less blood flow and retains sodium, eventually resulting in peripheral edema into tissues such as the legs and ankles. Congestive heart failure can lead to failure of both sides of the heart and may linger or result in sudden death.

Inflammation, a major category of disease, is the reaction of the body to various stimuli or injurious agents, living or nonliving. Inflammation can be caused by infectious agents. An infection is defined as an invasion of the body by pathogenic microorganisms and the reaction to them or their toxic products. Infections may be caused by viruses, bacteria, protozoa, and helminths. Inflammation is characterized by heat, redness, swelling, pain, and loss of function (see Chapter 3). Through inflammation and immunology the host can cope with both living and nonliving foreign agents. Both involve complex interactions of bloodborne elements and cellular elements that are brought forth to combat the offending agent. Not only does the host respond in an overwhelming manner to the injurious agent, but it also sets the stage for repairing the injury by producing new cells rapidly (proliferation).

Repair of tissue is the replacement of the injured area with scar tissue (connective tissue cells). Regeneration is the replacement of damaged tissue with the same type of tissue that was damaged. For example, damaged heart muscle cannot regenerate and is replaced by scar tissue. On the other hand, surface epithelium or bone regenerates rapidly. However, if the destruction of tissue is extensive, even tissue with a good ability for regeneration heals by repair (dense connective tissue).

Growth of tissue is another way the host can respond to injury. This proliferation of cells may or may not be associated with inflammation. The changes involved include hyperplasia, hypertrophy, and metaplasia. Hyperplasia is the increase in the number of normal cells of an organ or tissue with a consequent increase in size of the tissue (see Fig. 2.2). Hyperplasia can be physiologic, such as the response of glands to a demand for more secretion. Usually, however, the increase in the number of cells is a protective mechanism against a constant source of irritation. The oral epithelium undergoes hyperplastic changes to injury, which will be discussed under mucous membrane pathology in Chapter 6. Quite often, the underlying supporting tissue undergoes hyperplasia along with the surface tissue. An example of this is seen in denture hyperplasia caused by a poorly fitting denture.

Hypertrophy (see Fig. 2.2) is the increase in size of a tissue or organ caused by an increase in the size of the cells of the part involved. This is seen particularly in muscle fibers. For example, in a patient with heart failure, the heart muscles may undergo hypertrophy as a means of compensating for the original damage. Hypertrophy occurs physiologically in exercising of muscles and accounts for enlarged body contours. The masseter muscles may be prominent due to hypertrophy seen either genetically or in individuals who constantly clench their teeth together (Fig. 2.5).

The opposite of hypertrophy is atrophy (see Fig. 2.2). In a paraplegic, there is loss of nerve supply to the musces of the legs and therefore loss of function. With loss of function, the muscle cells undergo atrophy. They decrease is size below normal, and ultimately the whole muscle mass and leg become smaller. Atrophy can also be seen in the oral cavity. For instance, a defect in the hypoglossal nerve that innervates the tongue muscles can cause the tongue muscles to become atrophic. The muscles on the side affected shrivel. The tongue does not

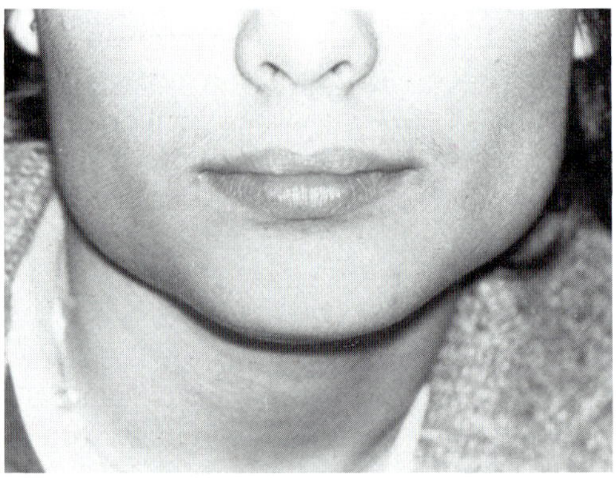

Figure 2.5. Hypertrophy of masseter muscles causing swellings at angles of the mandible.

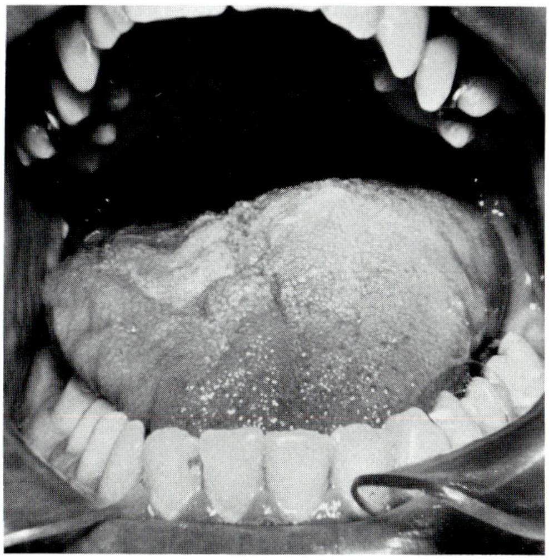

Figure 2.6. Hypoglossal nerve defect. Right side of tongue is atrophied and flaccid.

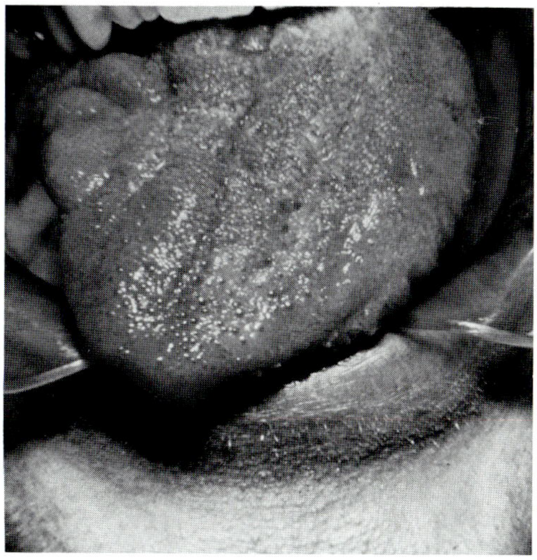

Figure 2.7. Hypoglossal nerve defect (same patient as in Fig. 2.6). Tongue deviates to the affected side when protruded.

look full and is flaccid (weak and soft) (Figs. 2.5 to 2.7).

Metaplasia is the microscopic change in which cells of one type are transformed into or replaced by cells of another type that normally would not be located in the particular site. For instance, in smokers, the ciliated epithelium that lines bronchioles transforms into stratified squamous epithelium. This transformation is a protective mechanism in the sense that stratified squamous epithelium is more resistant to injury. However, the ciliated epithelium is itself a natural protective mechanism, so that metaplasia in this instance is an abnormal response. This same type of change is seen in ducts of accessory salivary glands in the oral cavity (Fig. 2.8).

Metaplasia is noted in the connective tissue cells as well as in the epithelial cells (Fig. 2.8). For example, bone or cartilage may form within connective tissue in an area that usually does not have bone or cartilage within it. The transformation of normal connective tissue cells into the cells and substance constituting bone is metaplasia.

This concept of metaplasia is difficult to grasp, because it cannot be appreciated at the clinical level. Whereas the increase in cells of hyperplasia causes an increase in the overall size of a structure so as to produce a clinical lesion, the changes seen in metaplasia are microscopic only. For instance, a swelling on the gingiva is a hyperplastic response. However, on examining the tissue of this lesion by the microscope, one may seen bone forming in the connective tissue (metaplasia). Metaplasia and pathologic hyperplasia contribute to cellular turnover and may predispose the tissues to neoplastic change.

Neoplasia is the last category to be considered. The term neoplasia refers to a new growth of tissue that arises from existing tissue but grows independently of it and at its own rate. This abnormal new tissue is called a neoplasm technically, but more commonly it is called a tumor. Strictly speaking, a tumor is any swelling of tissue and as such may represent a lesion that is developmental, inflammatory, or neoplastic. By common usage the word tumor has become synonymous with a neoplasm, specifically, cancer.

Clinically, a neoplasm may present as a

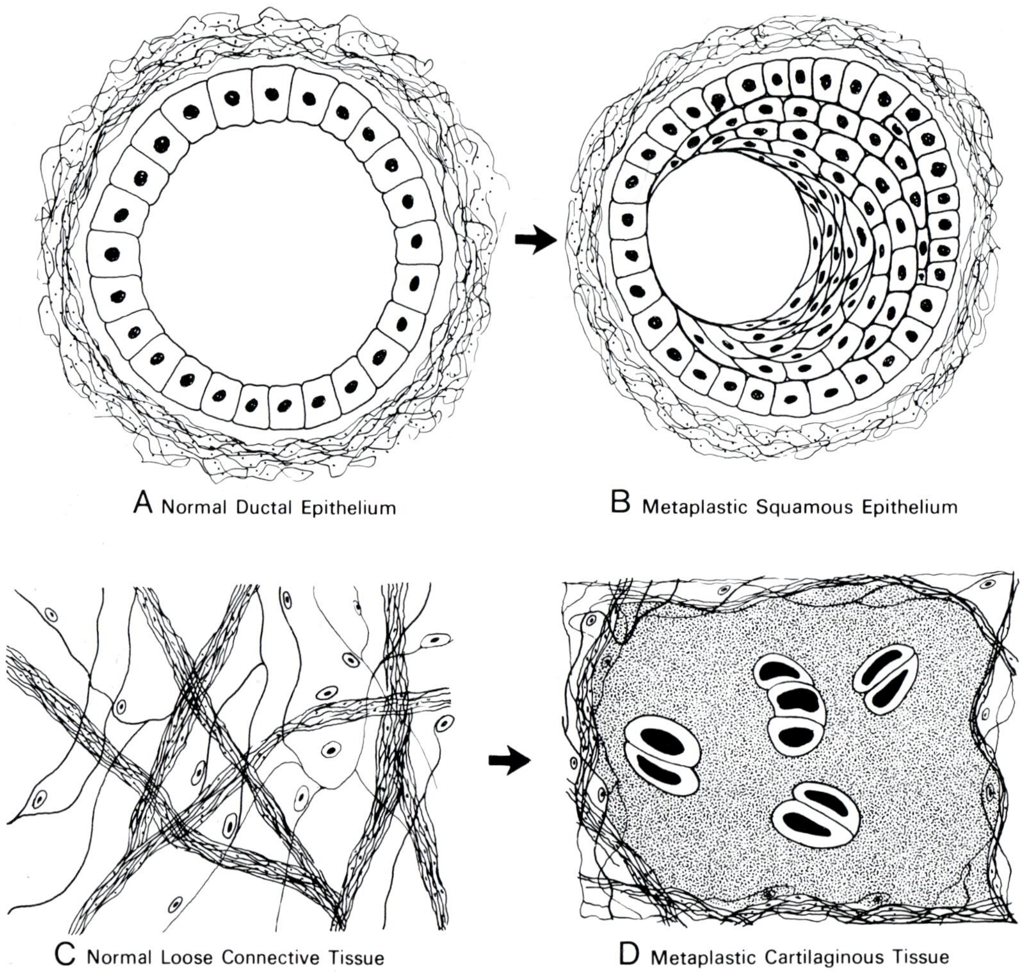

Figure 2.8. Diagrammatic representation of metaplasia. *A* and *B*, metaplasia of ductular epithelium to stratified squamous epithelium. *C* and *D*, metaplasia of normal loose fibrous connective tissue to cartilaginous tissue.

swelling. Only by microscopic examination of the tissue can the nature of the lesion become known. By the cellular characteristics, the growth is designated as benign or malignant. Those neoplasms that resemble the tissue of origin in cellular details and in behavior are called benign. These are slow-growing, localized lesions that may cause injury to the host by expansion against normal tissue or by releasing hormones.

By contrast, those neoplasms that present a marked difference in cellular details from the tissue of origin and are a threat to life or health because of their behavior are called malignant. The word cancer refers to any malignant neoplasm. Cancer of epithelial cells is a carcinoma. Cancer of connective tissue cells is a sarcoma. Cancers do not remain localized and can spread in many ways. The cells can grow in finger- or clawlike projections and infiltrate the underlying tissue (Fig. 2.9).

The cells may also spread by way of the lymph channels or bloodstream. If a second growth of the malignancy occurs at the distant site, the cancer is said to have metastasized. Metastasis is a characteristic feature of malignancy. For example, a

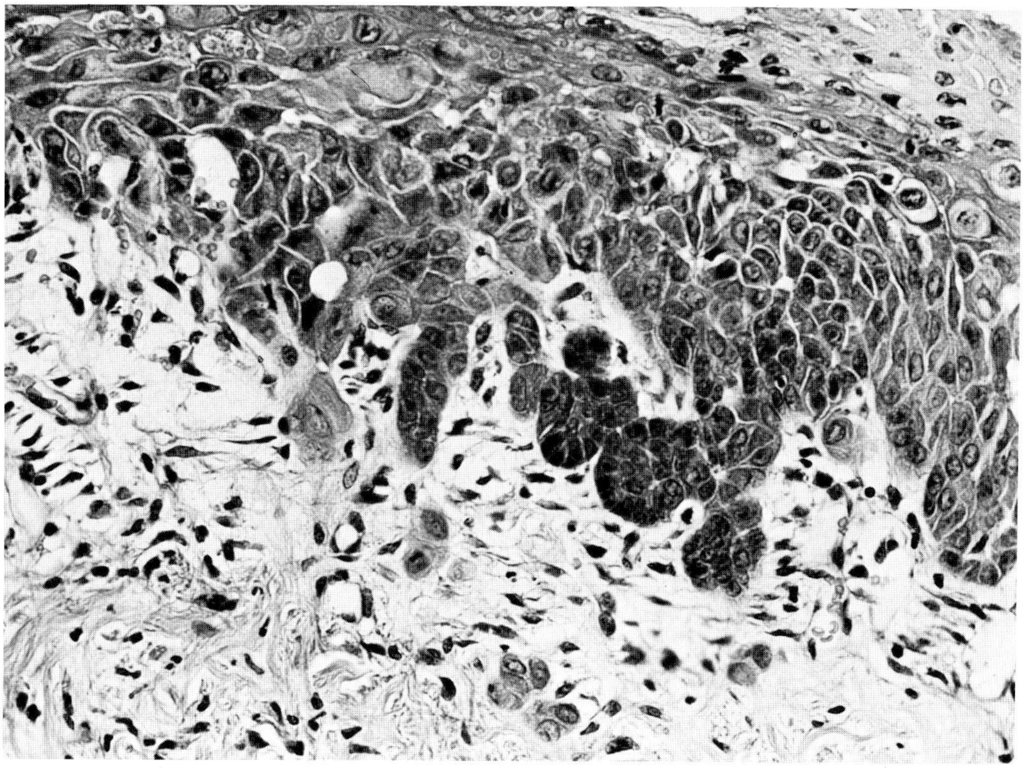

Figure 2.9. Squamous cell or epidermoid carcinoma. Atypical neoplastic epithelial cells extending and invading in clawlike extensions into underlying connective tissue.

female patient may have a primary cancer of the breast. This cancer often spreads to the bones. Not infrequently one may see on the radiograph a radiolucency or dark shadow in the mandible near a tooth. On investigation, the tissue from this area of the jaw may reveal the same cancer cells that originated in the breast. The cancer in the jaw has grown at a distant site and is therefore a metastasis.

Neoplasia can occur anywhere in the body. Developing from different tissues in different areas, cancer is more than a hundred different diseases. In the oral cavity it is a serious disease because, despite the ease with which it could be diagnosed, the cure rate and survival rates are poor. Neoplasia is covered in Chapter 7.

In summary, there are numerous causes both known and unknown for disease, but the responses by the host are limited. Some agents may cause minimal injury, whereas others may be overwhelming and cause severe damage. The extent of damage and the response depends on the resistance of the host. Given the same injury, each host reacts differently; the injury may be slight to one but severe to another. The responses of any host to an injury as presented in this section may also be used at the clinical level. When one is contemplating a disease, it is convenient to ask what category of disease one has at hand. These categories are developmental, metabolic, inflammatory (infectious), hyperplastic, and neoplastic.

Chapter 3
INFLAMMATION, IMMUNITY, AND REPAIR

The category of inflammation-immunology is extremely important in pathology and oral pathology. Inflammation is a common, favorable response of the body to irritants or microorganisms. Without inflammation, wounds would not heal, and without the immune response, bacteria and other organisms would flourish and eventually cause the death of the host. With inflammation the host has a nonspecific reactive process that not only walls off the area of injury but also sets into motion the process whereby the tissue may be healed. With an intact immune response, the host has a specific response to microorganisms and foreign substances.

The cause of the injury can be mechanical, such as trauma, tear, or laceration; it may be thermal or electrical and produce a burn; or it may be biological, such as viral, bacterial, or fungal. Whatever the cause, cells at the site of injury are damaged, and chemicals from these cells set into motion the continuum of events called inflammation.

Inflammation is designated by the attachment of the suffix "itis," meaning inflammation of, to the name of the area that is affected. Thus, inflammation of the colon is colitis; of the veins, phlebitis; of the gingiva, gingivitis; of the pulp, pulpitis. Regardless of the location, the events of inflammation are the same.

The events seen in inflammation are complex and should be considered as an ever-changing and dynamic picture. For convenience the components of the reaction are: damage to the tissues, a local change in circulation (alteration), infiltration of cells and fluid into the area (exudation), and the local proliferation of cells and growth of new tissue (granulation and repair).

Immediately following injury there is a brief moment in which the blood vessels in the area constrict. Test this by scratching the skin of the inside aspect of the wrist with a sharp point. You will observe that the line of the scratch blanches almost immediately due to the constriction of the blood vessels. Then the blood vessels, particularly the postcapillary venules, dilate and become quite prominent (Fig. 3.1). This vascular change brings more blood to the area by both active and passive hyperemia. It also causes the flow of blood within the vessels to slow down (stasis). The red blood cells and the white blood cells move from the center of the venule to the edges (margination). Because of the vasodilation, there are gaps created between the endothelial cells. Lipid, salts, and water leave in greater than normal amounts. Proteins, normally held back by intact endothelial cells, also leave the vessels. The red blood cells leave by a process called diapedesis, leaving between the cells of the intact blood vessel. The more damage there is to the vessel, the greater the number of red blood cells (hemorrhage) in the injured area. Clinically, if the site of injury is observable, such as the scratch, a redness appears and increases over the hours as more blood comes to the area. Heat may also be noted and is due to the increase in the flow of blood to the area. The sluggish circulation is necessary for the next event, which is the migration of cells (Fig. 3.2). Polymorphonuclear leukocytes or neutrophils are the first white blood cells called to the area by a chemical (chemotaxis) that is released by the injured cells. The summoned cells line

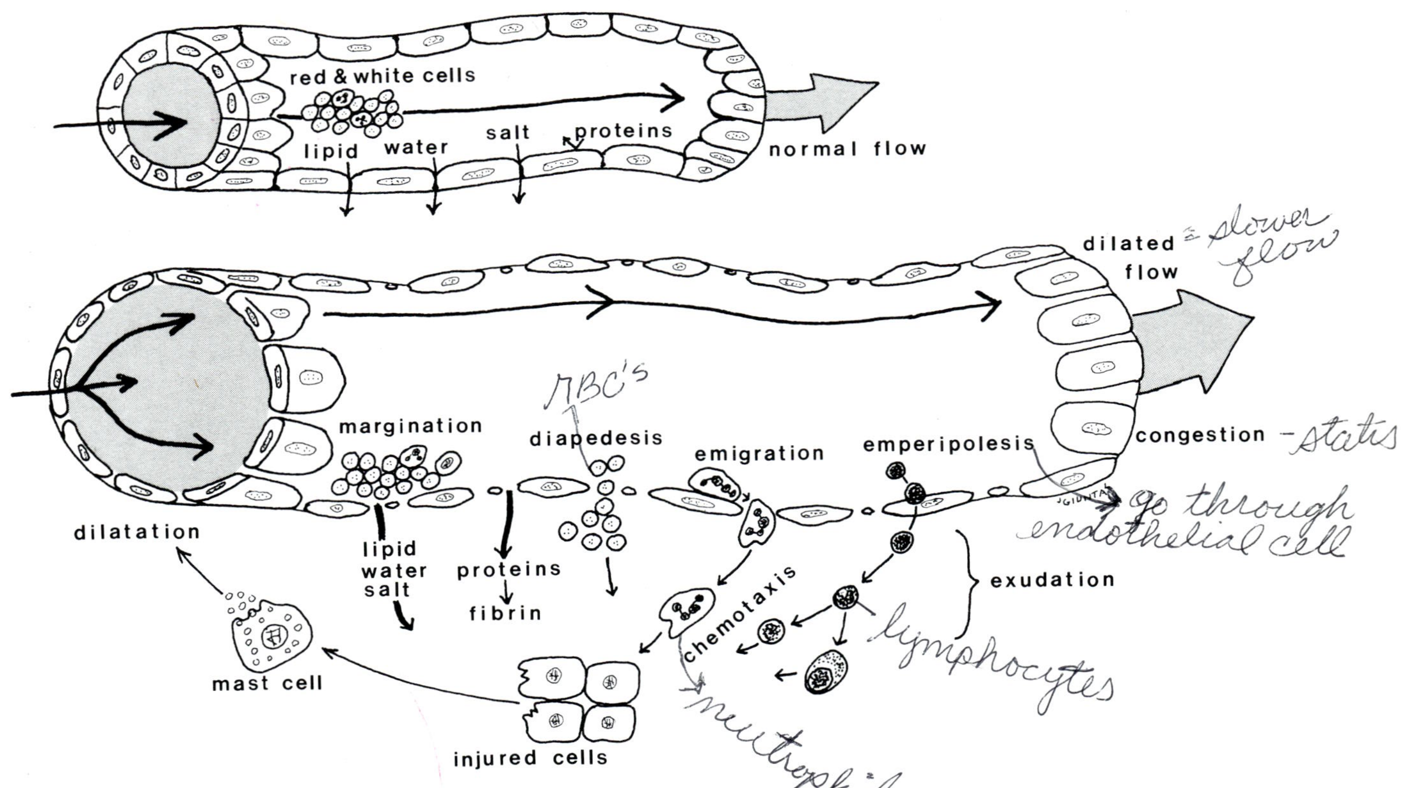

Figure 3.1. Diagram depicting particularly the early events of inflammation, vascular dilatation, fluid exchange, and cellular passage into the injured area.

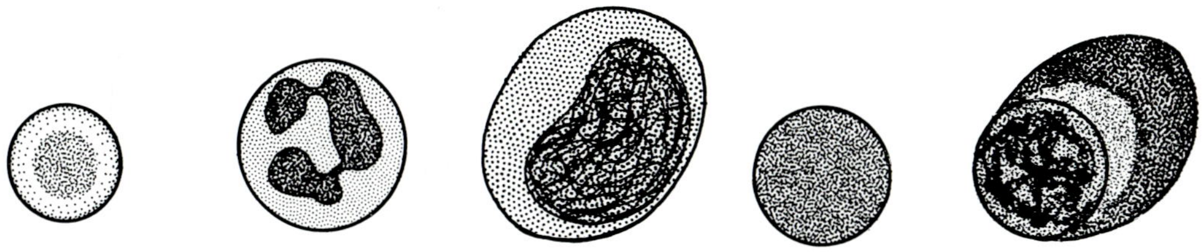

Figure 3.2. Diagrammatic representation of cells involved in inflammation, drawn to scale to illustrate relative size.

up along the sides of the dilated blood vessels and by ameboid motion emigrate between endothelial cells into the injured area within a few hours after the injury. Monocytes are the second white blood cells to emigrate. Lymphocytes usually enter much later, but in some diseases, such as viral ones, they are the first to enter by crossing through the endothelial cells (emperipolesis).

Neutrophils are cells with many lobes of the nucleus which can assume multiple shapes and are therefore called polymorphonuclear cells. They are phagocytic cells, meaning that they can ingest microorganisms, other cells (like necrotic cells), and foreign matter. In the cytoplasm are numerous granules that stain on microscopic sections with neutral dyes and account for the name "neutrophil." These granules contain enzymes capable of digesting cellular tissue including bacteria.

Fluid in more than normal amounts (edema) also accumulates in the tissue. This fluid from the plasma of the blood contains fibrinogen. By the activation of the clotting mechanism in the tissues (see Fig. 2.4), fibrinogen is converted to fibrin, a large strandlike protein that forms a spongelike mesh. The fibrin temporarily walls off the area and blocks drainage to lymphatic channels.

The intercellular fluid, with the many proteins from the blood and parts of the injured cells, is called an exudate. There are different types of exudate depending on the predominant product of the inflammatory response. A mucinous or catarrhal exudate has large quantities of mucin, as in upper respiratory infections, colds, and bronchitis. A fibrinous exudate has mostly fibrin and can stick two apposing surfaces together, as in the pleura of the lung or the pericardium. A serous exudate has mostly watery fluid high in protein with limited fibrin, as in the peritoneum. A hemorrhagic or sanguineous exudate has high numbers of red blood cells and is seen where vessels are intensely dilated or ruptured. A purulent exudate is characterized by an accumulation of pus with prominent liquefaction necrosis, as in a cellulitis or tissue abscess. Acute inflammation is usually characterized by a purulent exudate due to high numbers of neutrophils and dead cells. The exudate accounts for many signs and symptoms of acute inflammation.

The classic signs of inflammation are explained by the efflux of fluid and cells from the vessels at the injured site. The redness (rubor) and heat (calor) are due to the increased blood flow into the area. The swelling (tumor) is due to the exudation filling the interstitial spaces. The pain (dolor) is due to pressure from the swelling against nerve endings and from some of the chemical mediators such as prostaglandins that make local nerves more sensitive. The fifth classic symptom is loss of function and depends on the site and the extent of injury; e.g., fracture of a leg bone leads to not using the leg.

Certain factors or chemical mediators are responsible for altering the permeability of the blood vessels and allowing extra fluid and cells to diffuse into the injured area. Generally, there is a biphasic response, with different chemicals responsible at each phase. The first phase is short, lasting only up to ½ hour. After it peaks and falls, the second phase of increased permeability starts and lasts for several hours. If the insult or injury is severe, there is only an immediate, prolonged single phase of permeability. Histamine from mast cells in tissue or basophils and platelets in the blood, and serotonin from platelets mediate the initial phase. Several other chemicals, whose action is antagonistic to the constrictor epinephrine, mediate the second phase. These include blood peptides, kinins and complement fragments, and some prostaglandins (PGE). PGEs, kinins, and leukotrienes, another mediator, cause an increase in pain. Clinically, aspirin and nonsteroidal anti-inflammatory medications inhibit prostaglandin production. There are many other chemical mediators that increase permeability and may also activate the accumulation of neutrophils and macrophages into the tissue. These cells attempt to localize, to destroy the agent, and to clear the damaged tissue.

Neutrophils are capable of ingesting and destroying some but not all bacteria. If the number of bacteria is such that the enzyme system of the neutrophil can digest them, then the area is soon cleared of bacteria and neutrophils. Besides digesting bacteria and other small foreign particles, the lysosomes of neutrophils can dissolve the neutrophil itself if it dies, as well as liquefy local cells of the host and the insoluble fibrin wall that was laid down. If the number of bacteria are overwhelming or contain toxins to the neutrophils or if the resistance of the host is decreased, neutrophils accumulate, die, and in the process liquefy more host tissue, forming pus (suppuration). Pus is the liquefied material containing dead and dying neutrophils and host cell debris. When it is localized or walled off in a cavity, it is called an abscess. It is usually eliminated by the body by drainage to an exterior surface such as skin or mucosa or diffuses by the blood or lymphatics where it is carried off for destruction elsewhere. A suppurative process may be seen in either acute or chronic inflammation.

The build-up of fluid, fibrin, and neutrophils is the hallmark of acute inflammation which, clinically speaking, usually lasts only for a short time (hours to days). Within hours, but more noticeable from 1 to 3 days, other cells begin to appear and to proliferate.

Macrophages, important in acute and chronic inflammation, appear after the neutrophils. Macrophages, also known as histiocytes, are derived from the white blood cells, the monocyte. They respond more slowly to chemicals liberated by injured cells (chemotaxis). They are also phagocytic or scavenger cells but are larger and are capable of ingesting larger particles. In fact, it is common to see an ingested neutrophil within the cytoplasm of a macrophage. In certain instances the cytoplasm of several macrophages merge to form a large cell with multiple distinct nuclei, the foreign body giant cell. This type of cell can be seen in reactions to a wood splinter, to a suture, and to microorganisms such as fungi and the tubercle bacillus. Oftentimes, giant cells are seen in longstanding inflammation.

Macrophages phagocytize foreign material, dead cells, and debris at the site of inflammation and set into motion the immune response and repair. They release many factors including growth factors. Because of their time of appearance and function, they are considered the second line of defense. In most instances the neutrophils and macrophages can readily contain the injurious agent. However, if they fail, there is another system of cells called the reticuloendothelial system (RES) that can carry on. These cells resemble macrophages and are scattered in connective tissue and particularly in the liver, the spleen, and the lymph nodes.

The lymphocyte is another cell that appears later in the inflammatory process. This is a small cell with a densely stained round nucleus and very little cytoplasm. There are several types of lymphocytes whose prime function is to recognize foreign material (antigens) and to elaborate an immune response. Some of these cells are phagocytic and are capable of attaching themselves to an antigen. Other lymphocytes transform into plasma cells that produce antibodies. Plasma cells have a nucleus, similar to the lymphocyte but eccentrically located in a cytoplasm housing the machinery for producing the antibody. The antibody is expressed into the fluid surrounding the cells; it seeks out the foreign proteins and inactivates them by binding them to form antigen-antibody complexes. These complexes themselves can elicit an inflammatory response.

Another cell that is involved in antigen-antibody responses, particularly relating to allergy, is the eosinophil. An eosinophil resembles a neutrophil with a lobulated nucleus but has prominent granules that stain red with the dye eosin. The granules contain enzymes capable of digesting antigen-antibody complexes. This may be the reason for the appearance of these cells in allergic diseases such as hay fever and contact allergies.

Fibroblasts and new capillaries also begin to appear within the first few days of the inflammatory response. The fibroblasts are young connective tissue cells that can produce collagen fibers. The new capillaries, triggered by a macrophage factor, bud from existing capillaries in large numbers, increasing the blood supply to the area. Collectively, the fibroblastic and new capillary response is called granulation tissue. The longer the granulation tissue remains, the more collagen fibers are formed and the greater the amount of scar.

Both the macrocytic-lymphocytic infiltrate and the granulation tissue, a proliferation of cells and new tissue, are hallmarks of a chronic inflammatory response that clinically exists for an extended period (days to months or even years). If the injurious agent persists, then this response may linger without resolution and, with time, dense connective tissue (collagen) would replace the original tissue.

If the injurious agent is overcome, the inflammation subsides and the tissue undergoes repair. There are two types of repair. Restitution is the replacement of the injured area with the same tissue that preceded the inflammation. Repair with scarring (fibrosis) is the other form. A scar represents dense bundles of collagen fibers that have been produced from the granulation tissue to replace the injured tissue. At first the scar may appear red to the surface because of the increased capillary supply from the granulation tissue. But over many months these capillaries disappear and the avascular scar remains white due to the dense bundles of collagen. Thus the end of inflammation is heralded by a return of the tissue to its normal state or to a state of repair with a scar (Fig. 3.3).

An excellent example of the inflammatory response is seen in wound healing of ulcerations of the oral mucosa (Figs. 3.4 to 3.9). An ulcer is any break in the epithelial surface that exposes the underlying connective tissue. With this break, the energies of the local cells are involved in reuniting the surface. Wound healing takes place with the formation of abundant granulation tissue and epithelial proliferation. This is called healing by secondary intention, because the wound edges are not approximated and because the inflammatory response must fill in the destroyed tissue with granulation tissue that ultimately is replaced. This type of healing is seen in ulcers, tooth extractions, and bone fractures. If, on the other hand, the tissue is wounded but the edges are touching or are brought into continuity with sutures, that healing is by first intention and does not require the exuberant cellular response seen in ulcerations (Fig. 3.10). Thus, there is less scarring when wounds are sutured.

In an ulcer there is activity at both the epithelial surface and deep within the under-

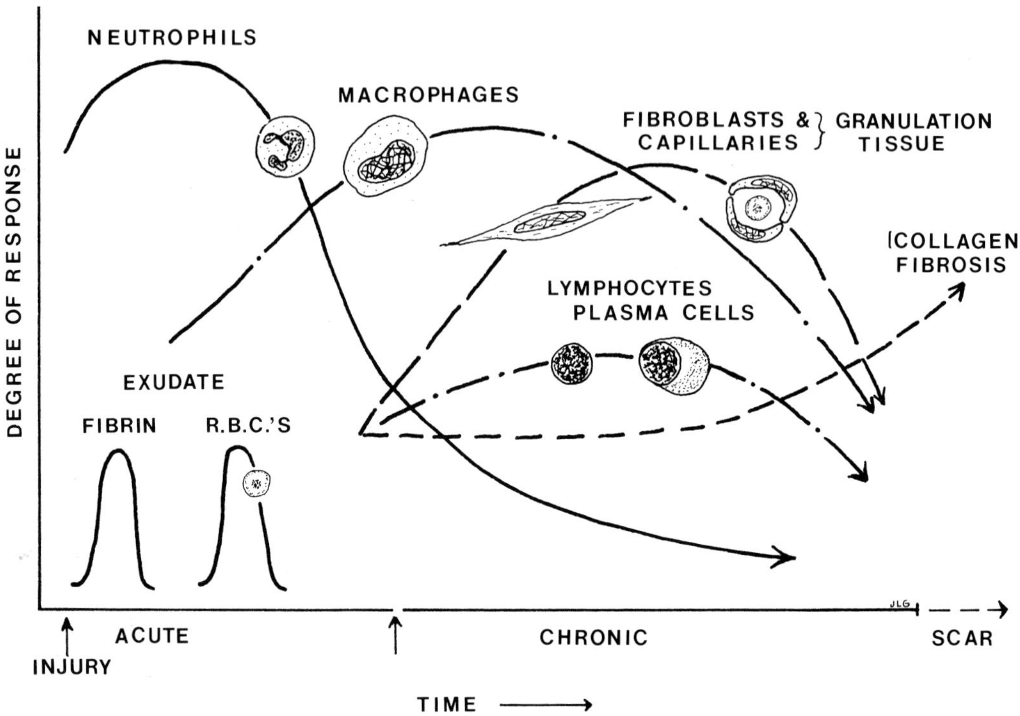

Figure 3.3. Schematic flow chart depicting events of the inflammatory response according to persistence of injury and time.

lying connective tissue. The destruction of the epithelial surface and some connective tissue initiates the inflammatory response (Fig. 3.11). If there is bleeding, a clot soon forms of fibrin and red blood cells. Within hours there is edema fluid, and neutrophils are seen in great numbers. The neutrophils begin to emigrate to the destroyed surface and ultimately build up the surface with a scab. The scab is composed of fibrin, red blood cells, and dead or dying neutrophils (Fig. 3.12). It is a necrotic plug and appears white or yellowish clinically. It protects the connective tissue until the epithelium can cover it again. At the same time there is cellular activity in the connective tissue. Macrophages soon appear and begin to phagocytize the necrotic cells and debris along with the neutrophils. In about a day, fibroblasts and capillaries begin to proliferate. On the surface at this time, the epithelial cells at the margins of the ulcer pile up slightly and begin to migrate toward the epithelium on the other margin. The epithelium extends itself between the scab and the tissue beneath it. In a matter of

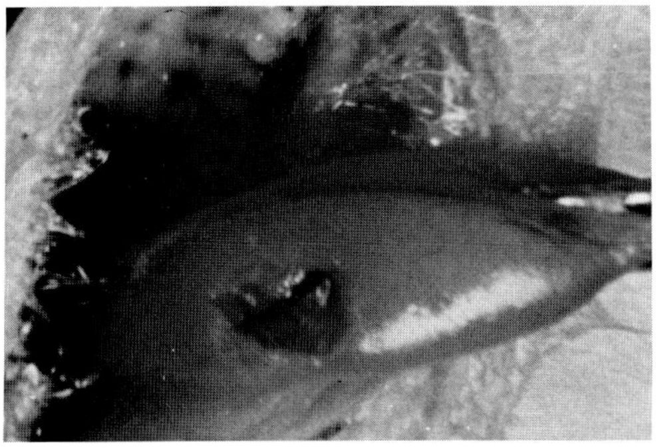

Figure 3.4. Figures 3.4 through 3.9 are a sequence following healing of experimental hamster. First figure taken at zero hours; fresh ulcer with bleeding.

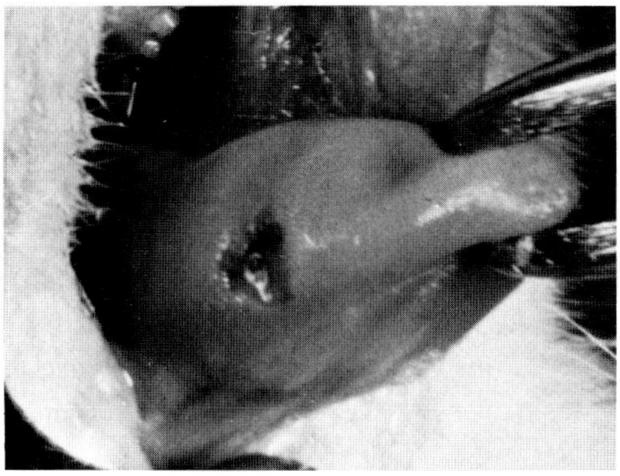

Figure 3.5. Five hours, early scab following clot.

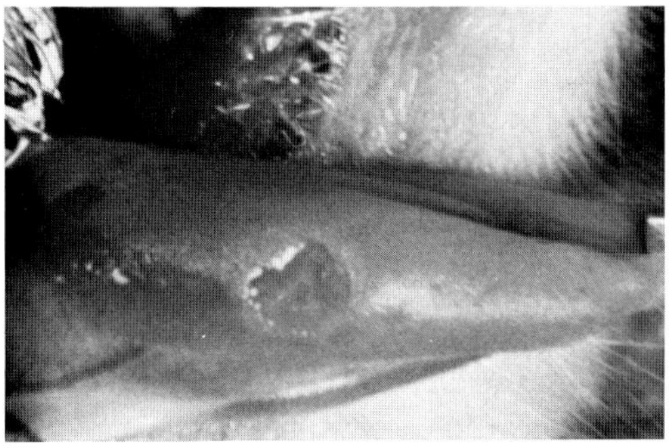

Figure 3.6. One day, scab is complete, appears white.

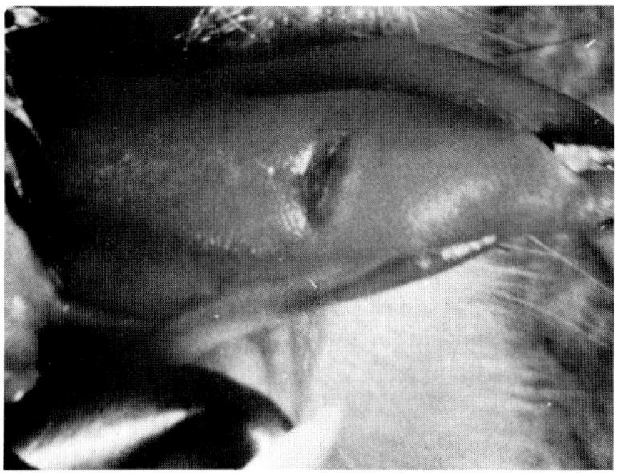

Figure 3.7. Three days, ulcer contracted, rolled borders.

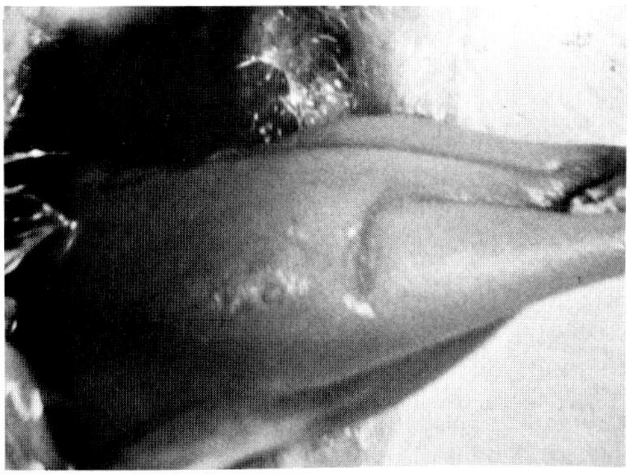

Figure 3.8. Seven days, epithelium healed, ulcer more contracted.

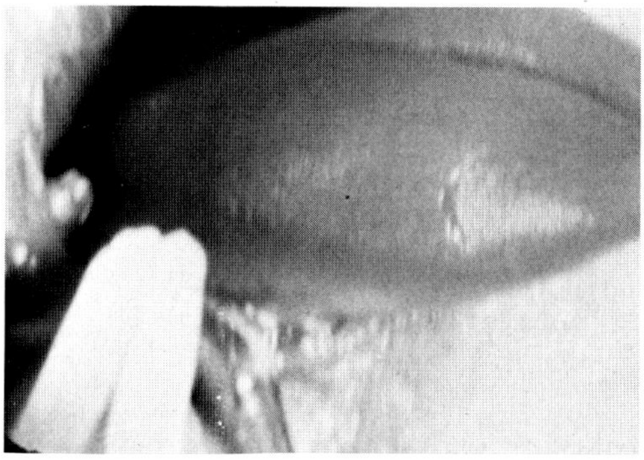

Figure 3.9. Fourteen days, only narrow defect remains, healing of connective tissue is continuing, contour of tongue is reestablished. At 21 days no evidence of an ulcer was seen.

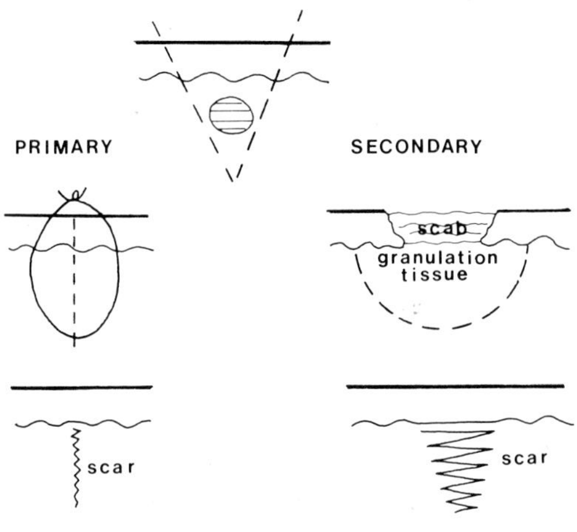

Figure 3.10. Diagram contrasting healing by primary intention versus healing by secondary intention. The wound is created by excisional biopsy of a lesion in the connective tissue. In primary healing the wound is closed with sutures, the edges coapt, and there is minimal granulation tissue and minimal scarring. In secondary healing, there is no wound closure, a scab is produced, and considerable granulation tissue yields a larger scar.

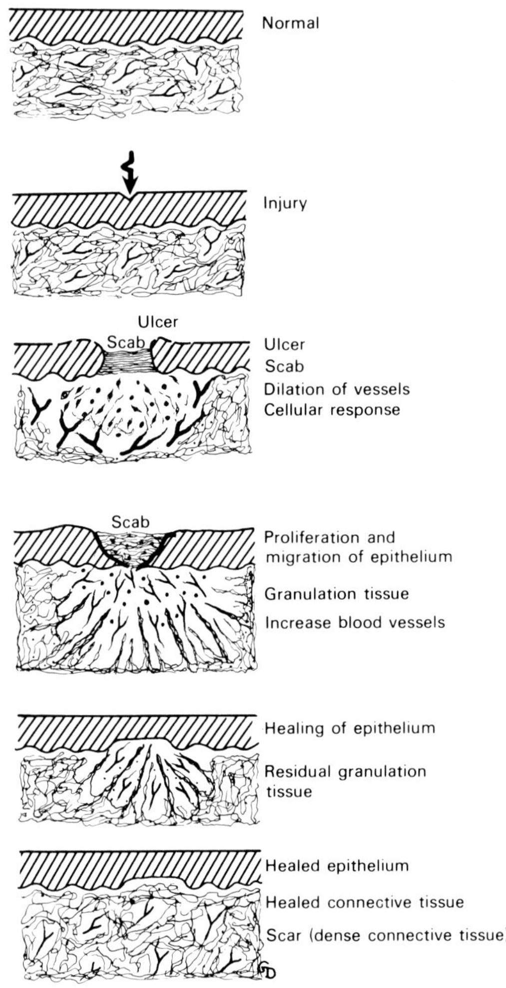

Figure 3.11. Reaction of mucosa to an injury that results in forming an ulcer. Schematic drawing depicting ulcer, scab formation, vascular and cellular response, formation of granulation tissue, proliferation, migration of epithelium, and healing by restitution of mucosal epithelium and connective tissue.

days when the epithelium meets with opposite margins at the center, the migration stops and the scab is cast off. In addition to the epithelial migration, open wounds close by a process of wound contraction in the connective tissue. Contractile elements in the granulation tissue, probably myofilaments in fibroblasts, cause the wound to be pulled in toward the center (Fig. 3.13). Factors such as excess corticosteroids and radiation therapy can interfere with the contraction, yielding a larger area of scar. After about 2 days there is abundant granulation tissue. The new capillaries and inflammatory response cover an area greater in width than the original ulceration and give the tissue a reddened hue or halo surrounding the ulcer (Fig. 3.14). Just as the epithelium migrates and regenerates, the connective tissue and skeletal muscle may regenerate in the connective tissue. The granulation tissue, which becomes infiltrated with chronic inflammatory cells, provides the vascularity with its nutrients so that new tissue can form. If the damage was not severe or longstanding, not much fibrosis occurs—particularly in the oral mucosa. Rather, the connective tissue reforms and muscle fibers and nerves regenerate. Inflammatory cells and vascularity subside and the tissue is restored.

The collagen in scar tissue is remodeled and reconstituted. The enzyme collagenase is responsible for removing excess collagen.

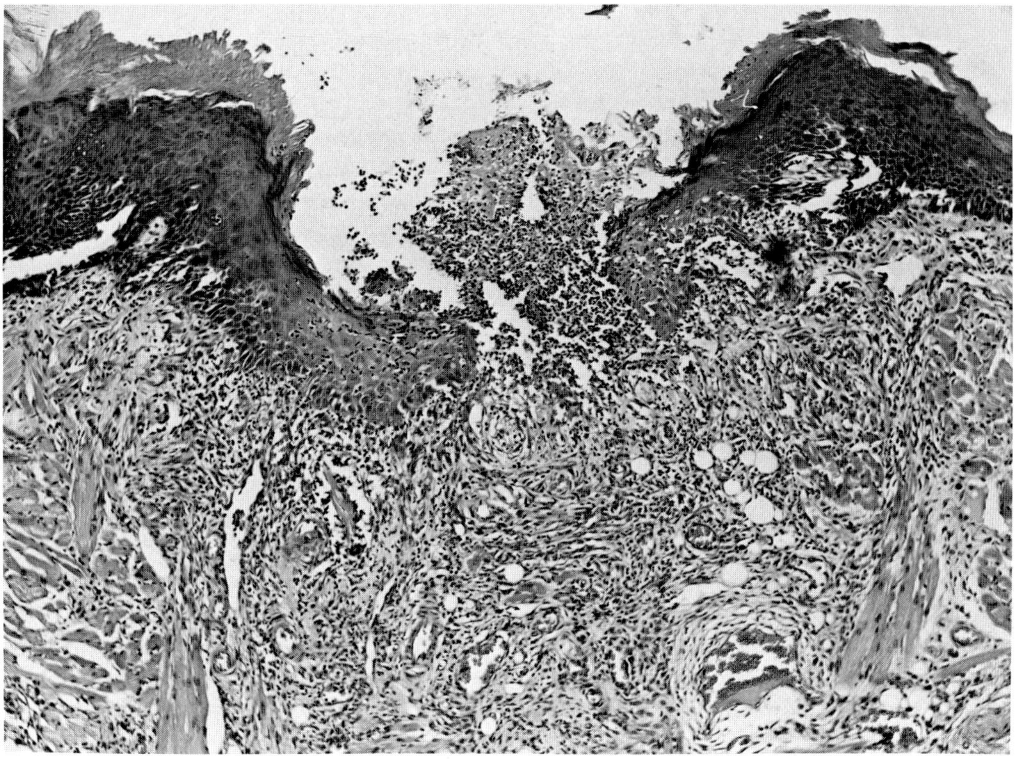

Figure 3.12. Healing experimental tongue ulcer, 4 days. Epithelium is migrating beneath scab. Margins of ulcer are rolled due to proliferating epithelium. Granulation tissue, rich in blood vessels and containing chronic inflammatory cells, is beginning to form new connective tissue and muscle.

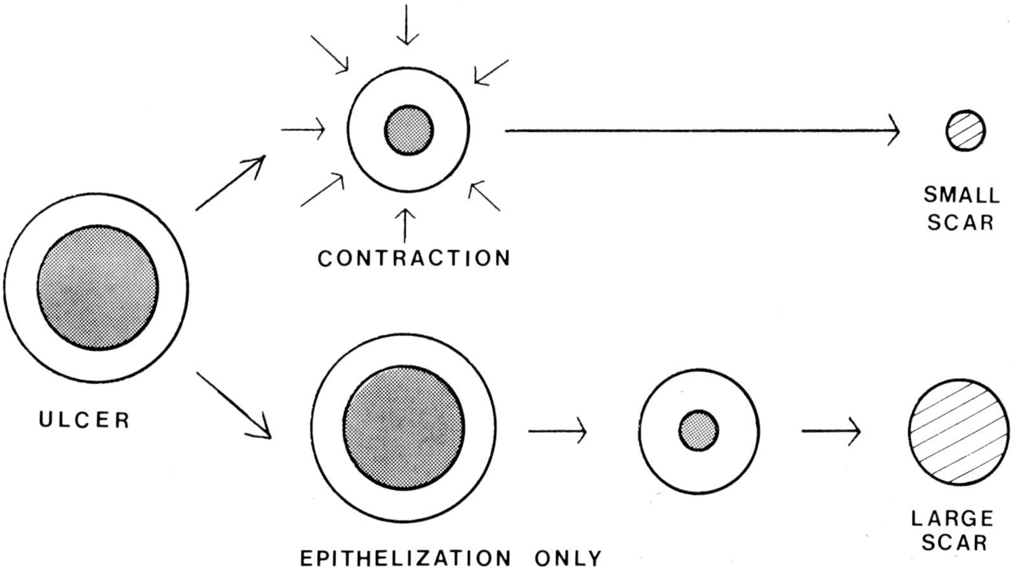

Figure 3.13. Diagram contrasting normal open wound (ulcer) healing with wound contraction and epithelial migration resulting in a small scar versus healing without contraction with only epithelial migration, yielding a large scar, as seen in irradiated tissue, excessive use of corticosteroids, and poor nutrition.

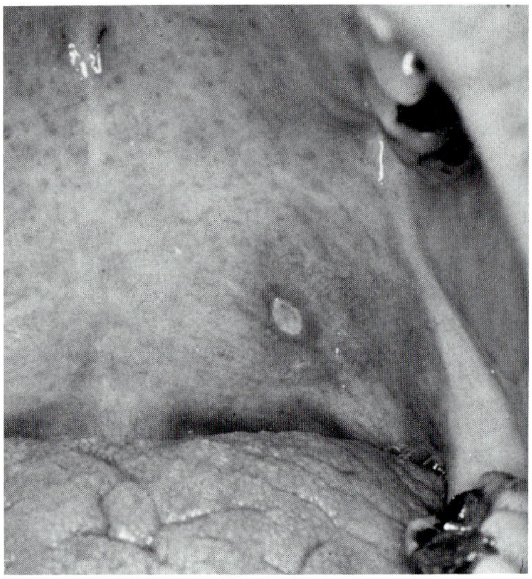

Figure 3.14. Ulcer on soft palate; aphthous stomatitis. Red halo surrounds clearly outlined oval white scab filling in ulceration.

In some individuals there is a deficiency of collagenase. During wound healing, they produce an excess amount of scar tissue called a keloid, producing a raised, often pigmented tissue at the site of injury.

The healing of an extraction socket site is similar, except that bone eventually forms from the granulation tissue (Fig. 3.15). After a tooth is extracted, there is bleeding followed by coagulation filling the socket, the surface forming a scab. Without the clot, there would be no healing, and a painful condition called dry socket would ensue. Next, growing into the clot is granulation tissue, and the surface heals as an open wound with the epithelium growing across and under the scab. Concurrently the clot is dissolved, and fibroblasts from the granulation tissue transform into osteoblasts. Osteoblasts also proliferate from the remaining bone edges and lay down a bone matrix (osteoid). At this stage, without calcification, the radiograph would show a radiolucent socket site. The next stage, several months in the human, is the calcification stage, in which the osteoid is calcified and becomes bone. At this stage, a radiograph shows the radiopaque bone spicules. The final stage is characterized by a remodeling and reshaping. The healed socket has less dense spicules of bone than the adjacent tooth-bearing bone, because there is no pressure from the tooth to cause there to be thicker plates of bone.

Inflammation is generally considered to be a favorable response, but there are occasions when its consequences or continued existence is not favorable. Inflammation of the cornea of the eye could lead to scarring and impairment of vision. That is why corticosteroid drops are used when the cornea is damaged. The corticosteroid as an anti-inflammatory agent diminishes the inflammatory response and consequent scarring. In the disease of poliomyelitis, which has been effectively abated by vaccination procedures, the complication of paralysis is a sign of inflammation that no longer exists. In poliomyelitis, important ganglion cells are infected by a virus and destroyed. Inflammation ensues and quickly heals the area. However, the area heals with scar tissue, because the specialized nerve cells cannot regenerate. Thus, without these cells to complete the proper synapses, the muscles lack control and, because of disease, undergo atrophy.

The Immune System

The human immune system exists to combat infection against alien organisms like bacteria, viruses, fungi, and parasites. Highly specific, it has the capacity to recognize self and nonself and, like the brain, can create and store information, can learn and memorize. For example, encountering an organism for the first time, cells and proteins in the blood and/or lymph system and in the tissues take time to mount a response sufficient to combat and kill the organism. However, on the second exposure by the same organism, there is immediate recognition and immediate response by specific cells and proteins to eliminate that organism before it can take hold. The body is then considered immune to that organism.

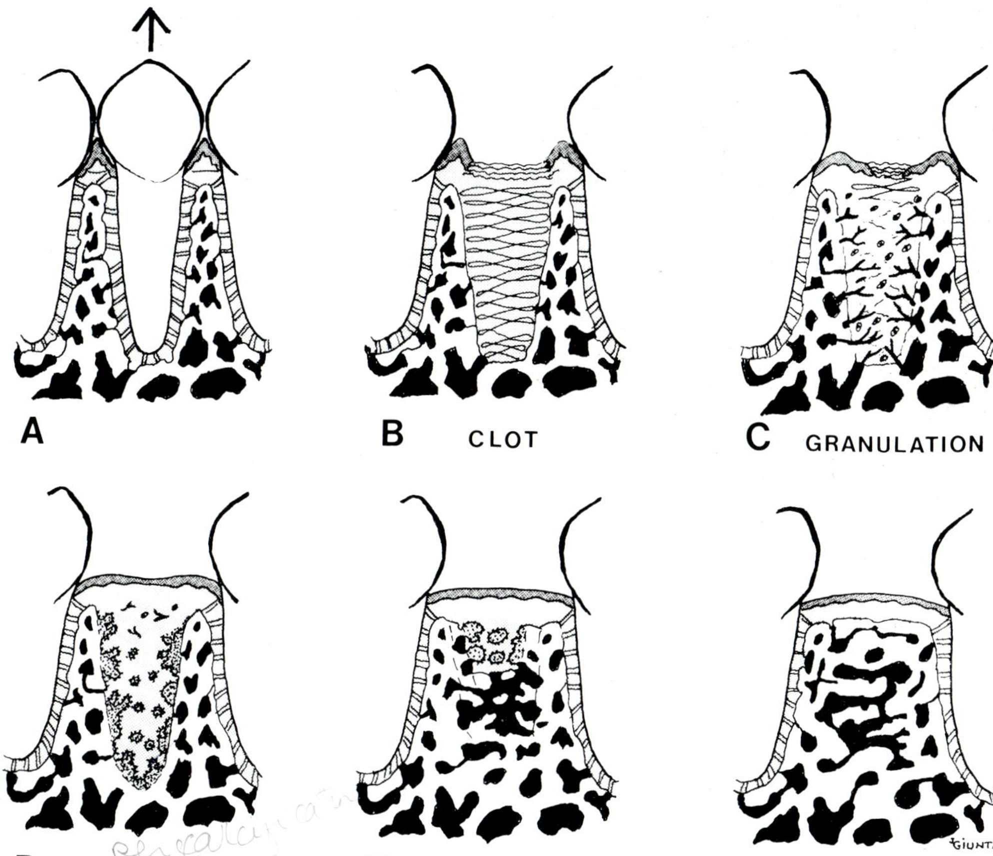

Figure 3.15. Diagram depicting the healing of a socket site after the extraction of a tooth, with the various sequential stages.

The cells involved with the immune response are phagocytes, T cells, and B cells. Immune dysfunction occurs when these cells are deficient in number or function, as in the disease of acquired immunodeficiency syndrome (AIDS), in which the macrophages and the T cells are affected. Or, dysfunction occurs when these cells or their functions proliferate, as in allergies, hypersensitivity states, and some malignant tumors, such as lymphoma.

The phagocytes, in particular the blood monocytes and tissue macrophages, act as early warning cells, constantly scavenging for foreign protein or carbohydrate, called antigen (Fig. 3.16). They also scavenge for damaged body cells. Also scavenging are cells that can recognize cancerous cells and signal the growth of specific killer cells to eradicate the cancerous cells. The macrophages are part of a nonspecific part of the immune system, in that they nonselectively engulf and destroy or try to destroy foreign organisms or debris. The phagocytic neutrophils are more primitive than the macrophages regarding immunity. Bone marrow derived, they live only a few days, do phagocytize organisms (usually bacteria), but may be overwhelmed and spill their contents, which can cause lysis and tissue damage of itself. Also aiding the process is the complement system, a group of proteins from the blood that are capable of adhering to the invader and having a

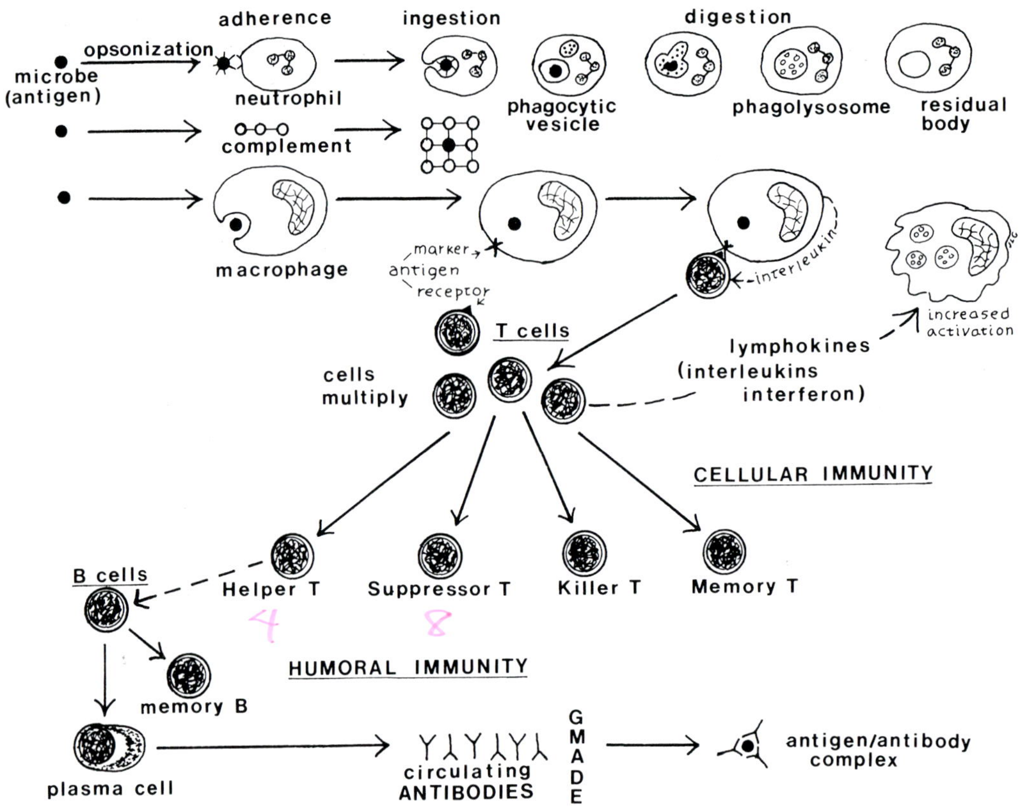

Figure 3.16. Diagram depicting nonspecific (neutrophils, complement) and specific (macrophages, T cells, B cells) immune response by the body after exposure to microorganisms (antigen). Cellular and humoral response (antibodies or immunoglobulins) are depicted along with the stages of phagocytosis as seen in a neutrophil.

reaction that can also kill the invader. The phagocytes and the complement system secrete substances that dilate blood vessels, a component of the inflammatory response.

Like all body cells, the macrophage has molecules on its cell surface that identify it as part of self (major histocompatibility complex—MHC). Once the macrophage ingests the organism, part of the organism's identity, the antigen, is displayed on the surface of the macrophage at the MHC. This antigen or marker then signals T cells that specifically recognize the invader. The macrophage then presents the antigen to the T cell, probably in a local node where there are many T cells to encounter. T cells control the immune response.

There are two major types of specific immune cells, the T and the B cells. Both are derived from embryonic bone marrow precursor cells that pass through either of two tissues to be specifically modified. Those passing through the thymus become "T" cells. Those passing through bursal lymph tissue, perhaps in the bone marrow, liver, spleen or gut, become "B" cells. (The bursa of Fabricius in birds is a small pouch of lymphoid tissue attached to intestine and is responsible for the name "B" cell.) Both the T and B cells circulate in the blood and in lymphoid tissues such as lymph nodes. There are several types of T cells, including helper, suppressor, and killer cells. The B cells evolve into plasma cells, which produce antibodies.

The helper T cell controls and turns on

the specific immune system and directs the other cells. Upon being presented the antigen by the macrophage, the T cell receives or locks onto the antigen by a specific receptor on its cell surface. Interleukin-1 is secreted by the macrophage, causing the T cells to divide and also causing a fever, which can boost the immune response by decreasing viral activity. The stimulated T cells secrete chemical mediators called lymphokines, including other interleukins and interferon. These mediators turn on a proliferation of many of the immune cells. This influx of cells is familiar in inflammation and accounts in part for the swelling.

The T cells couple with B cells and release a chemical that causes the B cells to become plasma cells. The plasma cells produce specific protein antibodies that bind to the causative agent, signaling and enabling scavenger cells and killer cells to annihilate the agent. The antibodies are called immunoglobulins, the most common being IgG, making up 80 percent of the antibodies. The gamma globulins are found in the serum and constitute the major humoral (fluid, not cellular) component of the immune system. The next most common antibody is IgA (13 percent), which is secreted by salivary glands and plays a major role in the defenses of the mucosal surfaces. IgM (6 percent) is an antibody that can activate the complement system. IgD (1 percent) may be involved in immune tolerance. The fifth class, IgE (<1 percent) is seen in immediate hypersensitivity reactions in which the antibody causes mast cells to release histamines in great quantity, causing severe vasodilatation.

The interferon released by the T cells causes the macrophages to be activated so that they can phagocytize better and kill the agents more efficiently. At the same time as the B cells are being activated, killer T cells are activated. They multiply and are capable of recognizing the antigen on the surface of cells that are infected by the agent. Coupling at the complex with the antigen, the T cells inject a protein into the cell's membrane that creates holes in the membrane, causing the cell's insides to leak out, thus killing the cell. In addition, the T cells release a message for the cell to denature the DNA of the cell and of the offender. Besides killing cells infected with organisms, particularly viruses, killer cells can kill tumor cells. Tumors can have antigens that differ from self, and the killer cells can attack them and are thought to be part of a constant surveillance system against tumor cells.

The immune system on first exposure to an organism reaches this frenzy of cellular and humoral activity after about 1 week and lasting as long as several weeks. With the organism's being killed there is less need for a full-blown attack. The suppressor T cells turn off the system by sending out chemical signals to suppress cytotoxic activity and antibody formation. They also suppress T cells, may themselves be cytotoxic, and may prevent the body from attacking itself.

Before the B and T cells disappear, they form memory cells that circulate in the blood and the lymph system for years. The next time the same organism invades, these memory cells immediately recognize the antigen and attack without delay. This attack includes antibodies in the serum and in mucus, saliva, and tears, so that the invader can be recognized from all portals.

Some diseases and conditions are characterized by a deficiency of part of the immune system.

AIDS is caused by the human immunodeficiency virus (HIV), which lowers the host's immune defense mechanism by infecting and altering key immune cells. The macrophages are the main target, with the virus living and reproducing inside the macrophages. The virus disrupts the many actions of the macrophage but does not kill it. In addition, the virus invades the T-4 (helper) cells either directly or from the infected macrophages. Among other functions, the T-4 cells normally activate the immune system, including the macrophages. The infected T-4 cells are killed, thus preventing them from signaling macrophages to fight certain infections. Meanwhile, the infected macrophages do not function properly to fight diseases even if they are signaled by the T-4 cells. Consequently, patients become vulnerable to organisms that normally would never make them ill (opportunistic pathogens). *Pneumocystis carinii* pneumonia, meningitis, Kaposi's sarcoma, and candidiasis, among others, are hallmark signs of AIDS. However, the virus may be latent in the host for several years before signs of the disease arise. Investigations on the mechanisms for the latency of AIDS suggest that AIDS is activated only when a genetic "switch" within the patient is thrown. Some patients may produce a substance that keeps the switch thrown off. When that substance is not produced, the switch is thrown and the effects of the HIV virus take place, producing opportunistic infection and cancers.

Once infected, the host is a carrier and can pass the virus on to others. However, the virus is not transmitted casually. It is transmitted through sexual intercourse, the sharing of drug needles, or to babies of infected mothers before or during birth. Sexually, it has been transmitted by anal intercourse among homosexuals and bisexuals, who account for the greatest numbers of AIDS cases. However, it may also be transmitted heterosexually. As a sexually transmitted disease, it is associated with *Chlamydia*, gonorrhea, syphilis, and hepatitis B. The oral cavity can signal the decrease in immune response with many manifestations. Patients with AIDS (including ARC or AIDS-related complex), have lesions in the head and neck area 50 to 95 percent of the time. All patients infected with HIV, with or without disease manifestations, are carriers of the virus.

Autoimmune disease results when the immune system makes an error and fails to distinguish self from nonself. In these circumstances antibodies are formed against the hosts own proteins or antigens. Antigen-antibody complexes arise and elicit a reaction. Among the autoimmunities are such diseases as rheumatoid arthritis, systemic lupus erythematosus, thyroiditis, rheumatic fever, glomerulonephritis, hemolytic anemia, myasthenia gravis, multiple sclerosis, and type 1 diabetes. In these diseases and others, the immune system mounts a selective, devastating attack against cells or cellular components of the body that it mistakes as foreign.

In type 1 diabetes, which affects 1.5 million young Americans, there is an insufficient supply of insulin. It appears that immune cells invade the pancreas and destroy the beta cells that produce the insulin. Without insulin, cells cannot convert sugar into energy needed for their function. The buildup of unconverted sugar in the bloodstream damages the lining of blood vessels, particularly capillaries. This leads to complications such as heart and kidney disease, poor circulation, blindness, and stroke. Systemic symptoms resulting from an inability to reabsorb water are frequency of urination (polyuria), frequency of eating (polyphagia), and excessive thirst (polydipsia). This last can lead to a complaint of dry mouth and burning tongue (see Chapter 8). There are many types of diabetes besides type 1. Type 2 is more common, is seen in older patients, is less severe, and is not insulin-dependent since it can be controlled by diet or antidiabetic drugs.

In rheumatoid arthritis, antigen-antibody complexes against joint tissues accumulate and elicit an inflammatory response. The accumulation of fluid, cells, and mediators in the joint space accounts for the swelling and pain. Treatment is against the inflammation by using aspirin or aspirin substitutes to decrease prostaglandins.

The immune system can overreact (immunoproliferation). It does so in hypersensitivity (allergy) reactions. Antigens that produce an allergic reaction are called allergens. They may be foods, mold, drugs, pollen, dust, cosmetics, poison ivy (urushiol, an oil in the plant), and others. Allergic persons produce IgE antibodies that bind to basophils in the blood and mast cells in the tissues around the blood vessels. This binding of IgE to mast cells causes them to release their intracellular granules, which include the chemical histamine. The histamine dilates blood vessels, an action meant to bring immune cells to an area of injury. Instead, it causes the swelling and inflammation associated with allergies. In pollen sufferers, the sudden release of granules by the mast cells causes sneezing and watery eyes. Treatment is with antihistamines and corticosteroid inhalants to reduce inflammation. For life-threatening, anaphylactic-type responses that can cause circulatory shock and asphyxia, epinephrine is administered to counteract the effect of histamine. Hypersensitivity reaction types I to III involve antibodies. The type IV reaction involves T cells and is called a cell-mediated reaction. It is also called a delayed reaction, because it takes time for the cells to respond to the allergen. Typically, the reaction starts at least 24 hours or later after exposure. An example is the reaction to liquid monomer in a temporary crown, bridge, or denture (see Fig. 8.20). Several diseases are characterized by delayed hypersensitivity reactions, examples of which are tuberculosis and tertiary syphilis (see Chapter 6).

Also caused by a delayed hypersensitivity reaction to a microorganism is rheumatic fever. Weeks prior to the disease, the patient suffers from a beta-hemolytic streptococcal infection of the oropharynx or the skin. Some individuals mount a delayed hypersensitivity reaction to the organism or its toxin. This can involve the heart (carditis), the joints (arthritis), the kidneys (glomerulonephritis), the skin, and other sites, along with fever. The rheumatic heart disease affects the endocardium and the valves. The healing process results in scarring with calcifications. The mitral valve in particular may not close well (stenosis), causing a rush of blood to the heart (heart murmur). However, the damage may be silent. The valvular insufficiency and the stenosis strain the heart over the years, causing compensatory hypertrophy and possibly heart failure. Patients with valvular damage from rheumatic heart disease are prone to infective endocarditis.

Infective endocarditis (subacute bacterial endocarditis or SBE) is a microbial infection of the heart valves previously damaged by congenital anomalies, atherosclerosis, or rheumatic heart disease. It is produced by a bacteremia, the presence of bacteria in the bloodstream, and the settling and growth of the bacteria (vegetations) on the previously damaged heart valves. A serious disease, the patients may develop heart failure and can die. The organisms include streptococci, staphylococci, and gram-negative species. The oral cavity is a ready source of organisms, *Streptococcus viridans* being the common offender. Therefore, any procedure such as prophylaxis, restorative dentistry, periodontal therapy, and surgery can cause bleeding, and bacteremia and antibiotic prophylaxis should be given to the patient in hopes of reducing and controlling the number of organisms during the bacteremia. (Dental offices generally follow the recommendations of the American Heart Association for the appropriate antibiotic prophylactic regimen.)

Some Infectious and Inflammatory Diseases

Hepatitis refers to inflammation of the liver and can be caused by drugs, chemicals (carbon tetrachloride, xylene inhalation), drinking alcohol, and viruses, among others. The principal hepatitis is viral, with A, B, non-A, non-B, and delta being recognized types. Hepatitis A (infectious hepatitis), caused by the hepatitis A virus (HAV), is spread by fecal contamination of food, clothing, toys, or eating utensils by the fecal-oral route. With an incubation period of about 4 weeks, it generally affects children and young adults causing nausea, diarrhea, fever, chills, and ultimately jaundice. Lasting about 5 weeks, it does not cause lasting damage. It has no antigen markers and no carrier state. Hepatitis B (serum hepatitis), caused by the hepatitis B virus (HBV), is spread by blood transference and body fluids such as saliva, tears, and semen. The incubation period is between 2 and 5 months. Highly infectious and easily transmitted, the virus can produce chronic liver inflammation with recurring episodes and is associated with an increased incidence of liver cancer. There are surface markers for the virus: HBsAg or hepatitis B surface antigen, HBcAg or hepatitis B core antigen (serologic test not available for this), and HBeAg or hepatitis B e antigen. The presence of HBeAg indicates viral replication is active, the viruses are high in the serum, and there is significant liver disease. Antibody to HBeAg (anti-HBe) suggests a low level of HBV in the serum of a carrier of HBsAg and is associated with a good chance of recovery. HBsAg is the first serologic marker after contact with the virus and is used to diagnose the disease and the carrier state. Antibody to HB cAg (anti-HBc) is nearly always present in chronic carriers of the surface antigen but may not be protective against future HBV exposure. Antibody to HBsAg (anti-HBs) indicates past clinical or subclinical infection with HBV and may indicate recovery and immunity from infection. It can also indicate antibody produced passively after exposure by prophylactic measures or an immune response produced by the HBV vaccine. (The HBV vaccine is highly recommended for health care workers and staff because of the infectivity of the virus and the possibilities of cross-contamination.) There may be lifetime carriers of the active virus who are prone to cirrhosis of the liver. Cirrhosis refers to a distorted or scarred liver, resulting in nodules of attempted regeneration of liver cells surrounded by scar tissue. It can lead to jaundice, and the altered blood flow yields varices of the esophagus and fluid in the peritoneum.

The non-A, non-B hepatitis (NANB) cannot be traced to either the A or the B viruses. Clinically, it is similar to the B, is spread by blood transfusions, and accounts for more cases caused by transfusion than the HBV. Laboratory diagnosis is by exclusion of the other viruses.

Delta hepatitis is caused by an RNA-containing virus (HDV) that replicates only in the presence of HBsAg and thus causes acute infection in chronic carriers of the B virus. Antibodies to the virus can be demonstrated in the serum for a short time after the acute infection.

Two of the herpesviruses may also cause a hepatitis. The Epstein-Barr virus (EBV) is responsible for infectious mononucleosis. Contracted by direct contact, such as intimate kissing, it is common in adolescents and young adults and may present as a hepatitis as well as a tonsillitis. Tests include smears, a heterophil antibody test, and those for antibodies to EBV. The other herpesvirus is cytomegalovirus (CMV). This may yield mononucleosis-like symptoms, and the hepatitis may be found in transplant recipients who are immunosuppressed and in AIDs patients. Diagnosis is by using a culture, antibodies to the virus, or histopathology.

Pneumonitis or pneumonia is an acute infection or inflammation caused by microorganisms or aspiration of foreign objects or irritants. Usually caused by a *Pneumococcus* or *Staphylococcus* bacterium, it may be caused by viruses, fungi, or protozoans, as in the opportunistic *Pneumocystis carinii* in AIDS. It may affect a whole lobe (lobar), or parts of a lobe around bronchi (lobular). The alveoli are filled with inflammatory cells, or the alveolar walls are swollen with them. This leads to a decrease of air in the lungs and a decrease in the diffusion of oxygen. Antibiotics cure many bacterial infections that used to kill the patient.

Chronic obstructive pulmonary disease (COPD) refers to those diseases that have in common some degree of obstruction of the air passageways. Bronchial asthma is caused by an allergic reaction that causes spasm of the smooth muscle of the small bronchi so that less air can be exhaled and mucus builds up to add further impedance to air flow. Patients wheeze and have a hard time breathing. Bronchitis, whose principal cause is cigarette smoking, is characterized by a thickening of the lining of the bronchi. The seromucous glands and mucous goblet cells secrete thick sputum to produce a cough. Emphysema is characterized by the alveoli being filled and extended like balloons. Because of the metaplastic and hyperplastic lining mucosa there is a decreased airway and exhalation is impeded, thus causing the alveoli to expand. With time the alveoli burst, forming large spaces, and there is healing with nonbreathing scar tissue. Patients have extreme difficulty breathing even on the slightest exertion and develop a barrel-shaped chest from the compensatory usage of their intercostal muscles that work to expel the air from the lungs. Cigarette smoking, air pollution, and industrial dust are common causes. Behavioral change can prevent this very debilitating disease.

Gingivitis, inflammation of the gingivae, is characterized by a redness and/or blueness with loss of tone and swelling of the gingivae, which bleed upon probing. It is consequent to the accumulation of supragingival plaque in which there is a specific sequential colonization of organisms as the plaque matures. The removal of plaque can prevent or reverse the gingivitis. Gingivitis is associated with a change from predominant gram-positive streptococcal flora to a more complex flora of gram-negative and spiral forms. As the plaque matures, gram-positive rods of *Actinomyces* species increase at the expense of the cocci. Over time a bacterial succession of additional species occurs, with more gram-negative rods and cocci appearing, such as *E. corrodens*, *Fusobacterium* species, and *Capnocytophaga gingivalis*. The more motile the forms and spirochetes, the more redness there is. The flora differs for specific clinical conditions in that there are different organisms associated with regular gingivitis, pregnancy gingivitis, and necrotizing gingivitis. Gingivitis is important in the development of subgingival plaque and in the progression to periodontitis. Not all gingivitis sites in the presence of plaque develop into periodontitis, but all periodontitis is preceded by gingivitis (Fig. 3.17). The requirements for this seem to be bacterial succession, poor oral hygiene, systemic factors, and time. A buildup of bacteria that are pathogenic to the periodontal tissues and a decrease in the host's immune response to those bacteria are responsible for the periodontitis.

Periodontitis is now recognized to be several distinct diseases with separate etiologies. The forms of periodontitis are: adult, juvenile, prepubertal, rapidly progressive, and refractory adult. Each has different groups of associated organisms and affects different age groups. Only the adult type of periodontitis is mentioned here.

Adult periodontitis is the most common form, affecting individuals aged 35 years and older, usually with no known underlying systemic disease. Caused by a small number of specific organisms, mainly anaerobic, that colonize the subgingival area, tissue destruction ensues following periodic attacks. The end result is loss of periodontal support and the appearance of clinical evidence in the form of pockets and tooth mobility. The tissue destruction is not slow and continuous but is due to repeated, short, random attacks followed by remissions and attempts at repair. Aided by the protective supragingival plaque and nourished by gingival fluid and products of the supragingival plaque, the subgingival flora is complex and has an increase in motile, gram-negative, capnophilic, and anaerobic species. The primary organisms appear to be: *Bacteroides gingivalis*, *B. intermedius*, "fusiform" *Bacteroides* organisms, *B. capillus*; *E. corrodens*; *W. recta*; *Selenomonas sputigena*; *Eubacterium timidum*, *E. brachyii*, *E. nodatum*; *Lactobacillus minitis*; *Peptostreptococcus micros*; *Fusobacterium nucleatum*; *Actinobacillus* species; and spirochetes. When the host defenses cannot check their numbers, these organisms increase and cause tissue breakdown. As in gingivitis, there is a loss of attachment of the junctional epithelium between the tooth

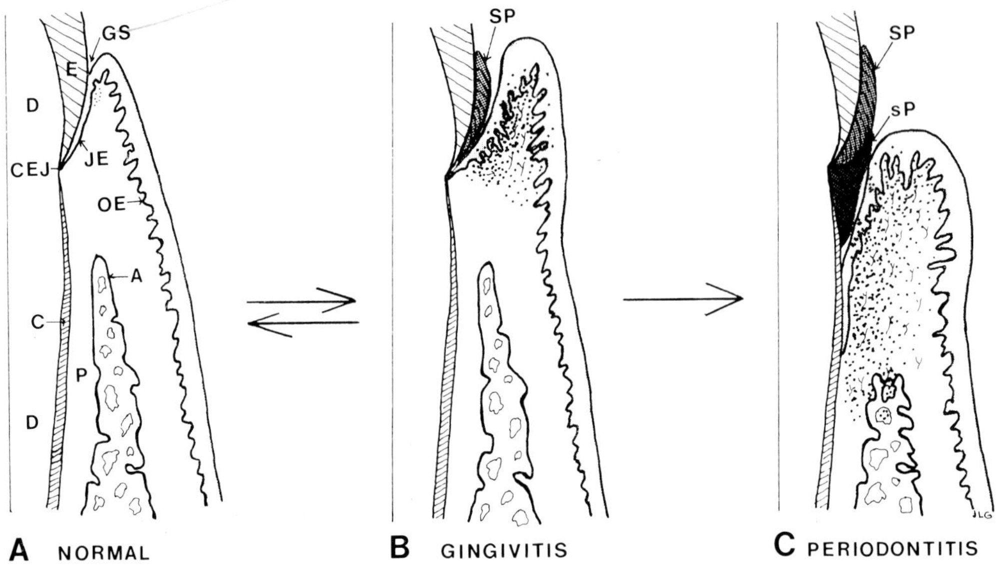

Figure 3.17. *A*, normal periodontal tissues. The gingival sulcus (GS) is minimal. The keratinizing oral epithelium (OE) of the marginal gingiva is continuous with the nonkeratinizing junctional epithelium (JE), which attaches to the cervical portion of the enamel (E) and terminates at the cementoenamel junction (CEJ). There are a few scattered inflammatory cells in the connective tissue beneath the sulcus. Alveolar bone (A), dentin (D), cementum (C), periodontal ligament (P). *B*, gingivitis. There has been a disruption of the JE and a deepening of the sulcus by the adherence of supragingival plaque (SP) to the pellicle-covered surface of the enamel. The created space between the JE and the tooth or plaque is a gingival pocket and can be probed. The gingival connective tissue is intensely infiltrated with chronic inflammatory cells, and the gingiva is swollen. The JE extends into the inflammation. There is no migration of the JE and no resorption of the alveolar bone. Gingivitis is reversible. Periodontitis is preceded by gingivitis. *C*, periodontitis. Subgingival plaque (sP) has formed beneath the SP. The response is an apical migration of the junctional epithelium from the CEJ along the root. The chronic inflammatory response has spread into the periodontal ligament and the alveolar bone, resulting in loss of attachment and resorption of bone. A periodontal pocket can be probed from the gingival crest to the attachment of the migrated junctional epithelium. The gingiva is swollen and is partially receded.

and the gingiva. This epithelium becomes ulcerative, and an inflammatory process follows, specifically with immunologic cells, e.g., macrophages, lymphocytes, and plasma cells. With time the attachment migrates beyond the cementoenamel junction, and a periodontal pocket is established. Collagen of the gingiva and of the periodontal ligament is degraded by enzymatic action through collagenase. The inflammation may spread along the periodontal ligament and into the alveolar bone. Factors such as osteoclastic activating factor are released from the inflammatory cells and cause loss of the alveolar bone. This attack is balanced by quiet periods in which there is healing. Loosened teeth may become more firm. Eventually the recurrent sporadic attacks account for substantial loss of support and, if left unchecked, as by treatment, lead to loss of the teeth. In adults, periodontitis is responsible for most tooth loss. Periodontal therapy seeks to eradicate pockets and to eliminate both supragingival and subgingival plaque. Preventing the plaque accumulation can prevent gingivitis and periodontitis.

Chapter 4
DEVELOPMENTAL ABNORMALITIES

Developmental abnormalities represent those disturbances in the pattern of human growth leading to external or internal changes. Some are so minor as to be merely a variation from the normal (e.g., mucosal tag). Others are more severe (e.g., cleft palate, cyst). Still others are devastating (e.g., monstrosities).

There are intrinsic and extrinsic factors responsible for the abnormalities. Sometimes, both are active. For example, identical twins can appear to be the same at first, but differences in their environment or upbringing can make them appear different despite the identical genes. The genetically determined abnormalities are due to inheritance or to mutations of the genes acquired from elements in the environment.

A birth defect may arise from a spontaneous mutation or through some alteration of the environment during uterine life. Sometimes there are lethal injuries and the fetus is aborted or is born dead. Other times there may be less severe injuries. The injury may be caused by a lack of oxygen (hypoxia). This is the leading cause of cerebral palsy and mental retardation. Malnutrition, hormonal disturbances, and chemicals such as thalidomide may cause malformations.

Congenital malformations are those developmental anomalies present at birth. Some disturbances, however, are determined in utero, yet they manifest later in life. Others may develop after birth and show up later in life.

Many of the developmental disturbances of the head and neck are minor, causing little or no disability. However, even two or three minor variations or malformations found in the head and neck (oral cavity) may be significant. They may be part of a syndrome (a set of symptoms or signs occurring together), which may be part of a more serious malformation. This book refers to only a few syndromes. There are several excellent texts enumerating and discussing them.

An example in which there is a known relationship of cause and effect is the injury caused by the virus of german measles (rubella) to babies. A pregnant woman, getting the disease for the first time during the first trimester, may deliver a baby with many malformations. Again, there are many possibilities of damage depending on the timing of the insult. The fetus may die when it is incompatible with life. There may be severe malformations such as cataracts and congenital heart disease. Or there may be minimal damage such as enamel hypoplasia of the deciduous teeth and delayed eruption of the teeth.

The following is a presentation of developmental abnormalities of the soft tissue, jaws, and teeth.

Soft Tissue Abnormalities

Cleft lip and cleft palate represent failures of fusion of islands of tissue during development. They occur commonly; 1 in 700 babies is born with one or the other, or both. More males are affected than females.

Cleft lip occurs on either side of the midline in the area corresponding to the maxillary lateral incisor and cuspid region. Most commonly it is unilateral, with the left side being involved more often than the right (Fig. 4.1). However, both sides may be affected, in which case the condition is bilateral; because of the resemblance to the lip of the rabbit, this may be referred to as a

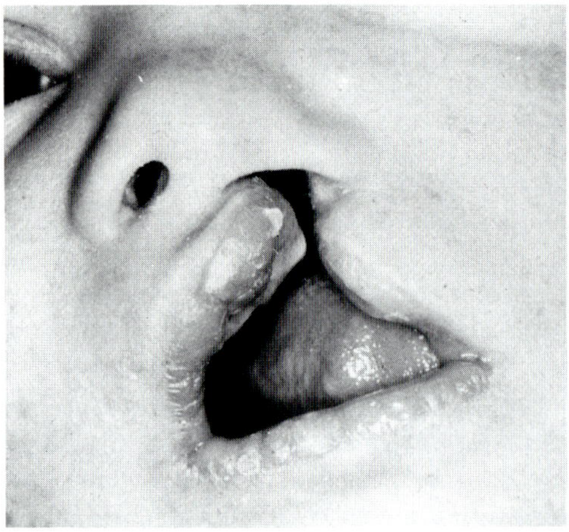

Figure 4.1. Complete cleft lip, unilateral.

harelip. The cleft may be complete, extending to the base of the nose; or incomplete, presenting as an indentation of the upper lip. It occurs between 4 and 7 weeks in utero, which corresponds to the time the lip normally develops. Because of this specific time of development, cleft lip may occur independently of cleft palate. However, cleft lip and cleft palate may occur together.

Cleft palate results from a failure of fusion of the developing palatine processes and premaxillary processes. It can vary in severity depending on the extent of the cleft from the alveolar ridge to the end of the soft palate. The variations seen reflect the sequence of development of the palate, which begins in utero at 8 weeks in the premaxillary region and ends at 12 weeks at the uvula of the soft palate. Thus, if the etiologic factor were at work from the eighth week, the cleft would occur anteriorly to posteriorly—including the alveolus, hard palate, soft palate, and uvula—resulting in a gross and serious defect. On the other hand, if the cause were acting near the end of the developing period (11th week), the cleft would be seen only in the posterior soft palate, resulting in a partial cleft or merely a bifid uvula (Fig. 4.2), a minor and innocuous defect that requires no treatment.

The cause of cleft lip and cleft palate is not definitely known. However, present theories favor both genetic and environmental factors. Treatment of the clefts is by surgical or mechanical closure. Usually teams of specialists from many disciplines work closely together to treat these young patients and to advise the parents.

Congenital lip pits are depressions on the lower lip and are rarely seen. The cause is unknown. No treatment is required.

Commissural lip pits are indentations that occur at the corners of the mouth.

Double lip is a pendulous fold of excess tissue on the inner aspect of the upper lip, usually seen on smiling. This can be surgically removed.

Macroglossia refers to an enlargement of the tongue. It may be developmental in origin, due to a hypertrophy of the tongue muscle. Because the tongue is large, it pushes against the teeth, and indentations can be created on the lateral borders of the tongue, yielding a scalloped appearance (Fig. 4.3). Macroglossia is seen in Down syndrome, a genetic disease with many other developmental disturbances (see Chapter 8).

Macroglossia may also be acquired. Besides being developmental, enlarged tongues can be seen because of tumors, inflammation, and hormonal changes (cretinism, acromegaly). Depending upon its severity and potential to cause other prob-

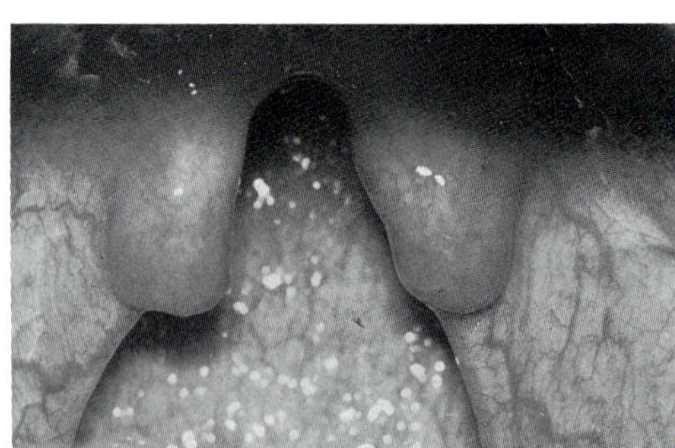

Figure 4.2. Partial cleft, soft palate, bifid uvula.

lems within the oral cavity, the enlarged tongue may be reduced to size by surgery.

Microglossia refers to a small tongue. It is extremely rare. In hemiatrophy of the tongue, half of the tongue is small. The cause may be a defect in the cranial nerve (hypoglossal) that innervates the tongue muscles. Without stimulation the tongue muscles atrophy, and the body of the tongue becomes smaller. In this instance the defect in the tongue reflects damage elsewhere.

Ankyloglossia (tongue-tie) refers to the partial or complete attachment of the tongue to the floor of the mouth (Fig. 4.4). The lingual frenum is attached too far forward and may be seen in various positions, the most severe being at the tip of the tongue. Mobility of the tongue may be hampered, and patients cannot touch the hard palate when the mouth is opened. Speech may be impaired. Mild cases require no treatment, and severe cases can be treated successfully with surgical removal of the misplaced frenum.

Bifid tongue (forked tongue) represents the rare failure of fusion of the lateral halves of the tongue. It is seen in the midline at the tip as a notch (Fig. 4.5). Usually, no treatment is required.

Central papillary atrophy of the tongue (Fig. 4.6), previously called median rhomboid glossitis, is an ovoid or rhomboidal rashlike area in the midline of the dorsum of the tongue anterior to the circumvallate papillae, occurring in 1 percent of the population. The filiform papillae are atrophic, yielding a reddened zone that may be flat or raised. Sometimes there are superimposed white lesions that may be scraped away. Originally, it was thought that the lesion was developmental, resulting from the persistence of the tuberculum impar of the

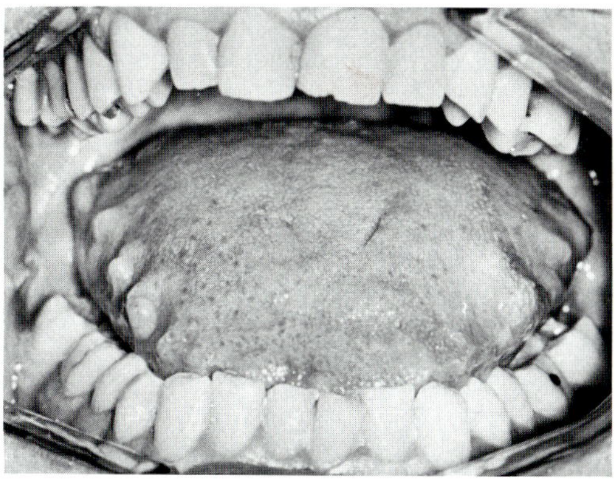

Figure 4.3. Macroglossia, scalloped borders of tongue correspond to embrasure spaces of teeth and are composed of tongue tissue.

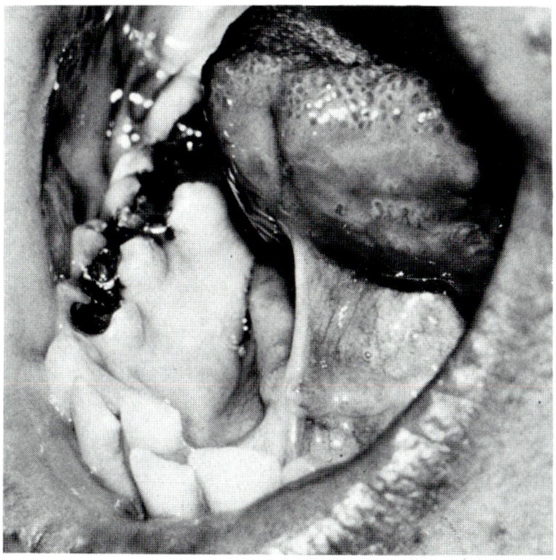

Figure 4.4. Ankyloglossia, broad lingual frenum attached near tip of tongue. Tongue is fully extended toward palate.

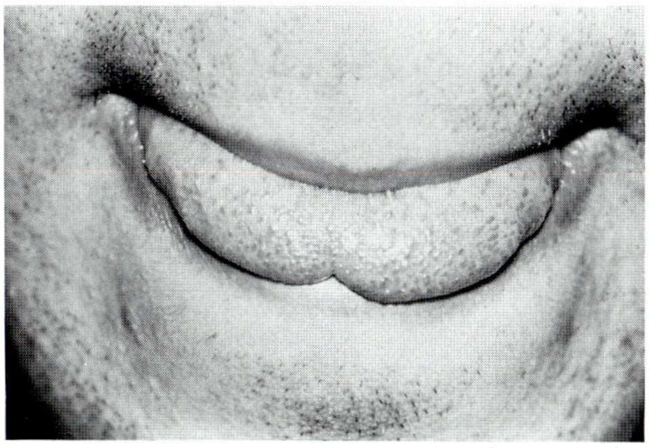

Figure 4.5. Bifid tongue.

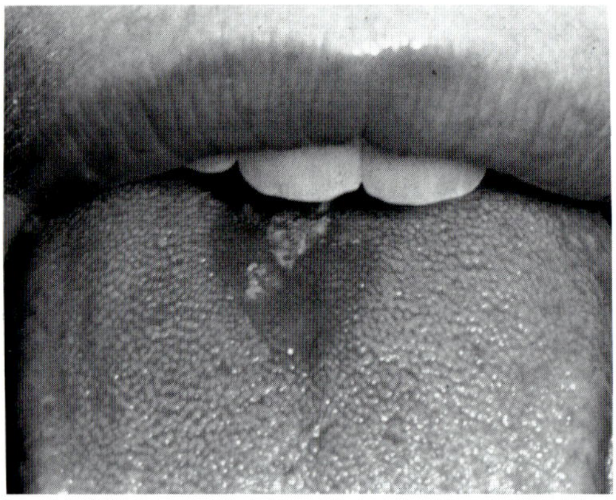

Figure 4.6. Central papillary atrophy of tongue (median rhomboid glossitis). This was due to *Candida albicans* infection. It disappeared with mycostatin treatment.

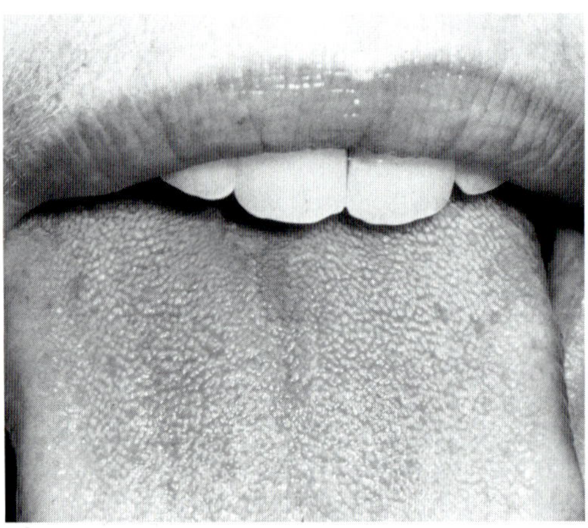

Figure 4.7. Normal tongue of patient in Figure 4.6 after 2 weeks of treatment.

tongue not being covered by the lateral halves of the tongue. However, it is rare to find this lesion in children. There is an association of this lesion with a fungus, *Candida albicans*, so it may be an inflammatory process secondary to candidiasis (Fig. 4.7). Interestingly, *C. albicans* is a normal inhabitant of the oral mucosa and has been cultured in greater numbers at that site even in normal-appearing tongues. Perhaps a change in the oral environment, triggered by a decrease in the immune response, allows the organism to flourish and cause the central atrophy. Smears of the lesions and biopsies yield the *Candida* organism. Antifungal medications can cause the lesion to disappear. However, because it may recur, treatment is used primarily for symptomatic lesions. Central papillary atrophy is a nuisance disease and is not a cancer, a fear of many patients.

Fissured or furrowed tongue is a common condition in which deep grooves occur in the dorsal surface of the tongue (Fig. 4.8). The fissures, resembling brain tissue, may be mild or severe and seem to deepen with age. In some instances, food and debris may lodge in the furrows and cause irritation with symptoms. In most cases there are no symptoms, and no treatment is required. Fissured tongue may be acquired, because it appears at older ages and is rarely seen in children.

Geographic tongue is an interesting condition that frequently occurs along with fissured tongue (Fig. 4.9). It is a common entity characterized by a loss of the filiform or white papillae in one or multiple areas of

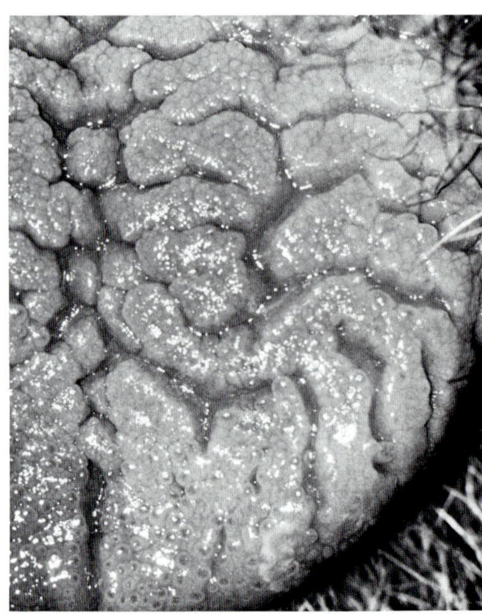

Figure 4.8. Fissured tongue, with deep grooves or crypts.

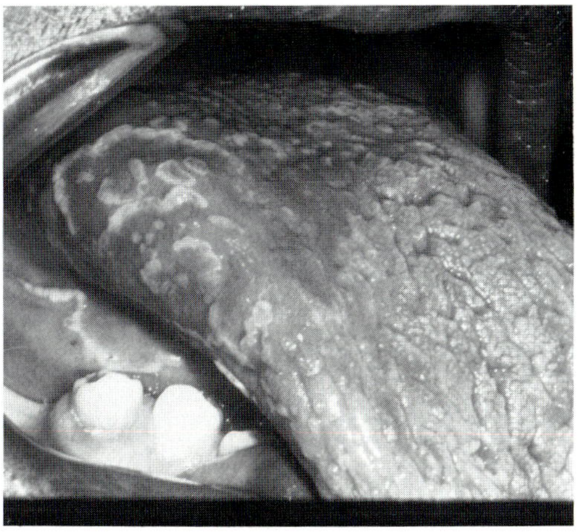

Figure 4.9. Geographic tongue and similar lesions (stomatitis migrans) of the adjacent floor of the mouth.

any surface of the tongue, particularly the dorsum. Red patchy areas are usually surrounded by a grayish white zone corresponding to the normal papillae, with a pile-up of some of the desquamated papillae. For this reason geographic tongue is considered as a white lesion. The rashlike areas assume many shapes, some of which resemble known geographic areas. Moreover, each time it is observed there is a different area with a different shape, because one area heals as new papillae grow while another area loses the papillae. Thus other names have been ascribed, i.e., wandering rash, glossitis areata migrans. Because the normal protective papillae are lost, the atrophic areas may be irritated, inflamed, and sensitive to certain foods. Usually, however, there are no symptoms, and it is discovered on examination or by self-observation. The patient who does observe it may fear cancer and should be reassured that it is not significant and is not cancer. The true etiology of geographic tongue is obscure. There is a strong emotional component, and therefore it may be of psychosomatic origin. It has been noted in association with the common cold, suggesting decreased immunity as a factor. This condition can recur. Lesions similar to geographic tongue may be seen in locations of the mucosa besides the tongue with or without the presence of tongue lesions. This ectopic geographic tongue has been called stomatitis migrans (Fig. 4.10). It seems to be psychosomatic in origin and interestingly, like geographic tongue and central papillary atrophy, microscopically it resembles psoriasis, a recognized psychosomatic disease of the skin. These lesions also may change, may disappear, and may recur. No specific treatment beyond diagnosis and reassurance is needed.

Hairy tongue is a condition, not specifically developmental, in which the filiform papillae elongate or undergo hypertrophy and do not desquamate or shed normally. Essentially the "hair" on the tongue is longer, particularly on the middorsal surface, although the lateral borders may be involved (Fig. 4.11). The color can vary from white to brown or black or other colors, depending on what produces the pigment. One cause is thought to be dehydration. For instance, in the common cold, the tongue appears white and "coated." Poor oral hygiene may be another

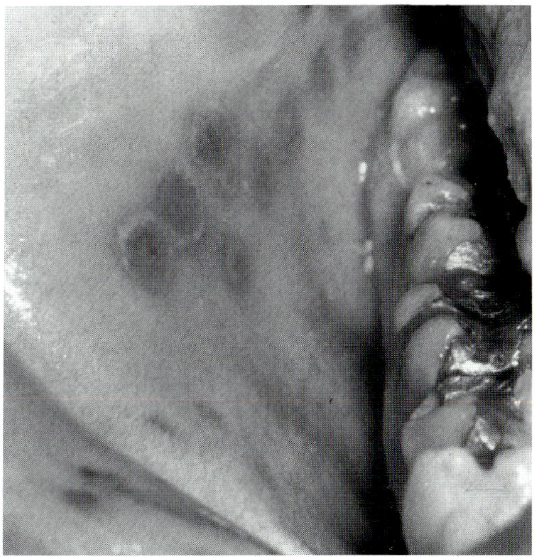

Figure 4.10. Stomatitis migrans of the buccal mucosa in patient with geographic tongue. The lesions are ringlike with red centers and a raised white border.

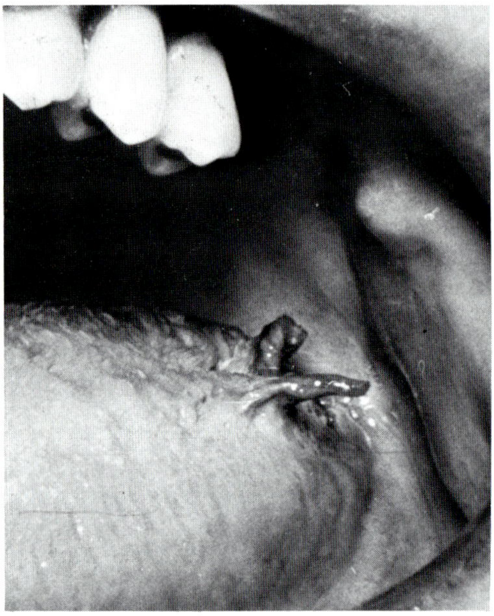

Figure 4.11. Hairy tongue, brown stain. Extremely long filiform papillae. Patient was a heavy smoker.

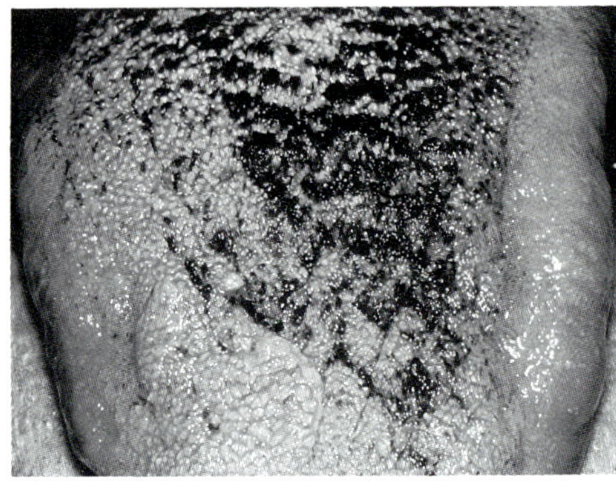

Figure 4.12. Black hairy tongue in 65-year-old who was taking penicillin for a tooth abscess. The filiform papillae are elongated and covered with chromophilic bacteria.

factor. Patients on antibiotics may get a black hairy tongue (lingua nigra) from the overgrowth of pigment-producing bacteria that are allowed to grow in excess because the normal oral bacterial flora is upset (Fig. 4.12). The condition disappears after stopping the antibiotic. The colors seen in hairy tongue, or even in the normal tongue, may be influenced by pigments in coffee, tea, tobacco, candy, and lozenges. Hairy tongue is benign. Better hygiene, such as brushing or scraping the tongue, may be suggested. Otherwise no treatment is required.

The tongue may assume different shapes and movements because of inheritance of the appropriate genes. It may be rolled into a tubelike structure with the lateral sides touching in the midline (Fig. 4.13). Some individuals can control the muscles at the tip of the tongue to form a cloverleaf pattern called a "trefoil" tongue (Fig. 4.14). Other individuals may inherit the capacity to move the tongue back and out of the oral cavity, called tongue swallowing. Such tongue gymnastics indicate genetic inheritance and do not represent disease but a normal state for those who can do them.

White sponge nevus is a hereditary disease in which several siblings and members of the same family exhibit excess folds of white, soft, spongy tissue. It can be seen anywhere on the mucosa but is common on the buccal mucosa and the lateral borders of the tongue. Mistaken for leukoplakia, it

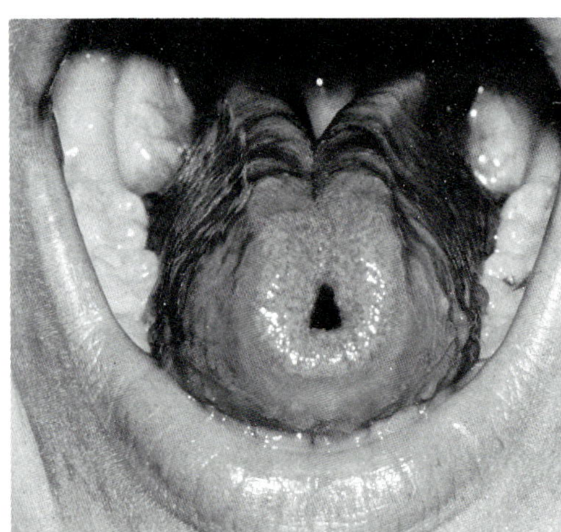

Figure 4.13. Voluntary folding of tongue that meets in the midline; an inherited trait.

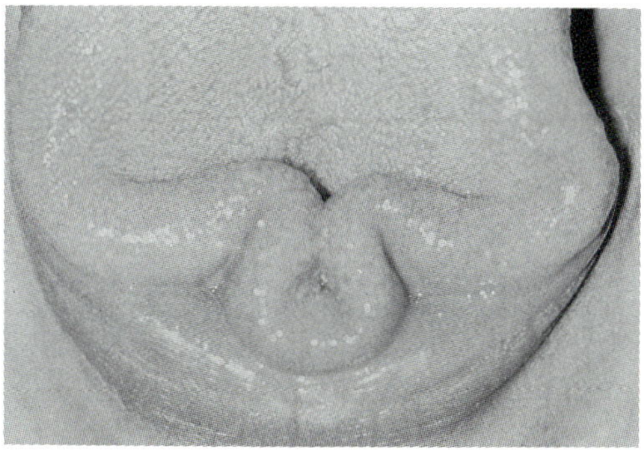

Figure 4.14. Voluntary folding of tongue into a cloverleaf or trefoil tongue; an inherited trait.

is similar to leukoedema. Adequate family history of the condition and biopsy confirm the diagnosis. No treatment is required.

Fordyce's granules or spots (Fordyce's disease) is not a disease but a developmental condition that is extremely common, occurring in 80 percent of the population. Fordyce's spots are multiple, small, yellow-white, submucosal papules that represent ectopic sebaceous glands without hair follicles. They can occur anywhere on the mucosa but are most commonly seen on the mucosal surface of the lips and on the buccal mucosa on each side (see Figs. 1.11 and 1.16). When they occur in other locations, or as single glands, the diagnosis is not so obvious (Fig. 4.15). They lie just beneath the mucosa and become more visible as the mucosa is stretched. They can vary greatly in number and may be so clustered in some patients that they evoke concern. They are of no clinical significance. They do not represent cancer. No treatment is required.

Fibromatosis gingivae (hereditary gingival fibromatosis) is a diffuse enlargement of the gingivae characterized by a growth in the connective tissue component (Fig. 4.16). It is inherited as a dominant trait and may be associated with other abnormalities. The gingivae are firm, normal in color, and may cover the crown of the teeth. Treatment is surgical removal of the excess tissue.

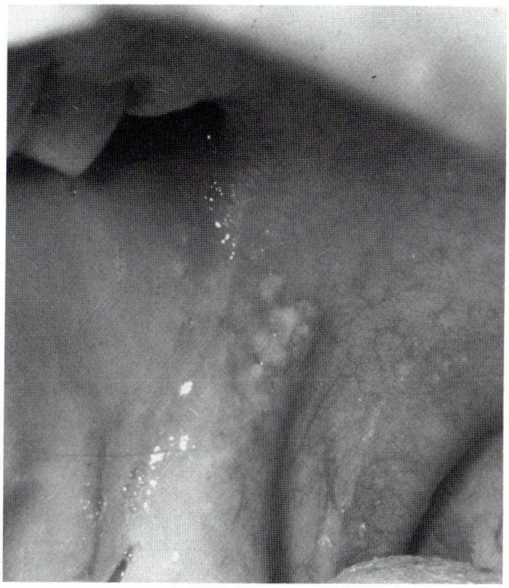

Figure 4.15. Fordyce's glands on retromolar pad. They are yellow submucosal clusters.

Tori are innocuous hard mucosal swellings that protrude from the jaws. They represent an excess of normal bone formation, appear radiopaque, and can occur in various sites. In the midline of the hard palate, one can occur as a single or multiple nodular mass and is termed a torus palatinus (see Figs. 1.18 and 4.17). In the mandible they usually occur as bilateral whitened masses lingual to the roots of the premolar teeth and are called tori mandibularis (Figs. 4.18 and 4.19). Similar projec-

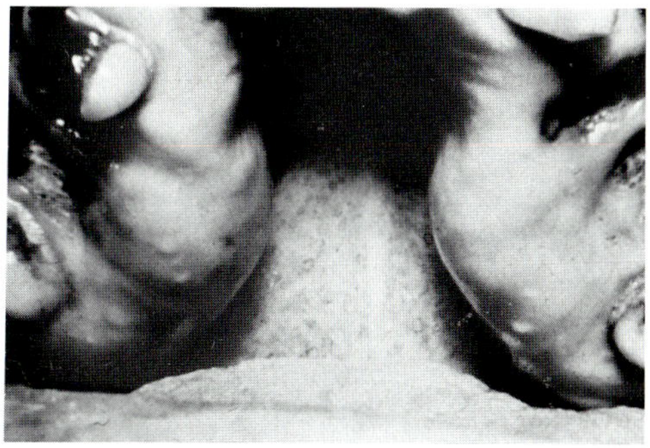

Figure 4.16. Gingival fibromatosis.

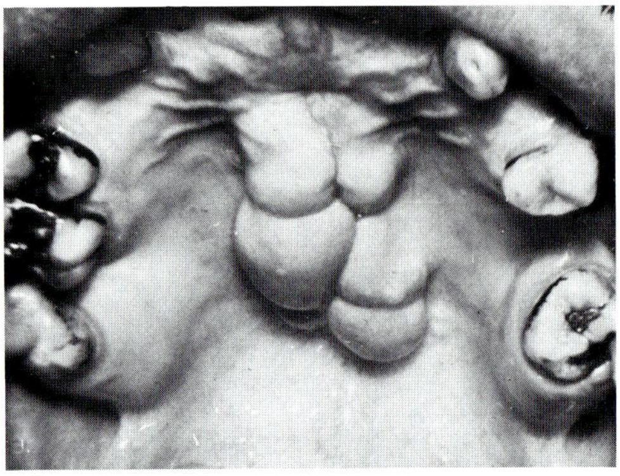

Figure 4.17. Torus palatinus, multiple bone projections in the midline of the hard palate covered by mucosa. Mucosa is exposed to traumatic insults.

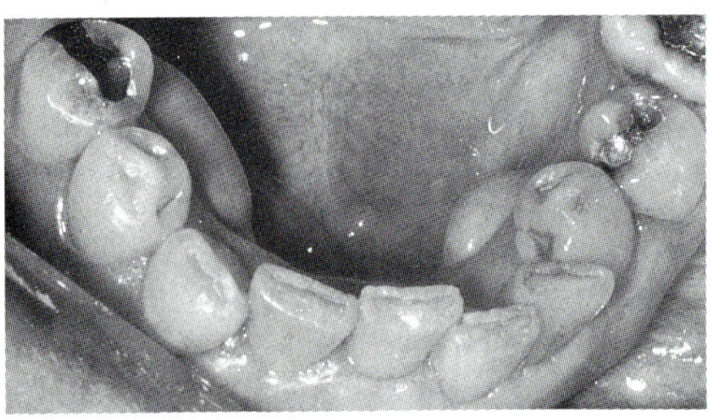

Figure 4.18. Bilateral lingual mandibular tori. Firm swellings behind bicuspid teeth.

tions of bone may appear on the labial or buccal surface of either the maxillary or mandibular alveolar ridges and are termed exostoses (bone outside of bone) (see Figs. 1.18 and 4.20). Tori are more common in females. Usually no treatment is required. If they interfere with dentures, other prostheses, or speech, they can be removed surgically.

Developmental Abnormalities of Jaws

Macrognathia refers to a large jaw. In the mandible this would result in a protrusion (class III, angle) with the chin being very prominent. It may be a congenital development that can be corrected by surgery. It may also be acquired through disease. In acromegaly, the patients have a tumor of the pituitary gland. This promotes continued growth at specific sites such as the fingers and the jaw bone of the mandible.

Micrognathia refers to a small jaw, usually involving the mandible. The chin may be severely receded or even absent (Fig. 4.21). The resulting prominence of the nose and upper lip has promoted the term "bird face." The cause is developmental or acquired. Injury to the condyle by trauma at birth or infection about the ears may cause the growth center of the condyle to be affected. This may be corrected by surgery.

If the jaws develop incorrectly, there may be crowding of teeth, and the jaws may fail to approximate each other so that the teeth do not meet properly or are in poor position for function or esthetics.

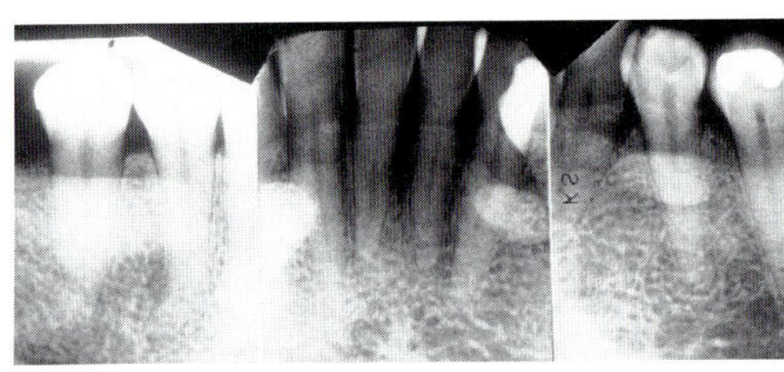

Figure 4.19. Lingual tori radiographically noted as opaque oval areas lingual to bicuspids. Same patient as Figure 4.18.

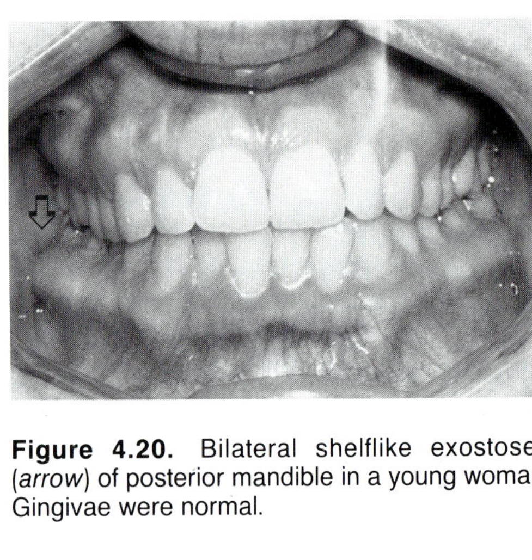

Figure 4.20. Bilateral shelflike exostoses (*arrow*) of posterior mandible in a young woman. Gingivae were normal.

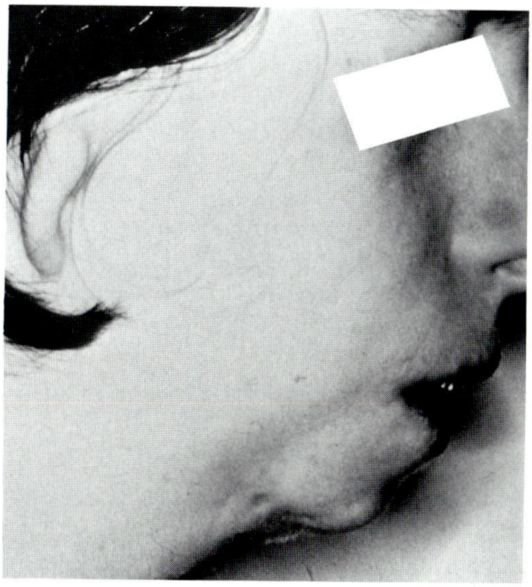

Figure 4.21. Micrognathia, retruded chin, low-set malformed ear, and malformed eye in patient with Treacher Collins syndrome.

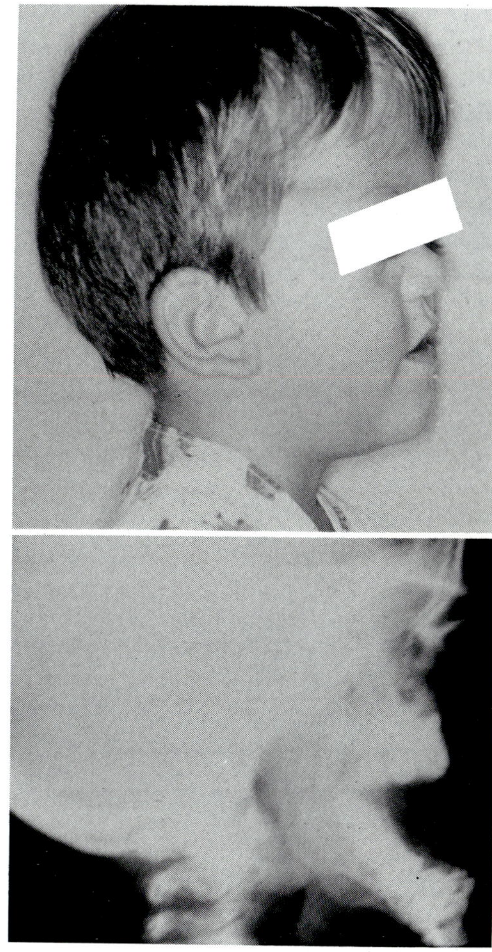

Figure 4.22. Patient with Crouzon disease. Note small maxilla, depressed nose, low-set ear. Radiograph shows small maxilla.

There are several disorders that affect the jaws as well as other areas. Some of these have a specific set of signs or symptoms associated with them and are called syndromes. An example, is Pierre Robin syndrome. These children are born with severe micrognathia of the mandible, drooping of the tongue, and cleft palate. Other defects such as deformities of the ear may also be present. Another example, is the Treacher Collins syndrome (see Fig. 4.21).

There are several developmental syndromes that present with micrognathia of the maxilla as part of the syndrome. Down syndrome, the most common genetic disease, is characterized by a small maxilla, among other features. In Crouzon's disease, a craniofacial synostosis related to Apert syndrome, there is a small maxilla and nose causing the face to be sunken inward (Fig. 4.22).

Developmental Disturbances of the Teeth

During the formation of a tooth, the tooth bud may be disturbed so that any or all of the components of the tooth are affected. The cause may be local, systemic, or hereditary. The clinical manifestation varies depending on the stage of development, the insult, and the length of time it persists. The formative cells are very sensitive to insults that may affect them until the tooth is calcified. There may be variations in number, size, shape, position, eruption, and structure. The disorder may appear independently or in association with some other condition.

If the tooth germ fails to initiate, *anodontia* occurs. Anodontia refers to the failure of teeth to appear or develop. Absolute anodontia or the failure of all teeth to develop is extremely rare. However, it can be seen in a hereditary disease called ectodermal dysplasia. In this condition, which affects mainly males, structures derived from ectoderm (from which the tooth is derived) are involved. These individuals are missing hair, sweat glands, sebaceous glands, and teeth—both primary and permanent. They may have complete or partial anodontia.

Partial anodontia is more common in the general population. Perhaps representing an evolutionary sign, the most common missing tooth is the mandibular third molar. The next most common congenitally missing tooth is the maxillary lateral incisor (Fig. 4.23).

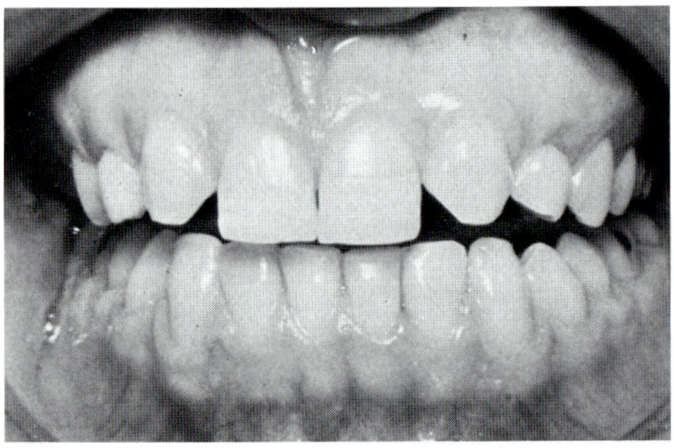

Figure 4.23. Congenitally missing maxillary lateral incisors.

Cleidocranial dysplasia is an autosomal dominant condition in which the clavicle fails to develop and the cranial sutures fail to close on time so that the eyes are wide apart (hypertelorism). In addition, the patient may show a clinical partial anodontia caused by faulty eruption. However, radiography reveals multiple impacted teeth and extra teeth.

Another hereditary condition that may feature multiple supernumerary teeth is Gardner's syndrome. Very significantly, these patients have hundreds of polyps, adenomas (benign tumors) of the colon, which predispose to cancer at an early age and lead to death if not diagnosed and treated. The dental team may arrive at an early diagnosis because of the oral manifestations. Besides multiple impacted supernumerary teeth, there may be multiple benign bony tumors called osteomas of the jaws, skull, or long bones, and/or multiple epidermoid cysts. Once diagnosed, these patients must be followed for malignant change of the many polyps.

Extra teeth or those that develop in excess of a normal complement are called supernumerary or accessory teeth. They can occur in either jaw but are seen most frequently in the maxilla in the midline of the anterior teeth and distal to the molar teeth. When the extra tooth occurs between the maxillary central incisors, it is called a mesiodens (Figs. 4.24 and 4.25). These teeth usually are small (microdontia), are peg-shaped, and do not resemble the teeth normal to the site. However, some supernumerary teeth may very closely mimic a normal tooth (Fig. 4.26). They may erupt or remain embedded in tissue or impacted in bone. A mesiodens that is impacted can cause a diastema or spacing between the maxillary central incisors. Supernumerary teeth may cause crowding of the normal teeth and may delay the eruption of permanent teeth. Treatment is surgical removal.

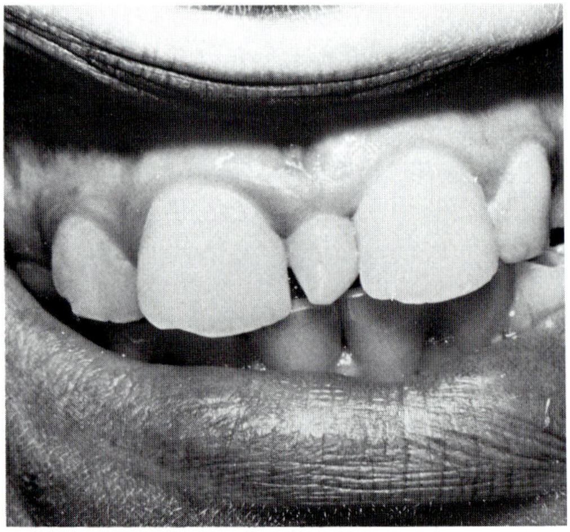

Figure 4.24. Mesiodens, supernumerary tooth between maxillary central incisors.

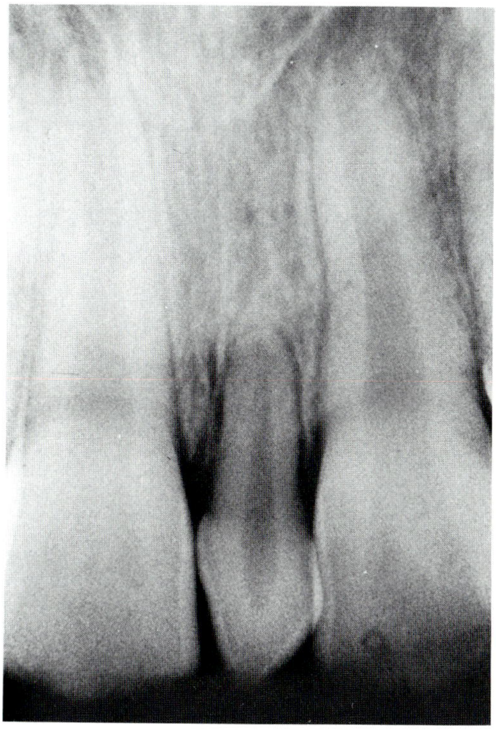

Figure 4.25. Radiograph of mesiodens. Note small size (microdontia).

Occasionally and rarely a newborn may have a tooth that erupts prior to birth (natal) or soon after birth (neonatal). Before removing them, they must be distinguished from a prematurely erupted primary tooth.

Macrodontia refers to a large tooth (Fig. 4.27). Some teeth may be quite large in width or height when compared to sizes that are known for normal teeth. Other teeth may be large because of some developmental defect other than just size.

Gemination results in a large tooth, because a single tooth germ attempts to form two teeth (Figs. 4.28 to 4.30). This twinning usually results in partial or completely separated crowns attached to a single root with one canal.

Fusion results in formation of one tooth from two separate tooth germs. This usually results in macrodontia with a large crown composed of the joined crowns (Fig. 4.31) and joined roots, usually with two root canals (Fig. 4.32). Fusion and gemination may be difficult to distinguish. A count of teeth present may be helpful because in fusion there should be one tooth missing.

Dens in dente means a tooth within a tooth. This describes the radiographic appearance of a dental anomaly caused by the invagination of the enamel into a deep groove in a tooth, frequently seen in the lingual pit area of the maxillary lateral incisor (Fig. 4.33). Because debris settles in the invagination, these teeth are prone to undetected decay, and periapical inflammation may be the first indication of the process.

Dilaceration (Fig. 4.34) refers to an abnormal angulation of the root with reference to the long axis of the crown. Usually it is very sharp and almost at a right angle. Trauma may be a factor so that the crown is displaced, and a twist or bend results in the root that develops after the trauma. Dilaceration creates a problem on extraction of the tooth.

There may be disturbances in the position of teeth. Inadequate space for teeth results in crowding. These irregularities are common. Some teeth may be completely rotated so that the buccal cusp is toward the lingual or palatal side. Other teeth may be transposed such that two teeth may seem to have changed positions (Fig. 4.35). Or, teeth may erupt in an abnormal position.

Although the pattern of eruption of teeth is normally quite variable in that no two individual patterns are alike, there are times in which the eruption may be premature or delayed. The cause for this is usually obscure; however, in some instances it can be related to certain events or systemic influences. Trauma with the loss of a primary tooth may cause the early eruption of the corresponding permanent tooth. In hyperthyroidism the teeth often erupt prematurely. Conversely, in the disease of hypothyroidism, with diminished metabolic activity, the eruption of the teeth is usually delayed. An impacted tooth represents an eruption pattern that is remarkably delayed.

Text continues on page 57

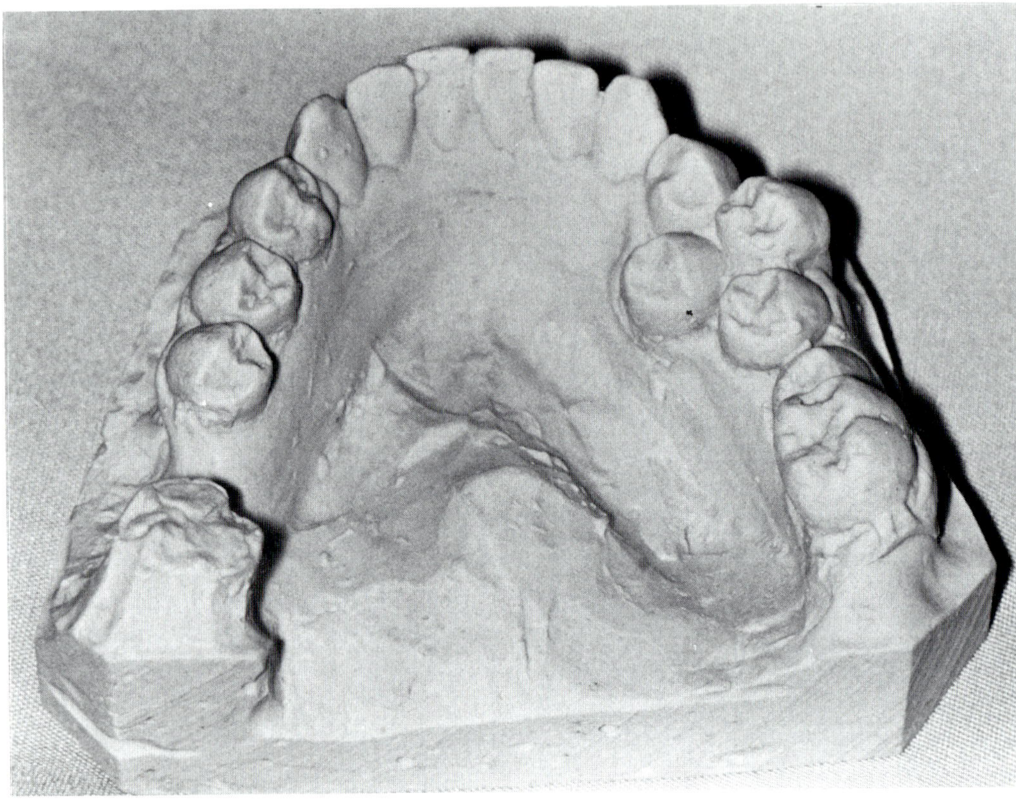

Figure 4.26. Study model showing several supernumerary bicuspid teeth.

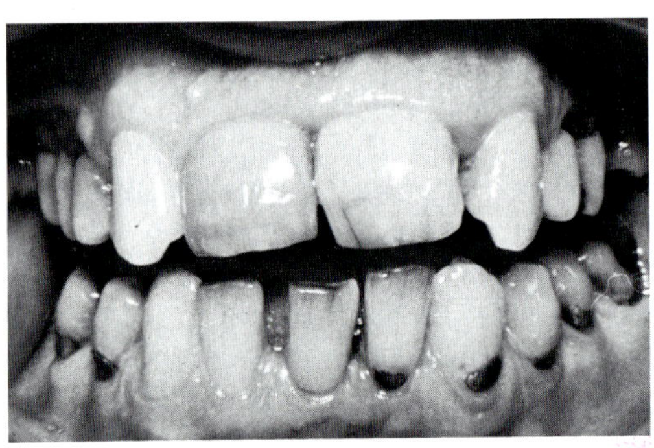

Figure 4.27. Macrodontia of central incisors. Lateral incisors were missing.

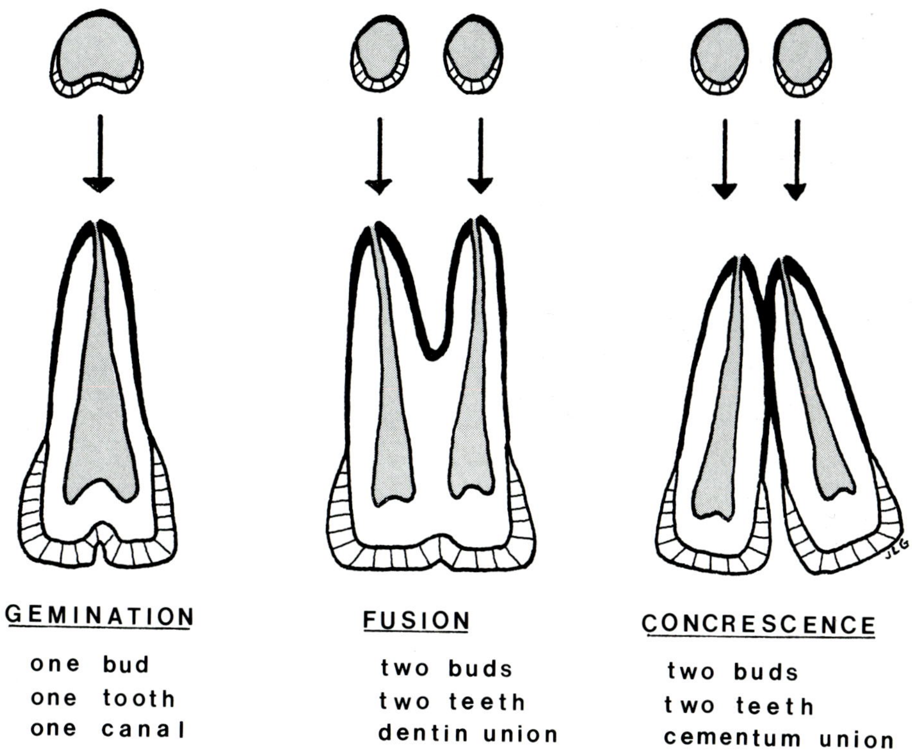

Figure 4.28. Diagrams of gemination, fusion, and concrescence. All three present clinically as macrodontia.

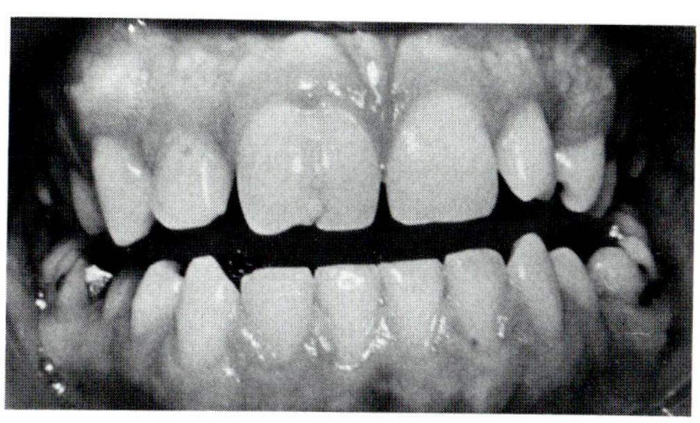

Figure 4.29. Gemination. The maxillary right central incisor appears to be two teeth (macrodontia). The lateral incisor is present.

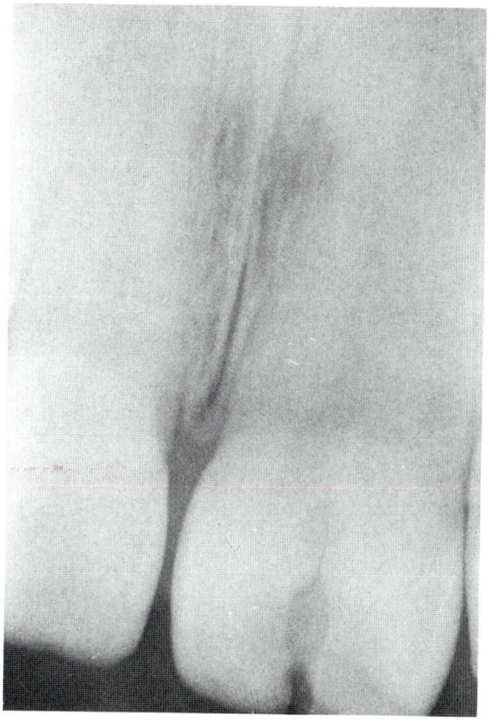

Figure 4.30. X-ray of gemination seen in Figure 4.29. Note two pulp chambers and single root canal.

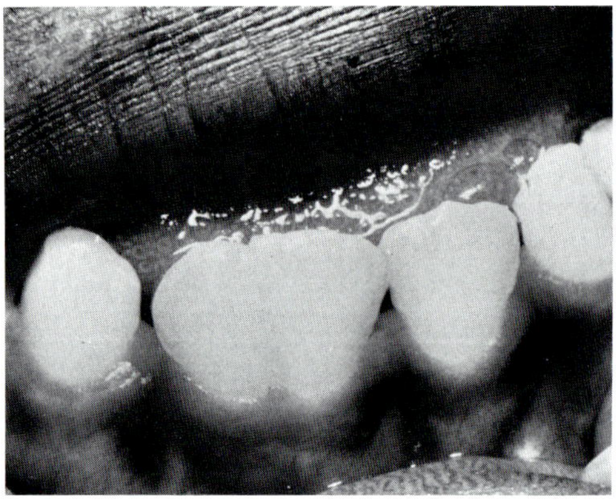

Figure 4.31. Fusion of mandibular right central and lateral incisor, creating a large tooth (macrodontia).

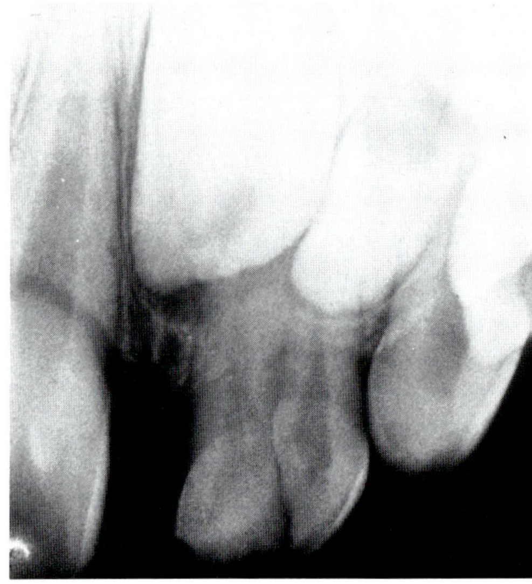

Figure 4.32. Radiograph showing fusion of deciduous central and lateral incisors. Note the separate root canals.

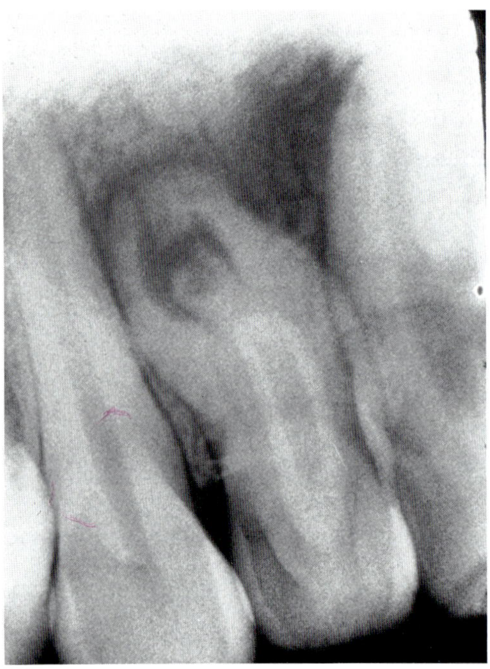

Figure 4.33. Dens in dente of maxillary lateral incisor associated with periapical radiolucency.

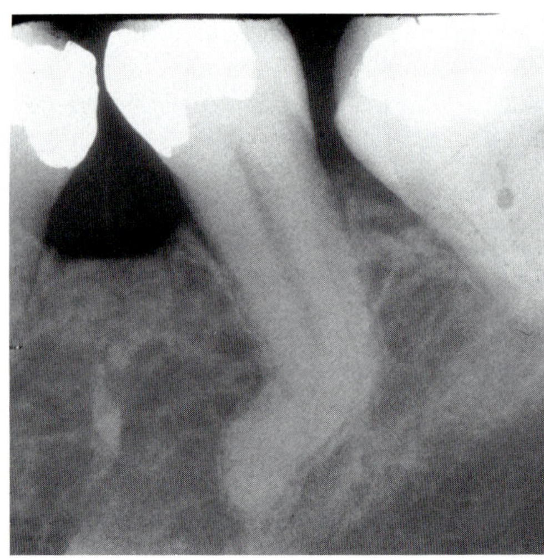

Figure 4.34. Dilaceration of root of mandibular bicuspid.

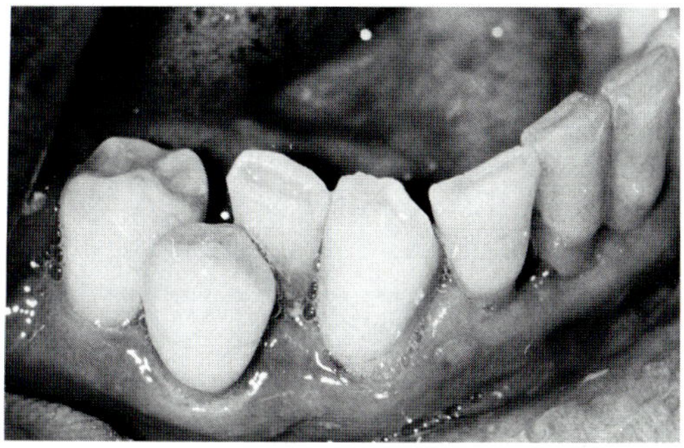

Figure 4.35. Transposition of mandibular right lateral incisor and cuspid teeth.

Enamel Hypoplasia

If the ameloblasts are damaged during the period of tooth formation in which they are forming enamel matrix, the tooth will have defects in its form or shape. Enamel hypoplasia is the term used for the incomplete or defective formation of the enamel with resulting gross defects or change in form. Enamel hypoplasia may involve the primary and permanent dentition. It is quite common and occurs in about 10 percent of the population.

Clinically, there is a wide variation of appearances. Hypoplasia may appear as small pits, as rows of horizontal grooves or pits, or simply as missing enamel. If the insult was systemic, the hypoplasia involves the contralateral teeth with a pattern that corresponds to the time during which the teeth were forming. Because teeth follow a specific incremental development, the time of injury can be determined. For example, in permanent teeth, the majority of cases of hypoplasias occur between 1 and 10 months of age. During this time, the crowns that are developing and that would show defects are the first molars, the incisors (except the maxillary laterals), and the canines. If the maxillary lateral incisors and the premolars are involved, the timing of the insult occurred between 11 and 34 months. Thus, enamel hypoplasia provides a permanent record of an injury that occurred at a specific time. If the injury was of short duration, the pits, grooves, or lines involve only a narrow portion of the teeth. On the other hand, an extended period of injury results in more tooth structure being defective, and a broad band may result (Figs. 4.36 and 4.37). Two bands, one at the incisal third and one at the cervical third of an incisor, for example, indicate two separate periods of injury (Fig. 4.38).

There are various factors, known and unknown, that can injure the ameloblasts and cause hypoplasia. Nutritional deficien-

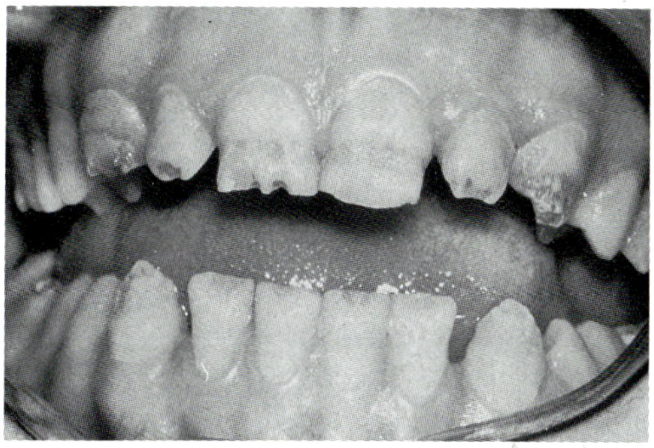

Figure 4.36. Systemic (environmental) hypoplasia, 17-year-old. The first molars, central and lateral incisors, and canines show hypoplasia of the incisal third corresponding to the timing of matrix formation for these teeth. The hypoplasia is chronic because the patient was ill from birth through 18 months.

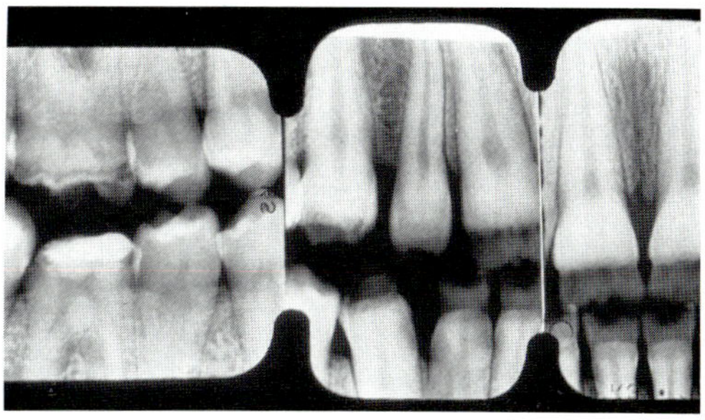

Figure 4.37. Radiographs of teeth with systemic (environmental) hypoplasia due to continuous respiratory infections from birth through 18 months of age. The bicuspids are not affected. Same patient as Figure 4.36.

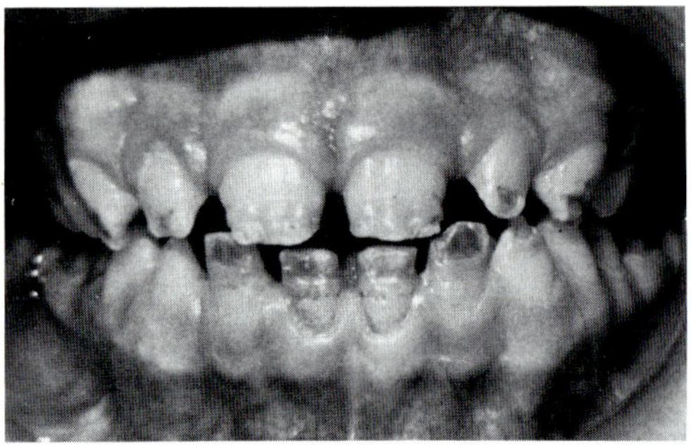

Figure 4.38. Systemic enamel hypoplasia. The broad areas with less enamel from incisal edges to junction of middle third indicate the child was ill enough to damage ameloblasts from birth through about 18 months. The separate linear defect in the middle third corresponds to tonsillitis at about 2½ years of age.

cies of vitamins A, C, and D can result in systemic hypoplasia. Patients with a history of rickets (vitamin D deficiency) often display severe hypoplasia. Diseases associated with high fevers, particularly measles and chickenpox, cause horizontal pitting. These pits accumulate debris and bacteria that can stain a deep brown.

Another cause of hypoplasia is congenital syphilis. In untreated pregnant women infected with syphilis, the causative spirochete invades the fetus after the 16th week, and the tooth germs may be affected. In some of these children characteristic changes (stigmata) may be seen in the permanent anterior teeth and/or posterior teeth. Essentially, there is a reduction in the mesiodistal dimension of the teeth affected (Fig. 4.39). The anterior maxillary incisors are narrowed at the incisal third. The central incisors may resemble a screwdriver, may have a central notch, and are called Hutchinson's incisors after the physician who first attributed the change to syphilis. The lateral incisors usually are conical and are called peg-laterals. The first molar teeth are narrowed and may have numerous rounded cuspal structures on the occlusal surface. Resembling a mulberry, these teeth are called mulberry molars. Although these types of hypoplastic teeth are frequently associated with congenital syphilis, similar changes may be seen without such a history, and more information would be required before the definitive association is made. For instance, peg-laterals, an example of microdontia and hypoplasia, are commonly seen but the cause is usually unknown.

Hypocalcemia is a decrease in calcium and can cause pitting of the teeth. This may be seen in the disease of hypoparathyroidism, as well as in vitamin D deficiency. The

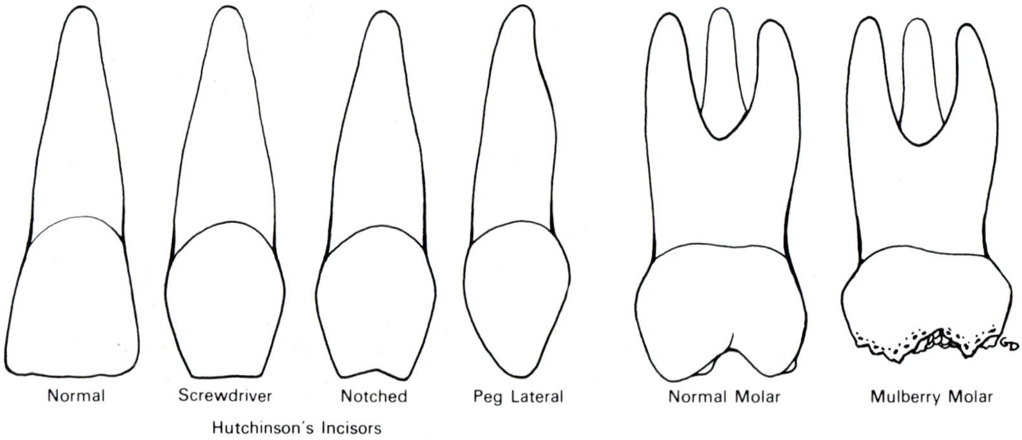

Figure 4.39 Changes noted in teeth in patients with congenital syphilis. Basic change is hypoplasia with a loss of tooth structure in the mesiodistal diameter at the incisal or occlusal third of the teeth.

changes are the same as those seen in systemic hypoplasia.

Birth injury or premature delivery may cause a definite horizontal or mesiodistal defect, seen as a line. This neonatal line is usually seen at the gingival third of the primary incisors and the tips of the first permanent molars.

When local factors are responsible, the condition is called Turner's hypoplasia. Usually only one tooth is involved and this can be called a Turner's tooth (Fig. 4.40). There is no symmetrical pattern, and the time of injury is reflected only on the tooth involved, usually the permanent maxillary incisors or the premolars. The cause is trauma to the primary tooth or infection about the root of a primary tooth that affects the developing crown of the permanent tooth.

Chemicals may cause hypoplastic defects. Excessive amounts of fluoride can produce mottled enamel; the condition is called dental fluorosis (Fig. 4.41). Mottling is the discoloration of the enamel in irregular areas. There are two types of defects that can be noted, and the severity of the defects increases as the fluoride concentration increases. There may be white flecks or opacities (hypocalcification), pitting with loss of normal shape (hypoplasia), or both (Fig. 4.42). The spots are white on eruption, but with time they acquire the brown stain that characterizes mottled enamel. The optimal level of fluoride in drinking water is considered one part per million, because below that level there is little benefit in decreasing decay and above that level the dental fluorosis becomes prominent. Thus, in communities with natural fluoride in the drinking water at five parts per million, teeth have little decay but may be severely mottled.

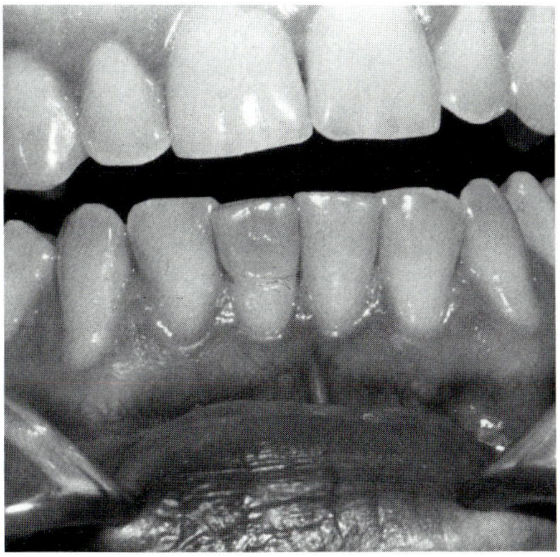

Figure 4.40. Turner's hypoplasia of mandibular right central incisor. Note horizontal indented line in middle of tooth.

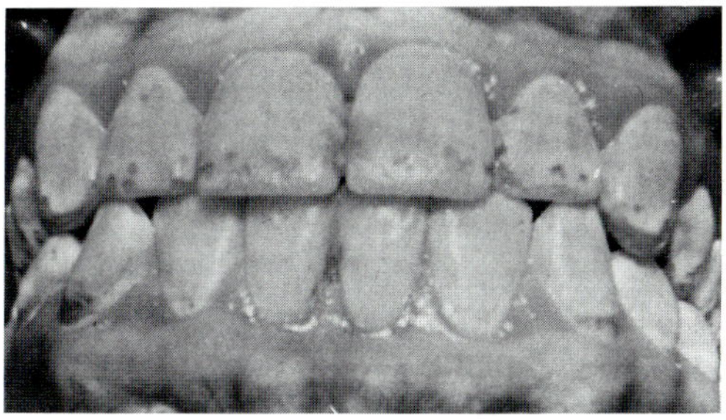

Figure 4.41. Dental fluorosis, mottled enamel. White variegated pattern of teeth is due to excessive quantities of fluorine in natural drinking water.

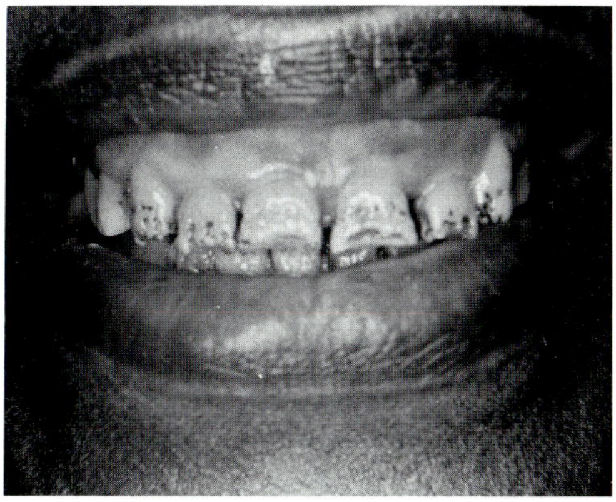

Figure 4.42. Severe dental fluorosis. Pitted hypoplastic defects due to high concentrations of fluorine in drinking water.

Probably the most common cause of hypoplasia is idiopathic, a term meaning "cause unknown."

Enamel Opacities (Hypocalcification)

Enamel opacities are white opaque spots that appear in permanent and primary teeth (Fig. 4.43). These are common and may be seen in 25 percent of the population. The maxillary central incisors are the teeth most commonly involved. Local or systemic factors similar to those in enamel hypoplasia are responsible. In this condition, however, the factor injures the tooth germ during the calcification stage. Thus, the defect is represented as a white spot because of the decrease of calcium at that time of injury. The shape and form of the teeth are normal in enamel opacities. It is likely, though, that a tooth may exhibit both enamel opacities and hypoplastic defects so that, at times, the specific entities may be difficult to distinguish.

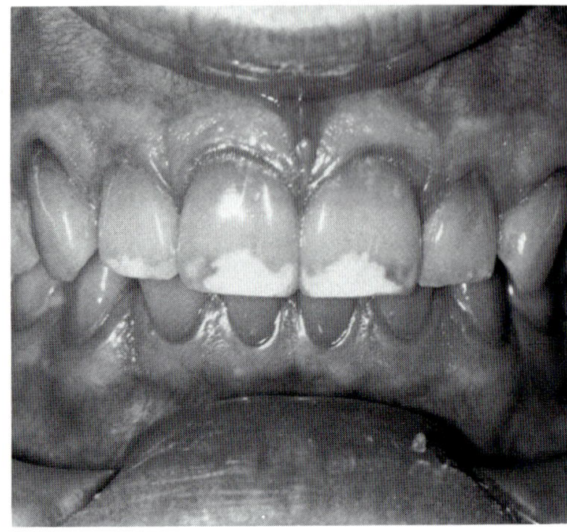

Figure 4.43. Enamel opacities of maxillary central incisors in a patient with dark teeth caused by tetracycline staining.

Hereditary Disorders of Teeth

There are hereditary disturbances of the teeth that can affect the enamel, dentin, or pulp. The most common are those affecting the enamel and dentin.

Amelogenesis imperfecta is an inherited disorder that reflects alterations in regulatory and/or structural genes associated with enamel, which may feature hypocalcification, hypoplasia, or both. The dentin and pulp are normal. Both the primary and the permanent teeth are affected. Incidence of the disease is 1 in 15,000 individuals. Many patterns of inheritance have been noted. Some are autosomal dominant, some recessive, some X-linked, so the number of individuals affected in a family can be variable.

A major form is X-linked, which is of interest because it appears that X-linked genes regulate tooth size and form in humans. A family history for the trait may reveal that several members of a family in several generations have had the disease. The gene defect causes the enamel to be hypocalcified or hypoplastic. Clinically, there may be a variation with pits, grooves, and defects occurring in horizontal or vertical patterns with no relationship to chronologic development. The most common type is the hypocalcified variety in which the teeth are originally normal in thickness, brown, friable, and soft. Calculus may build up heavily on the defects that occur as the enamel fractures away from the dentin (Fig. 4.44). Once the enamel fractures, the exposed dentin can be ground down rap-

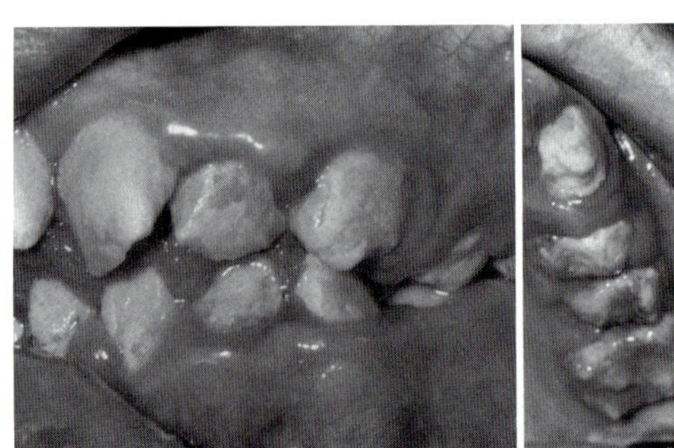

Figure 4.44. Amelogenesis imperfecta. All teeth were hypoplastic and hypocalcified. The enamel chips easily and is worn away. Other family members had a similar dentition. There are heavy calculus deposits on teeth.

idly, leaving only the roots. Radiographically, the enamel is barely visible and appears ghostlike or absent (Fig. 4.45). The treatment is to cap the teeth with full crowns or to extract the teeth and make dentures.

Dentinogenesis imperfecta (hereditary opalescent dentin) is more common than amelogenesis imperfecta and is characterized by irregular dentin formation in both the primary and permanent dentitions reflecting alterations on chromosome 4 of regulatory and structural genes associated with dentin formation. It is a dominant inherited or sporadic genetic defect and is seen in 1 in 8,000 individuals in the population. Clinically, the teeth are normal in contour on eruption. Characteristically, their color is blue, gray, or violet and may have an opalescence (Fig. 4.46). The enamel chips away readily because of a defective dentinoenamel junction. This may lead to severe attrition similar to that seen in amelogenesis imperfecta. Radiographically, the characteristic changes noted are the obliteration of the pulp chamber, short roots, and constriction of the cementoenamel junction that gives the crown a bell-shaped appearance (Fig. 4.47). Dentinogenesis imperfecta is also seen in many cases of osteogenesis imperfecta, another hereditary disease characterized by imperfect formation of type I collagen resulting in fragile bone and blue sclerae of the eyes.

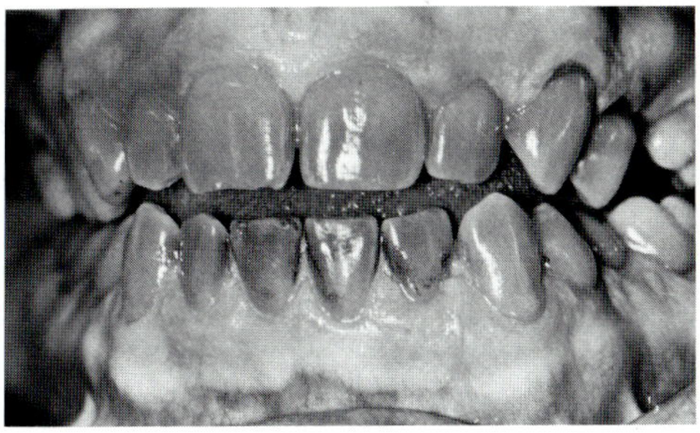

Figure 4.46. Dentinogenesis imperfecta. Teeth have gray color and opalescent hue. Patient's primary teeth were similarly affected. His mother had the same condition.

Acquired Teeth Defects

Certain defects of teeth are not developmental in the sense of being congenital. After the eruption of teeth, various factors can cause teeth to acquire characteristic lesions of the calcified surfaces. These are attrition, abrasion, and erosion.

Attrition is the normal wearing away of the biting surfaces of the teeth by mastication. This occurs in all individuals but may be more pronounced in some, depending on personal habits and diet. The mamelons on newly erupted teeth are quickly worn away, except in individuals with an anterior open bite because their anterior teeth never meet. Some individuals clench and grind their teeth unconsciously (bruxism) and may

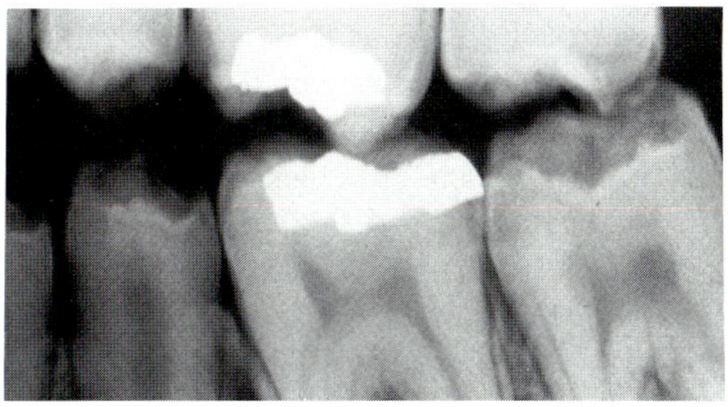

Figure 4.45. Amelogenesis imperfecta. Note absence and ghostlike appearance of enamel. All teeth are affected. Same patient as Figure 4.44.

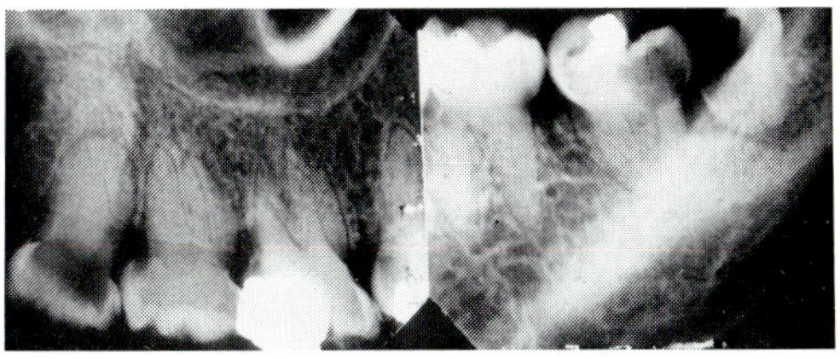

Figure 4.47. Radiographs of molar teeth of patient shown in Figure 4.46. Note bell-shaped crowns, constriction at the cementoenamel junction, lack of pulp chambers, sclerosed canals, and short roots. Patient presented with toothache due to extensive caries.

speed the process of attrition. Rough, gritty food is another factor related to attrition. In severe cases the dentin is exposed, and in some instances the teeth appear to be cut in cross-section with a central darker area of secondary dentin appearing where the pulp originally was (Fig. 4.48). The dentin, when exposed, tends to stain brown by absorbing debris or tobacco stains. The worn surfaces (facets) are shiny and firm. In some cases, the pulp may become exposed. Pulpitis and periapical disease may then follow.

Abrasion is the pathologic wearing away of external tooth surfaces by mechanical means. Various abrasive agents may be responsible and can usually be determined by a careful history or astute observation. Because of the diversity of causes, the tooth defects assume various shapes and forms. The surface of the defects are hard and smooth. Several examples are noted. A patient with a full upper denture with porcelain teeth can wear away the natural teeth that remain in the lower jaw. Toothpicks, dental floss, bobbypins, nails, or any other item that is habitually and excessively used against the teeth can cause abrasion at the site of use. Pipe smokers frequently hold the stem only in one position. After years, there is significant wearing, and the teeth conform in shape to the pipestem (pipestem abrasion) (Fig. 4.49). Toothbrushing may cause abrasion at the cervical labial margins, particularly if a back-and-forth motion is used. The resulting grooves in the cementum simulate erosion, but the defects are usually more severe on one side depending on the dexterity of the individual.

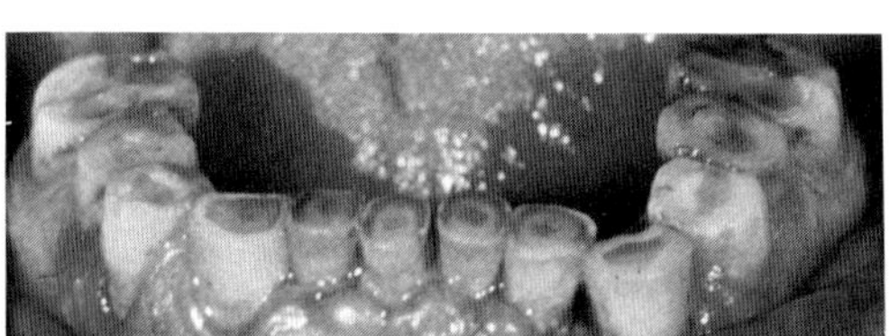

Figure 4.48. Severe attrition of mandibular teeth. The surfaces are flat, hard, and shiny. Secondary dentin fills the pulp chamber area.

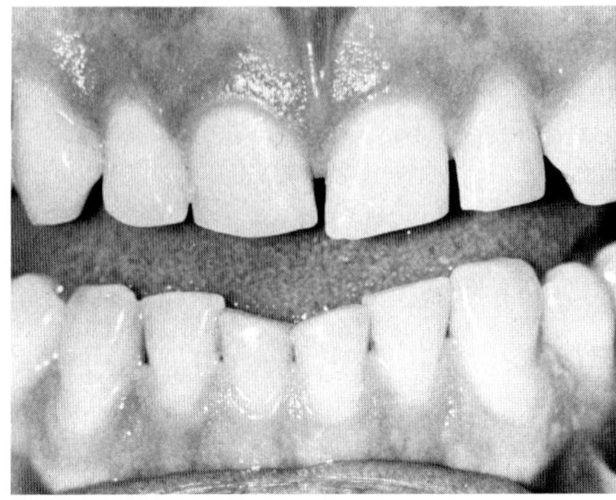

Figure 4.49. Pipestem abrasion of teeth. Pipestem has abraded mandibular central incisors.

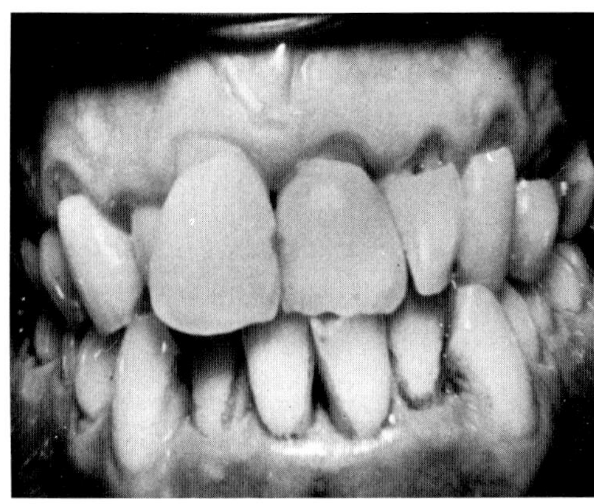

Figure 4.50. Dental erosion. Smooth, hard defects occurring at cervical margins of the teeth.

Erosion of teeth refers to the dissolution of the tooth by chemical means or by frictional intraoral forces not defined as yet. Characteristically erosive defects occur at the labial or buccal surfaces, particularly of the incisor teeth, at the cementoenamel junction; the biting surfaces are not involved. They appear as hard, smooth, shiny, ditchlike areas (Fig. 4.50). Other patterns of erosion may be seen such as on the lingual aspect or around the entire circumference of some teeth. Perimolysis, the loss of enamel and dentin on the lingual surfaces, is a marker in bulimic and anorec-

Table 4.1
Causes of dental erosion

Dietary
Fruits and food with citric acid
Lemons, oranges, grapefruits, tomatoes, bananas
Fruit juices
Acid (carbonated) beverages
Soft drinks; nondietetic and dietetic
Vinegar—pickled foods
Candy—sour balls, mints
Cordials
Vitamin C (chewable)
Medicinal
HCl replacement
Iron tonic
Vitamin C
Acid drops (tablets)
Aspirin
Regurgitational
Anorexia nervosa
Vomiting—bulimia
Stress—reflux phenomenon
Occupational
Industrial acids
Gas chlorinated pools
Idiopathic
Acid saliva

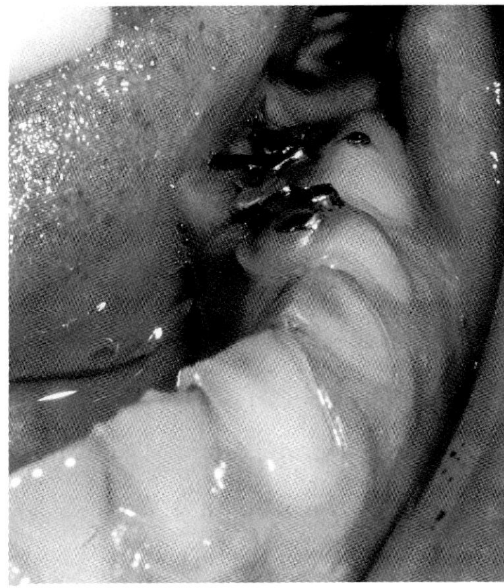

Figure 4.51. Severe dental erosion. Note the missing enamel and dentin and the fillings standing above the surface. The patient was diabetic and drank 15 sugar-free colas a day.

tic patients. Erosions are primarily idiopathic; however, some are associated with acids from foods, beverages, or gastric disturbances (Table 4.1). Patients who suck on lemons or drink large quantities of orange juice develop erosions on the labial surfaces (Fig. 4.51). Erosive patterns can even be noted on restorations that are placed in teeth. Treatment is difficult because the erosion progresses even after the area is restored, although restorations do retard the process.

Chapter 5

CARIES AND DENTAL PULP DISORDERS

Dental Caries

Dental caries (tooth decay) is a progressive disease of the hard dental structures. It is characterized by decalcification, proteolysis, and microbial invasion, and it results in the destruction of the hard structures to form a cavity. It follows the interaction of three main factors, namely, the host (susceptible teeth), bacteria, and food (diet).

Dental caries is one of the most prevalent worldwide chronic diseases of humans. Over 95 percent of the population have decay or will have had it before they die. Very few individuals are immune to it. However, current measures to control the disease, especially through the use of systemic fluoride and topical applications, are causing a decrease in occurrence.

Problems arise because of the complications stemming from decay. The hard dental structures are unique. Enamel is 97 percent mineralized (calcified). Dentin is about 70 percent mineralized, and 30 percent of it is organic (cellular and pericellular material). Cementum is about 60 percent calcified. However, the teeth are not protected as are other systems by epithelium. Moreover, once the destruction process begins, it generally is progressive. Fluorides and remineralization procedures offer hope in controlling caries. The only means to date of repairing the destruction is by restorative dentistry, which is usually time-consuming and expensive. The challenge, then, is to overcome the complications of dental caries through prevention.

Dental caries is an infectious disease with a multifactorial etiology involving endogenous bacteria, food, and a susceptible tooth. The bacteria are normal to the mouth, and there are differences in some organisms for the different types or areas of caries on the tooth involved. *Streptococcus mutans*, capable of converting food breakdown products into large amounts of lactic acid, is the primary pathogen for all types of dental caries. *S. mutans* produces sticky substances called dextrans that promote the adherence of the bacteria to the tooth surface. It is the primary organism for smooth-surface or interproximal caries and, coupled with other organisms, is responsible for pit and fissure and root surface lesions. *Lactobacillus* species, *A. viscosus*, and *Actinomyces* species, although producing much less acid than *S. mutans*, contribute in conjunction with *S. mutans* to the etiology of dental caries.

The stagnation of food is related to decay. Food stagnates in pits and fissures (occlusal surfaces), beneath contact areas of teeth, at the cervical margins, beneath clasp arms of dentures, beneath overhanging margins on restorations, around orthodontic appliances, about crowded teeth, and in many other conditions. With the stagnation of food, bacteria can proliferate and yield metabolic products—some of which are acids. The acids are capable of demineralizing the tooth, and if the circumstances are proper (i.e., if the tooth is susceptible), the hard structure begins to disintegrate and decay. Thus, there appear to be two processes, the production of the cariogenic agent (acid) and the production of a susceptible tooth surface on which the agent can act. A simplified schema for the pathogenesis of dental caries is:

$$\text{food} + \text{bacteria} \rightarrow \text{acid}$$
$$\text{acid} + \text{tooth} \rightarrow \text{caries}$$

There are many factors that alter this

process. The types of food most incriminated are the carbohydrates. Within 15 minutes of their ingestion, the pH level of the saliva drops to a point that may cause demineralization if it is not buffered. Not only are sweet foods, such as caramels, chewy fruit-flavored candies, and fat-rich chocolate cookies responsible for producing an acid environment, but starchy foods such as crackers, breadsticks, potato chips, raisins, and other "natural" foodstuffs also produce acids and are cleared away more slowly than the sweet foods. The length of time the food is present and the type of food is important. Sticky foods, such as toffee candy, are more cariogenic than hard candy. However, hard candy is usually held in the mouth longer and therefore causes more acid production by the bacteria. Confoundingly, the bacteria may not consistently consume the sugar meal and may produce bursts of acidity that may not damage the teeth. Nonetheless, the longer the food is present, the longer there is a potential acid tooth-wearing environment. The frequency of eating is therefore important and in the snack-oriented United States continues to be a major factor in promoting caries. The kinds of food, how they are eaten, when they are eaten, and with what they are eaten are all separate factors. Some foods, like cheddar cheese, reverse the rise in acidity. Eating aged cheese along with carbohydrate snacks or meals increases the protective acid-lowering saliva. Unsweetened chocolate has a chemical that is anticariogenic. Chewing sugarless gum following a meal quickly reverses the acidity by stimulating the saliva. The kinds of food are important, in that some foods produce less damaging acids than others. Thus, the food factor is complex, and research is still unfolding its mysteries. A diet history can reveal what foods may be contributing to caries and which ones are to be avoided or reduced. In the absence of food residue, a mouth bathed in saliva is free of acidity.

Saliva is a major defense against dental caries. Normally neutral or slightly alkaline, saliva has buffers to counteract acidity. In addition, it contains antimicrobial molecules, including IgA, and ions, such as calcium and phosphates, which are important in remineralization mechanisms. It serves as a lavage to wash away carbohydrates. Patients whose normal flow of saliva is diminished or lacking, as in xerostomia (dry mouth), can develop dental caries in just a few months. Causes of xerostomia are medications that reduce saliva, diseases such as Sjögren's syndrome or diabetes, and radiation damage causing atrophy of the glands. In Down syndrome there is less caries but more periodontal disease, attributable to a more alkaline saliva. If a person eats just three meals per day and no snacks, there is adequate time for the mouth to return to neutral and for the teeth to regain any lost minerals due to the salivary ions. With frequent eating, as in snacking, there are constant food residues, and the steady acid production cannot be balanced by the minerals in the saliva, causing the tooth to decalcify and to create dental caries.

Teeth are more prone to caries when they first appear in the mouth. This accounts for the fact that the decay rate is greatest during the years of eruption, falls after 25 years of age, and increases again in older age. The occlusal surface is the most susceptible to decay, followed by the mesial, distal, buccal, and lingual (except on the maxillary teeth, where lingual surfaces decay more than buccal). The posterior teeth present more decay than the anterior teeth. The lower incisors appear to be the least susceptible but are usually involved in cases of severe or rampant caries. This order of susceptibility is a clinical fact and definitely relates to the order of eruption and the areas of stagnation that occur as the teeth erupt. The increase in decay in older age relates to the fact that more root surface is exposed as the gingiva recedes and the recession promotes the stagnation of food. Characteristically, the caries most prevalent in older age is cemental, whereas the caries of youth is mostly pit and fissure and smooth surface.

The fluoride content of teeth affects the

susceptibility to caries. If the fluoride content of drinking water is one part per million during the formation of teeth, those teeth will be less susceptible to decay. Once the crown is calcified, systemic fluoride is of no benefit but topical application is, and remineralization of the outer surface may take place. Above one part per million, the teeth may develop fluorosis or mottled enamel. In this case there is still a reduction in decay despite the fact that there is hypocalcification and hypoplasia. Teeth with hypoplastic defects are not more prone to caries but can collect more debris that may promote the carious process.

Dental caries starts at the external surface of the tooth and progresses toward the pulp. The process in the enamel is mainly demineralization, because the enamel is mostly calcified tissue. In the dentin demineralization, proteolysis (breakdown of the protein organic matter), and microbial invasion occur. The pattern of decay can best be classified according to its clinical location, i.e., pit and fissure, smooth surface, and cemental caries (Fig. 5.1).

Pit and fissure caries is seen in areas normally considered self-cleansing. Food may stagnate in grooves and crevices of the occlusal surfaces of molars and premolars, buccal surfaces of mandibular molars, and lingual surfaces of maxillary molar and anterior teeth. The pattern is one of a spreading cone following the enamel rods. In sections, the apex is at the occlusal surface and the base is toward the dentinoenamel junction. When the dentin is reached, there is a lateral spread along the dentinoenamel junction, undermining the enamel. As the process advances toward the pulp, it follows the course of the dentinal tubules in a conical pattern with its base at the dentinoenamel junction and its apex toward the pulp. Because of this pattern, the pit and fissure caries looks deceptively small at the surface. There may be only a pinpoint defect on exploration, but considerable other destruction must be assumed.

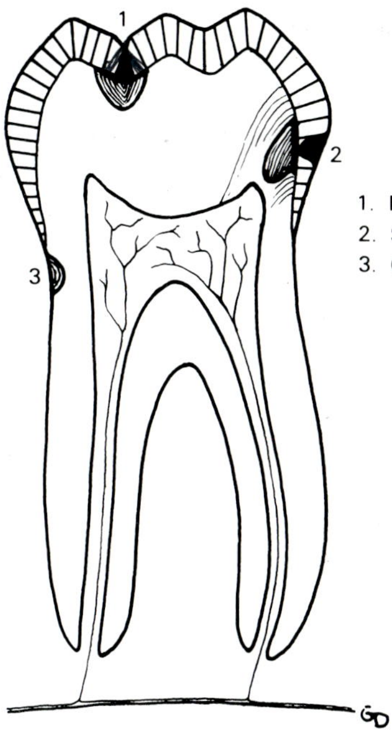

Figure 5.1. Dental caries. Patterns of dental caries in enamel and dentin according to surface involvement. 1, pit and fissure caries; 2, smooth surface caries; and 3, cemental caries.

Smooth surface caries occurs in those areas of the tooth that are not self-cleaning. Usually this is at the interproximal area just below the contact point of adjacent teeth, where food debris stagnates. These areas are associated with plaque. Plaque is an invisible film of bacterial colonies and food debris that sticks to the tooth surface by gummy substances called dextrans. Streptococcal organisms are primarily responsible for producing these dextrans and for the production of the acids that can demineralize the tooth surface. The plaque covers a broad area, and the carious lesion is therefore broader at the surface than pit and fissure lesions. The external surface outline is elliptical with the length of spread being in the buccolingual direction. In sections, the process follows the direction of the enamel rods in a triangular pattern with the base at the smooth surface and the apex toward the dentinoenamel junction. When the dentin is reached, there is lateral spread similar to that seen in the pit and fissure lesions. The decay involves more tubules and following the tubules spreads pulpally in a conical or triangular pattern with the apex toward the pulp (Fig. 5.2).

As the caries progresses in the dentin, there are two protective mechanisms that can take place. The odontoblastic processes within the dentinal tubules degenerate, and the empty tubule becomes plugged with calcium salts and forms a harder or sclerotic dentin. This temporarily stops the advance of the process in those tubules. Unfortunately, the process can affect other tubules and continue toward the pulp (Fig. 5.3). Ultimately the calcified dentin is demineralized, bacteria invade the tubules, and the dentin decomposes and becomes softened.

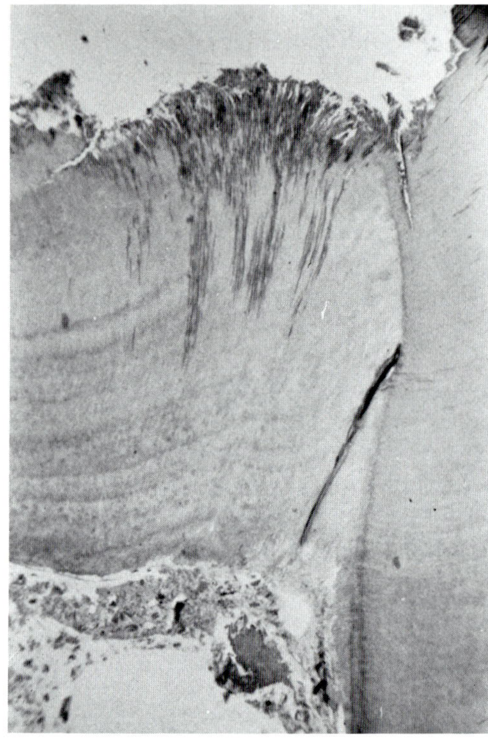

Figure 5.3. Decalcified section of molar tooth with extensive decay. Dark linear streaks represent bacterial colonies within dentinal tubules of reparative dentin. The pulp below is necrotic.

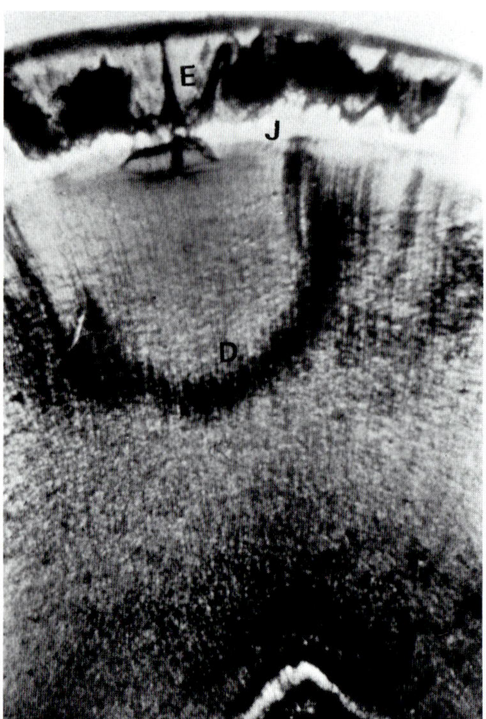

Figure 5.2. Ground section of tooth with smooth surface caries. E, multiple lesions in enamel; J, lateral spread along dentinoenamel junction; and D, pattern of decay in dentin, with apex toward the pulp.

The other protective mechanism is the formation of reparative or tertiary dentin. In the area of the pulp corresponding to the dentinal tubules involved with caries, the odontoblasts move toward the pulp and lay down new dentin behind them. This is to protect the pulp and reflects the fact that the best protection for the pulp is an adequate thickness of dentin. Therefore, early treatment of caries is essential in order to maintain this thickness of dentin.

Cemental or root surface caries presents a pattern similar to that of dentinal caries. However, the lesion starts on the root surface secondary to recession of the gingiva and the accumulation of plaque, particularly with *Streptococcus mutans* and *Lactobacillus* species acting concurrently. Root caries is associated with poor dental health habits, infrequent dental visits, use of sweets in beverages, and xerostomia, and is more common in men. The caries starts at Sharpey's fibers (a type of collagen fiber in the cementum) and spreads in a broad pattern in the dentinal tubules with a triangular pattern in cross-section with the apex toward the pulp. As the lesion expands, the enamel may become involved and is undermined. The spreading lesion can be difficult to treat by restorative procedures. If the lesion extends around the tooth, the crown can be lost. Preventive measures, such as fluorides and antimicrobial rinses and behavioral change in dental health habits are helpful.

Clinically, the naked eye cannot detect the initiation of the carious lesion (Fig. 5.4). As decalcification occurs the enamel may appear chalky white. With an explorer this may feel smooth, so cavitation is no criterion for judging the extent of the lesion. With time cavitation may occur, and bacteria penetrating the cavity and dentin cause a brown stain (Fig. 5.5). Because of the undermining of the enamel, it may fracture easily. The demineralized dentin may be easily removed with an excavator.

The dental radiograph is an adjunct in determining caries, particularly interproximal lesions. On the radiograph, the hard tooth structure appears gray-white and is radiopaque. The pulp appears dark and is radiolucent. Dental caries is seen as a radiolucent lesion; the pattern mimics that previously described (see Fig. 5.1; Figs. 5.6 and 5.7). The radiograph, however, is merely a shadow. In fact, the carious process on a radiograph usually underestimates the actual extent of involvement (see Fig. 5.4). Despite this caution, the radiograph is most useful in detecting interproximal caries that clinically may be undetected by explorer because of lack of a

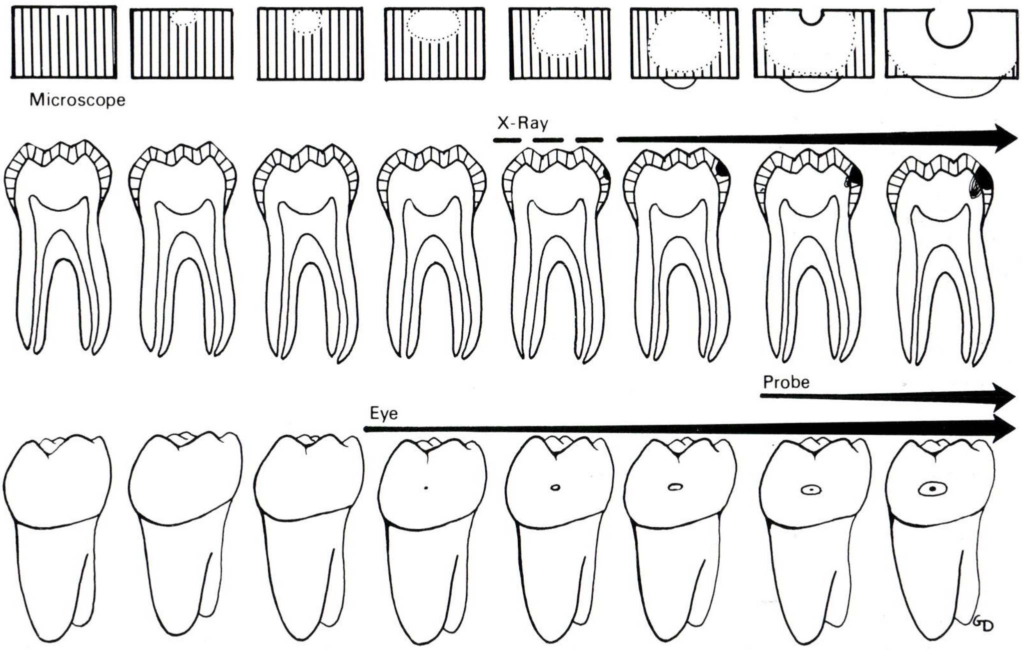

Figure 5.4. Schematic diagram tracing the progression of dental caries on the distal aspect of a mandibular molar. *Top*, line indicates microscopic appearance in enamel (*vertical lines*) and then dentin. Lesion starts at surface long before it can be detected by eye, x-ray, or probe. *Middle*, drawings depict cross-section in mesiodistal dimension. *Bottom*, drawings depict distal view of tooth. Once decalcification is well established in enamel, the eye can detect a white lesion clinically. The x-ray is not as sensitive as the eye but is essential for proximal lesions. The probe can palpate a lesion only when a cavitation or surface breakdown has occurred.

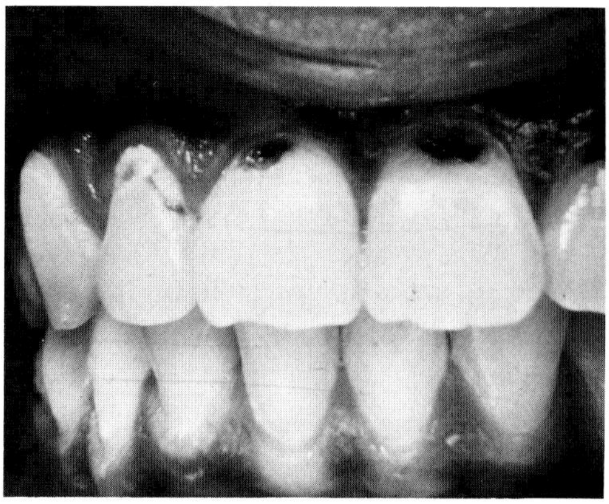

Figure 5.5. Cervical enamel dental caries. Note progression from left to right of opaque lesion to cavitation with deep staining. An earlier opaque lesion appears on the cervical third of the mandibular cuspid.

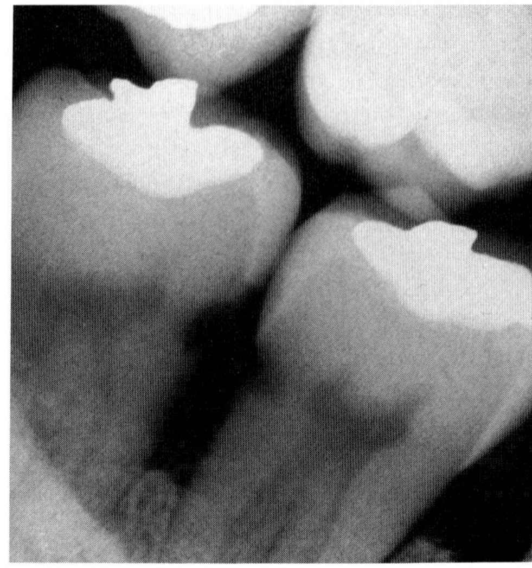

Figure 5.7. Bitewing radiograph showing cemental caries of second and third mandibular molars.

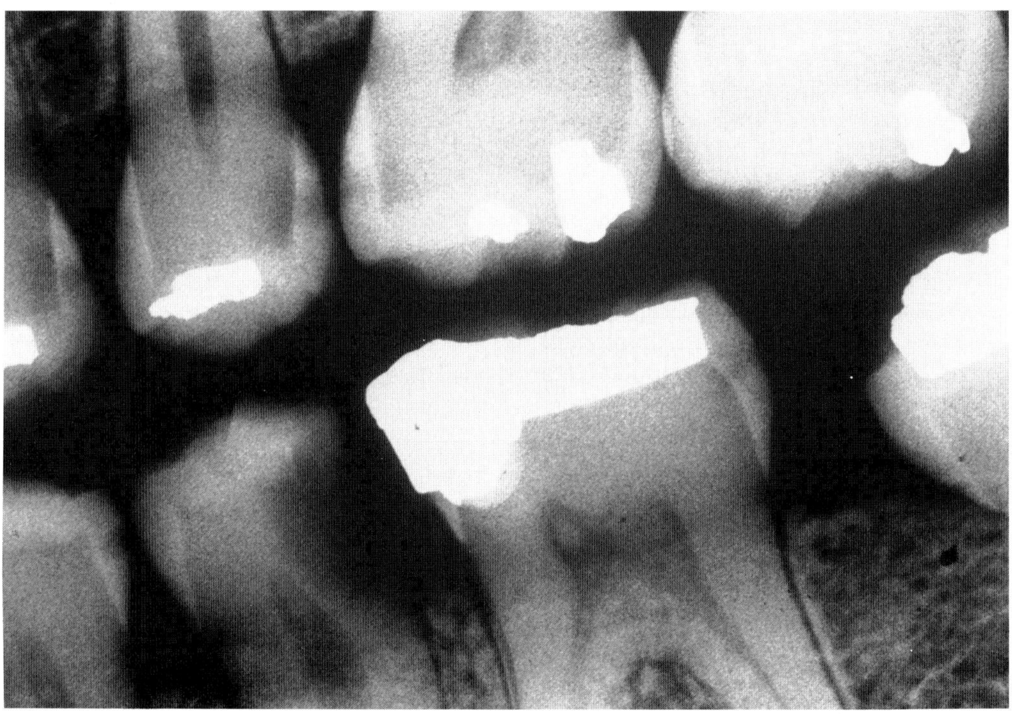

Figure 5.6. Bitewing radiograph showing multiple smooth surface carious lesions.

rough enamel surface or cemental caries hidden beneath the gingiva.

Usually there are no symptoms of dental caries. There may be slight pain stimulated by heat, cold, or sweets that disappears when the stimulus is removed. But most often caries is progressive, yet symptomless.

Although most decay is chronic and progressive, there are two other types recognized in terms of activity, these being considered extremes of the basic chronic type. One is acute caries which, as the term implies, runs a rapid and painful course. There usually is no defensive activity, and the pulp is quickly involved. The other type is arrested caries and indicates that the process is in a state of inactivity. Arrested decay is seen commonly in children with large occlusal lesions in which the decayed surface becomes essentially open and self-cleaning. In these instances the decayed dentin wears away and leaves a hard, brown-stained remineralized dentin. The same phenomenon is seen on proximal surfaces with caries exposed after the extraction of an adjacent tooth or on cervical or cemental caries exposed after recession of the gingiva (Fig. 5.8).

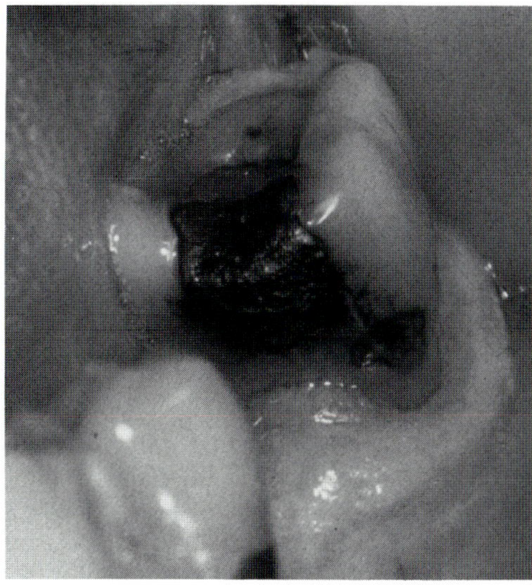

Figure 5.8. Arrested dental caries on exposed mesial root surface of mandibular molar. It is firm and very blackened.

The treatment for dental caries is multiple. Restorative dentistry, utilizing various materials, removes and replaces the lost tooth structure. Preventive dentistry utilizes plaque removal, application of fluorides, and acid-etch bonding to prevent and halt the carious process. Research is working on an immunologic approach in developing a vaccine against the carious organisms. A key to treatment is an understanding of the dynamics of demineralization and remineralization that occur naturally.

There is a demineralizing–remineralizing equilibrium between the saliva and the oral hard tissues (Fig. 5.9). Factors involved are pH or acid levels, mineral ion concentrations, complexing agents, fluoride, and the frequency and severity of cariogenic challenge. Remineralization is the replacement of mineral in teeth that was lost to cariogenic challenge. At a critical pH level (and there is no single level), enamel dissolves and the surface softens. With more acid in the environment, there is greater dissolution. With more ions including minerals, there is less dissolution. If there is sufficient Ca^{2+} or $HPO_4{}^{2-}$ in saliva or plaque and a high pH, there is crystal formation (remineralization). The duration of demineralization action is important. If it is long, the dissolved enamel diffuses into the saliva and is not available for remineralization, thus allowing the lesion to progress. The dental mineral is in equilibrium with its environment, and saliva has elements for hydroxyapatite crystal growth. However, remineralization is not always complete, because diffusion is necessary and, as the surface becomes filled, the deeper locations on the tooth are restricted to diffusion. Also, the pellicle on the tooth may be a natural diffusion barrier. Thus, the demineralization–remineralization process is complex. However, advantage can be taken of the process. For instance, active caries can be stopped by giving the patient concentrated solutions with calcium and

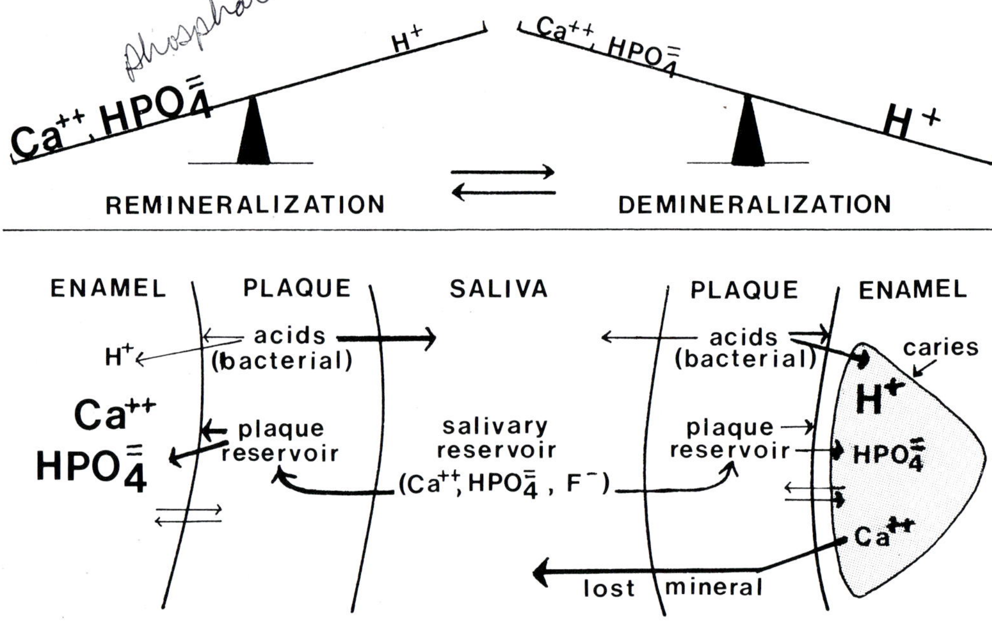

Figure 5.9. Diagram on remineralization balanced by demineralization. With more acid in the environment, there will be dissolution of the tooth and loss of minerals. Bottom of diagram contrasts a tooth surface without caries on the left and with caries on the right. Larger letters and arrows indicate the predominant constituents and direction of the reaction. Note constant interplay among the salivary and plaque fluids and the surfaces of the teeth.

phosphates and following up with fluorides to make the surface remineralize and harden.

Pulpitis

Pulpitis refers to inflammation of the pulp. The dental pulp is a loose cellular connective tissue with branching and anastomosing neurovascular channels. Pulp is unique in that it is surrounded by rigid dentin, and it has no collateral circulation because the dental arteries are end arteries. Specialized cells of the pulp are the odontoblasts that line the outer layer of the pulp and communicate to the dentinoenamel junction by long extensions of their cell bodies lying within the dentinal tubules. These cells are responsible for the sensitivity of teeth and for the formation of secondary or reparative dentin. Despite these unique features, inflammation of the pulp is like inflammation of connective tissue anywhere else in the body.

Pulpitis is somewhat difficult to understand, because the clinical symptoms and signs that occur cannot be correlated to changes that occur histologically. Therefore, it is discussed in relation to the various pulpal irritants and the possible pulpal responses that can occur. In general, the effect of the irritant is balanced by the resistance of the host. If the resistance is low, the result may be severe, with necrosis of the pulp. Conversely, the irritant may be severe but the pulpal response may be limited and quite favorable. In this circumstance, the damage to the pulp may be reversible and the pulp can be repaired. A severely damaged pulp is likely to be irreversible and can lead to further consequences, such as periapical disease.

The pulpal irritants are microorganisms, traumatic, iatrogenic, chemical, idiopathic, and systemic.

The most common cause of pulpitis is microbial, with the bacteria of dental caries being primarily responsible. Bacterial toxins, bacteria themselves, or products of degradation caused by their invasion can cause inflammation.

Other avenues for bacteria are dental erosion, attrition, fractures of teeth, and periodontal disease. Pulps may be affected in periodontal disease via lateral canals and through the apical foramen in cases of severe disease.

Trauma from fractures, blows, or bruxing (grinding) of the teeth can irritate the pulp.

Iatrogenic causes are those that are introduced by the person performing a treatment or service. Simply preparing a tooth for a restoration has an effect on the pulp. In this regard, a high-speed water-cooled drill with light pressure is least damaging to the pulp. Even polishing of the teeth can cause pulpitis. The rubber polishing cup is capable of generating sufficient heat to cause thermal changes that affect pulpal tissue via the odontoblasts. Restorations that replace destroyed tooth structures can cause similar changes. Amalgam and gold respond to thermal changes differently than dentin.

Chemicals cause pulpal changes. Various chemicals are applied to the dentinal tubules in the form of fillings, bases, and disinfectants. Unlined composite restorations may cause low-grade chronic pulpitis. The eugenol in the temporary dressing, zinc oxide and eugenol, is used to relieve the pain of toothache but is also a pulpal irritant.

Idiopathic causes are unknown or vague. Most pulpal disorders occur in or are associated with older pulps. Thus, aging appears to be a factor. An older pulp has fewer cells and more fibrous tissue, so resistance may be lowered with age because there are fewer cells available to respond favorably. Resorption of the dentin is another cause that can be listed as idiopathic.

Systemic causes reflect the fact that the pulp is not divorced from the general circulation. For example, diabetic patients are prone to bacterial infections. These patients commonly have multiple infected pulps. In patients with sickle cell anemia, with less oxygen available, there may be a pulpitis without caries or other irritants.

No matter what the irritant is, the pulp can respond basically in only two ways: clinically and histologically. There may be pain, no pain, reparative dentin formation, or a spectrum of inflammatory changes.

Eighty percent of toothaches are due to pulpitis or pulp-related periapical inflammation. Pain, then, is a major pulpal response. Pain results from the increase of pressure within the confined pulp and from the shifting of the fluid medium of the pulp. The stimulus for pain can be heat, cold, sweets, air, or inflammatory exudation. Regardless of the stimulus, the result is pain, which can be categorized in terms of duration, frequency, intensity, and character.

Pulpalgia refers to pain in the pulp. Generally speaking, pain of short duration that disappears on removal of a stimulus is favorable. That which lingers is unfavorable for the vitality of the pulp. Previous episodes of pain in a tooth (frequency) are also a sign of pulpal destruction and irreversibility. The pain may be acute, being of short duration but severe. This type is associated with pulp abscesses and pulps with partial necrosis; it is usually well localized, and the tooth may be sensitive to percussion (tapping or biting). Chronic pain, on the other hand, is usually vague and intermittent.

When a toothache occurs, one usually finds a carious tooth, a lost restoration, or a chipped tooth. Other pains mistaken for toothaches are the result of dental erosion or periodontal inflammation—usually due to food impaction and maxillary sinusitis. Another aspect to be considered is referred pain. For instance, a pulpitis in a lower right second premolar may refer pain to the right ear and the right temple.

There may be no clinical manifestations of pulpitis. That is, there can be pulpitis without pain. Clinically, painless pulpitis can be suspected. A tooth with an existing deep restoration of amalgam or a full crown probably has some pulpitis although there may be no history of pain.

Histologically, there are several possible responses. The most favorable response is the formation of reparative dentin. This occurs in the advance of dental caries and also in response to the preparation of teeth for restoration. So long as there are healthy odontoblasts, there can be dentin formation, the mechanism of the tooth to insulate the pulp from an irritant. If there is at least 1 mm of remaining dentin, the pulpal damage will be minimal.

In histologic pulpitis, the connective tissue is usually involved with a chronic inflammatory response. Assuming an irritant, the first change is the degeneration and necrosis of odontoblasts. As these die, there is undoubtedly an initial acute inflammatory response, but the typical neutrophilic response is rarely seen on microscopic sections. What is seen is a condition called hyperemia, which refers to blood vessels congested with red blood cells, but none of the red blood cells are seen outside the vessels. This may be the first sign of inflammation in the pulp. With time, chronic cells and fluid appear. The pulp can repair by forming new odontoblasts to lay down dentin, or it may remain in a state of chronic inflammation (Fig. 5.10). This may be confined to the coronal portion or, depending on resistance, may involve all of the pulp. If the pulp does not repair, and this can include the formation of dense connective tissue, it may undergo necrosis and death. In some pulps, a whole spectrum of inflammatory events can be seen. Clinically, it is a challenge to guess the histologic state of the pulp.

In a carious tooth in particular, there may be a pulpal abscess. One or more abscesses can occur in the pulp horn. As more and more bacteria or toxins invade the pulp, neutrophils try to engulf them. A collection of neutrophils, dead and dying, plus bacteria in a liquid state, forms and becomes encapsulated. This is a pulpal abscess and is associated with severe pain (Fig. 5.11). Most often there is normal pulp tissue below the abscess, so if the abscess or pus is removed for treatment (pulpotomy) the pulp is likely to heal. However, clinically one can only guess at the possibility of an abscess being present. A diagnosis of irreversible pulpitis is followed by endodontic therapy.

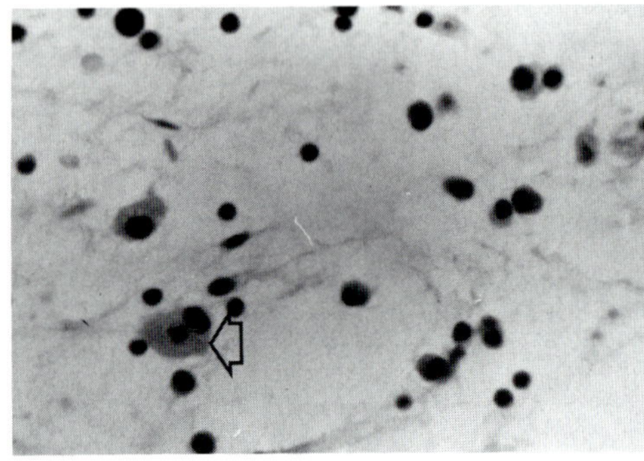

Figure 5.10. Chronic inflammatory cells. Lymphocytes, plasma cells, macrophages. Macrophage with phagocytized cell (*arrow*).

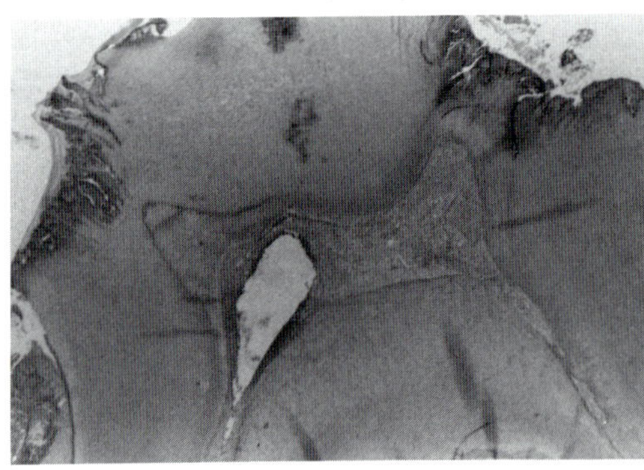

Figure 5.11. A pulpal abscess in decalcified tooth with extensive dentinal caries and reparative dentin of pulp horns. The cleared area in vivo was filled with liquified necrotic pulp and neutrophils.

Chronic hyperplastic pulpitis (pulp polyp) is a dramatic and relatively frequent type of pulpal response. It is seen in younger pulps, mainly in children and young adults, in primary molars and first and second permanent molars. Generally, the decay rate has been sufficiently rapid so that the crown disintegrates and the pulp becomes exposed. The pulp responds with chronic inflammation in the coronal pulp. However, there is a buildup of granulation tissue (hyperplasia), and with time this type of tissue grows toward the open space. It looks like a grape or polyp extending from the pulp (Fig. 5.12). It usually fills the defect of the crown and often mimics hyperplastic gingivae. Because of the new blood vessels in granulation tissue, the pulp polyp is a red-pink and tends to bleed readily when probed. However, there is no sensitivity because granulation tissue contains no nerve tissue. The underlying pulpal tissue often is intact and uninflamed, a sign of excellent host resistance. Therefore, the pulp polyp can be treated by pulpotomy if the tooth is restorable. Otherwise, root canal therapy or extraction must be done.

The complication of pulpitis is that the inflammation progresses beyond the root apex into the periapical area. The sequelae of pulpitis are the dentoalveolar abscess, cellulitis, periapical granuloma, or cyst.

The treatment of pulpitis depends on the determination—based on clinical signs and symptoms—of whether the damage is reversible or irreversible (ultimately leading to pulpal necrosis). There is no reliable means of determining the vitality of the pulp. Pulp testers and thermal responses are merely aids and in no way indicate actual vitality. Radiographically, there are no discernible changes. For reversible pulpitis the treatment is a pulpal dressing and new restoration or pulpotomy. For irreversible pulpitis, pulpectomy and root canal therapy or extraction are required.

Internal resorption or idiopathic resorption refers to the destruction of the dentin from the pulpal side toward the outside of the tooth. The cause is unknown; however, a history of trauma may be elicited. The dentin is whittled away by giant cells, and this process may continue rapidly or stop spontaneously. Internal resorption is asymptomatic and is noted on routine radiographs as ballooning radiolucent expansion of the pulp, usually in the root (Fig. 5.13). It may occur in the pulp of the crown in which case the pink tissue of the pulp shows through the enamel (pink tooth). The treatment is root canal therapy. If the resorption perforates the periodontal ligament, the tooth is treated by extraction.

External resorption of teeth is more common than internal resorption. It occurs naturally in the shedding of primary teeth and microscopically on most teeth. Occasionally, however, it is progressive. Exter-

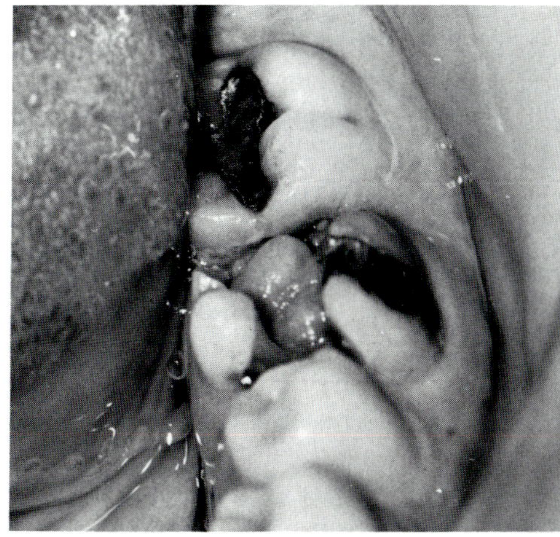

Figure 5.12. Pulp polyp. Inflamed tissue from pulp extends to fill space of crown lost by rapid decay.

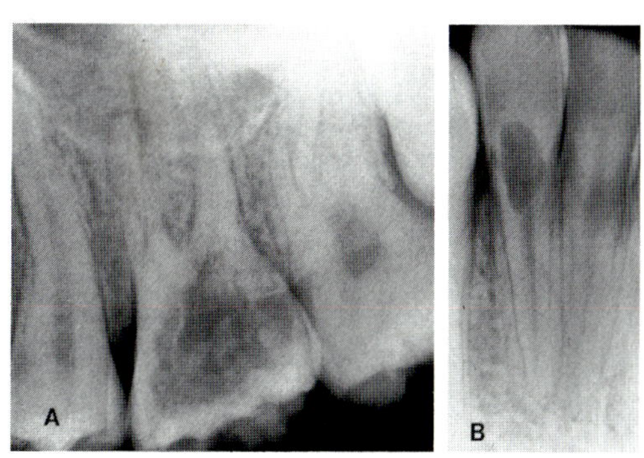

Figure 5.13. *A*, internal resorption of maxillary molar crown. The external surface of the tooth appeared normal but was pink. *B*, internal resorption of mandibular incisor. The pulp area is expanded.

nal resorption refers to the loss of cementum and dentin of a tooth from the external surface in toward the pulp. Radiographically it is seen as an irregular loss of root structures (Fig. 5.14). Known causes are periapical inflammation, reimplantation of teeth, tumors and cysts, excessive forces (orthodontic), impacted teeth, and idiopathic forces (Fig. 5.15). The treatment is to diagnose the cause and to remove it. The resorbed portion of the root does not heal but does not progress further after therapy.

Pulp stones are gross calcifications occurring in the pulp (Fig. 5.16). They are very common. Radiographically, they appear as small, rounded radiopaque (white) masses within the pulp chamber or canal (see Fig. 5.15). The cause is unknown. They are also referred to as denticles, because some of them are composed of dentin. They do not cause pain and may interfere with root canal therapy.

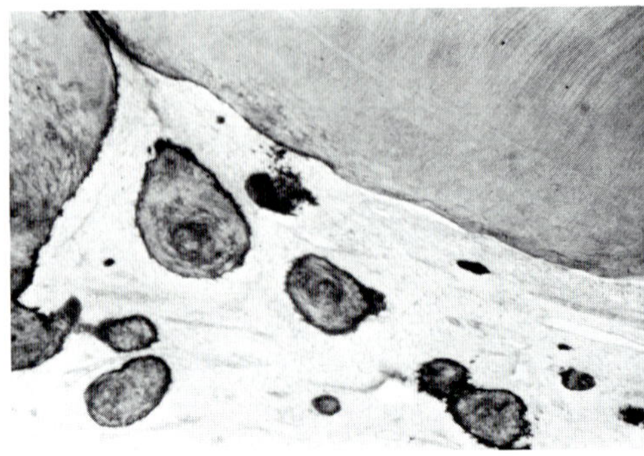

Figure 5.16. Numerous pulp stones within pulp of a tooth.

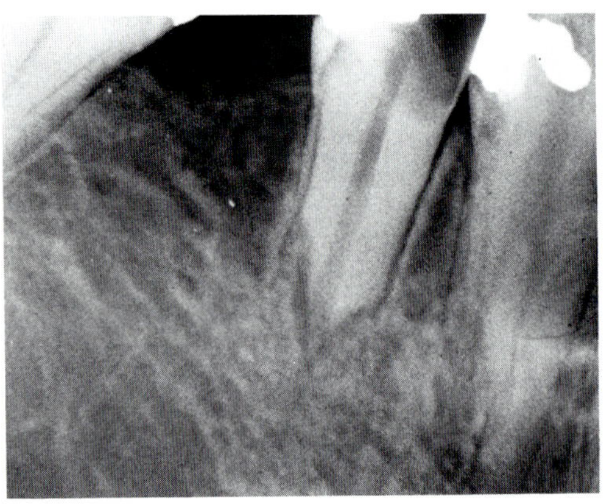

Figure 5.14. External resorption of root. Note irregular outline of apical end of root.

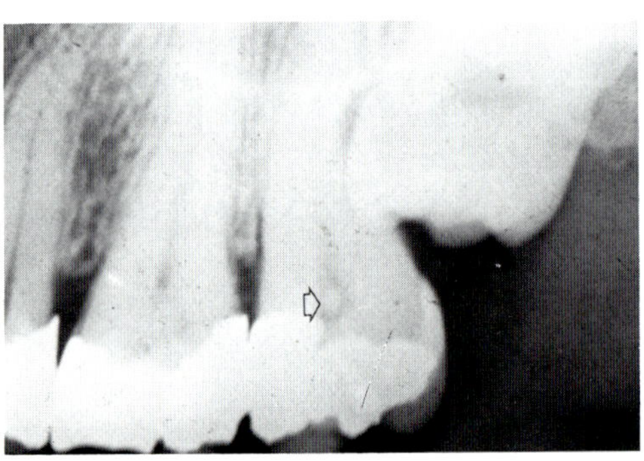

Figure 5.15. External resorption of root of second molar by pressure from impacted third molar. Also note opaque object within pulp chamber of second molar (pulp stone, *arrow*).

Sequelae of Pulpitis

The extension of inflammation of the pulp beyond the tooth into the periodontal ligament area represents periapical inflammation. In many instances the pulp is necrotic. However, periapical inflammation can be present despite the presence of vital tissue in the pulp. There are three common lesions that may follow pulpitis, namely the periapical abscess, granuloma, and cyst (Table 5.1).

The periapical or dentoalveolar abscess is an acute or chronic suppurative (pus-producing) process in the periapices or radicular area of the involved tooth. The usual cause is untreated dental caries, but a periodontal pocket or a partially erupted third molar may be other etiologic factors. Clinically, acute periapical abscesses are responsible for severe pain. The buildup of pus and edema at the root end causes pressure, which acts on nerve endings in the periodontal ligament and elicits pain. In addition the inflammatory exudate pushes against the root causing the tooth to

Table 5.1.
Periapical sequelae of pulpitis

	Abscess	Granuloma	Cyst
Clinical	Acute Severe pain Extrusion Parulis Cellulitis Chronic No pain Fistula	Little or none	None
Radiographic	Early: none Late: radiolucent	Radiolucent	Radiolucent
Microscopic	Acute Pus Chronic Pus Granuloma or cyst	Chronic inflammation Granulation tissue Fibrosis	Lumen Epithelial lining Chronic Inflammation Fibrotic wall
Treatment	1. Drain pus and 2. Root canal or 3. Extraction	1. Root canal, 2. Apicoectomy or 3. Extraction	1. Root canal, 2. Apicoectomy or 3. Extraction

extrude. The affected tooth then touches its opponent first and causes more pain. Diagnostically the tooth is sensitive to percussion, so tapping teeth can locate the offending tooth. If the abscess forms immediately following the extension of inflammation into the periapical region, there may be no indication on a radiograph of periapical destruction. In these acute abscesses there may be only a slight widening of the periodontal ligament at the tooth apex (Figs. 5.17 and 5.18). If, on the other hand, the abscess originates in a preexisting granuloma or cyst, there is a clearly defined radiolucent shadow about the root or beyond it, corresponding to the destruction of the granuloma or cyst. The pain, however, is a manifestation of the abscess.

The nature of pus within tissue is to find an exit or drainage. Consequently, the treatment is to establish drainage. This is done by opening directly into the pulp chamber of the tooth or by extraction. The pressure of the suppurative process is released and, dramatically, the pain is abated. Patients may have additional symptoms of fever and malaise, which should be treated on an individual basis. Often antibiotics are necessary.

If the tooth is not drained or removed, the natural course of the periapical abscess proceeds to establish drainage. The pus burrows through the alveolar bone forming a channel called a sinus or a fistula that eventually opens to an outer surface. Generally, it follows a pathway of least resistance. After exiting the bone buccally, labially, lingually, or palatally, the suppuration may form a painful red swelling beneath

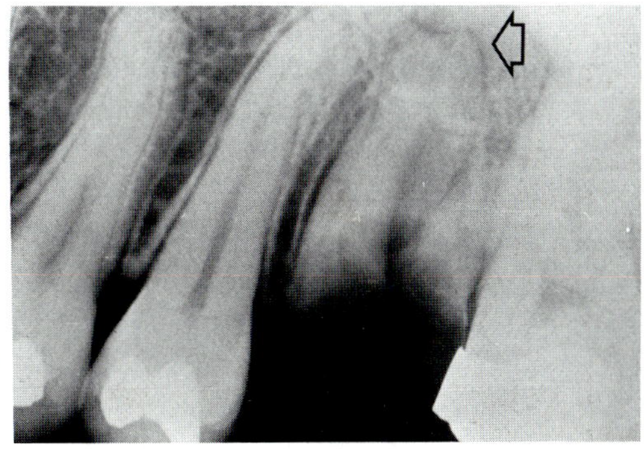

Figure 5.17. Acute dentoalveolar abscess, maxillary first molar. Note retained roots after loss of crown due to caries. Note widened periodontal membrane and loss of lamina dura at apices of roots (*arrow*).

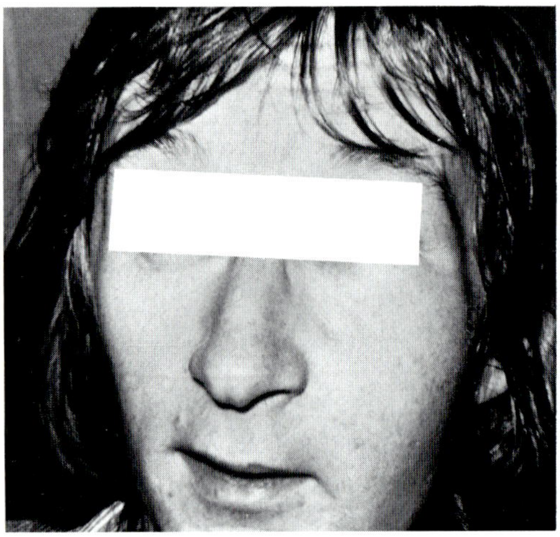

Figure 5.18. Acute dentoalveolar abscess. Same patient as in Figure 5.17. Note swelling obliterating nasolabial fold.

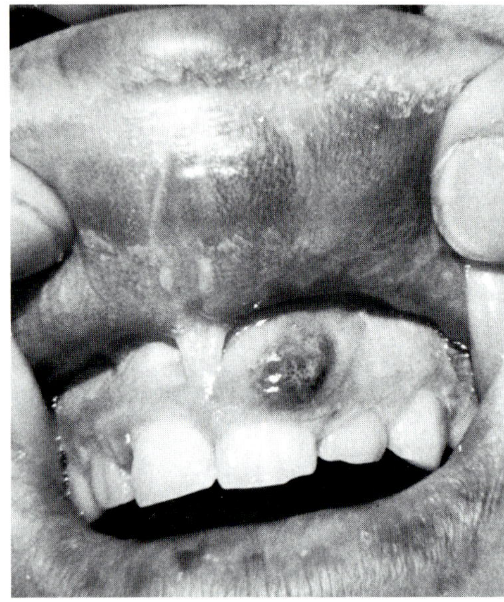

Figure 5.19. Gingival abscess or gumboil representing exit of inflammation originating at apices of maxillary left central incisor. Patient's lip was swollen with a cellulitis.

the mucosa called a gumboil or parulis (Fig. 5.19). A gumboil may result from periodontal disease or foreign implanted material as well. Ultimately the gingival or palatal abscess may drain spontaneously (Fig. 5.20). Clinically, this mucosal abscess may be drained by incision and drainage, often by starting the endodontic therapy. With drainage, the pain subsides. The patient may give a history of foul taste and no swelling or pain for a chronic dentoalveolar abscess. With spontaneous drainage, there remains a small red pimplelike lesion with a central fistulous opening. The fistula then connects the mucosa with the destruction at the end of the involved tooth (Figs. 5.21 and 5.22). This tract heals after treatment.

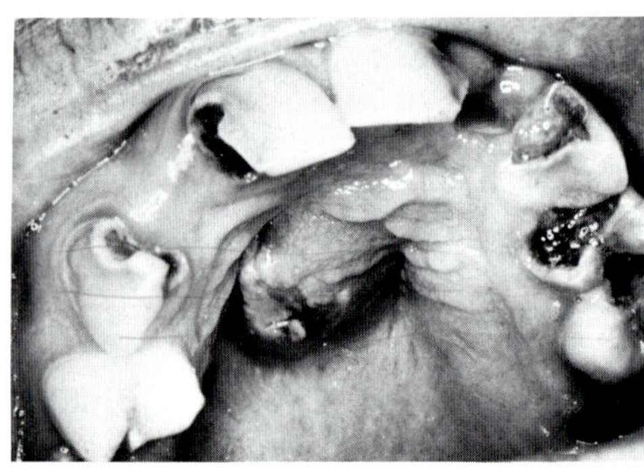

Figure 5.20. Palatal abscess with some drainage. Note many carious teeth that also had periapical involvement.

The pus may, in some instances, burrow through the bone deeper than alveolar bone and exit in areas other than mucosal surfaces. It can follow along sheaths of connective tissue that outline muscle and through the muscle itself. For instance, a lower molar may drain above the mylohyoid muscle of the floor of the mouth and present as a gingival abscess. But if it drains below the mylohyoid, a large hard swelling of the lower face may occur. This represents the spread of inflammation along the muscle and is termed cellulitis. It may be seen with or without a parulis being present. Patients with cellulitis are sick with fever and pain. The process may continue with spontaneous drainage onto the face, thus forming an oral-facial or oral cutaneous fistula (Fig. 5.23). Excluding

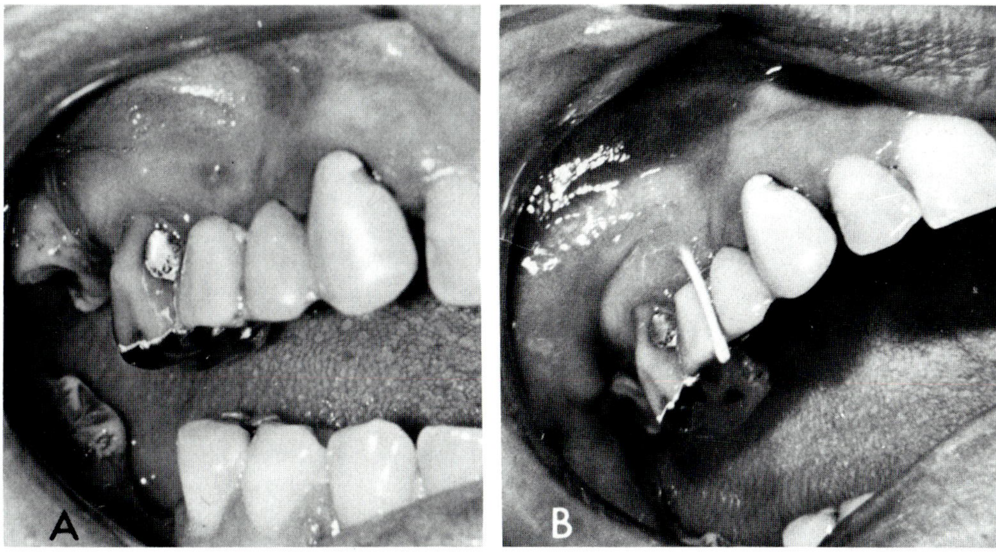

Figure 5.21. *A*, fistula on alveolar mucosa above second bicuspid pontic area of bridge in a patient with a chronic dentoalveolar abscess and no pain, but foul taste. *B*, gutta percha point inserted into fistulous opening, without anesthesia.

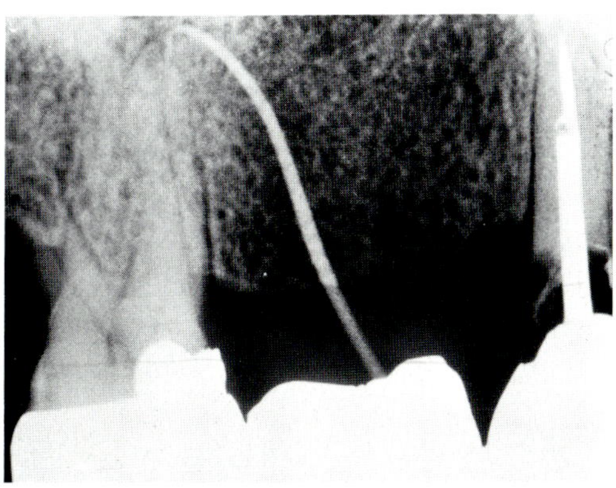

Figure 5.22. Radiograph showing gutta percha tracing fistulous tract or sinus, which extended from the first molar tooth (same patient as shown in Fig. 5.21).

trauma, the periapical or dentoalveolar abscess is the most common cause of facial swelling.

The periapical or dental granuloma is one of the most common lesions seen in a dental office. Inflammatory periapical lesions are a common sequela, being an inflammatory response to antigenic contents of the root canal system. It represents longstanding inflammation in the bone at the root end of the tooth. There usually is no clinical sign or symptom. The tooth may have had a prior history of pain or some slight sensitivity. Vitality testing usually indicates necrosis of the pulp. With the extension of inflammation into the radicular alveolar bone, a chronic inflammation is set up and persists. With time the periodontal ligament is destroyed and the bone is invaded by the extension of inflammatory cells. The process smolders without symptoms. Granulation tissue plus fibrous tissue replace the bone and its marrow. The plasma cells are from the local humoral immune reaction. The lymphocytes are from the cell-mediated reaction. Often, giant cells, cholesterol, and foam cells, all chronic cells indicating longstanding inflammation, also are seen. The process usually becomes self-limiting but never heals, and a circumscribed area of granulating tissue (thus, granuloma) remains until treatment is instituted. On a radiograph, the granu-

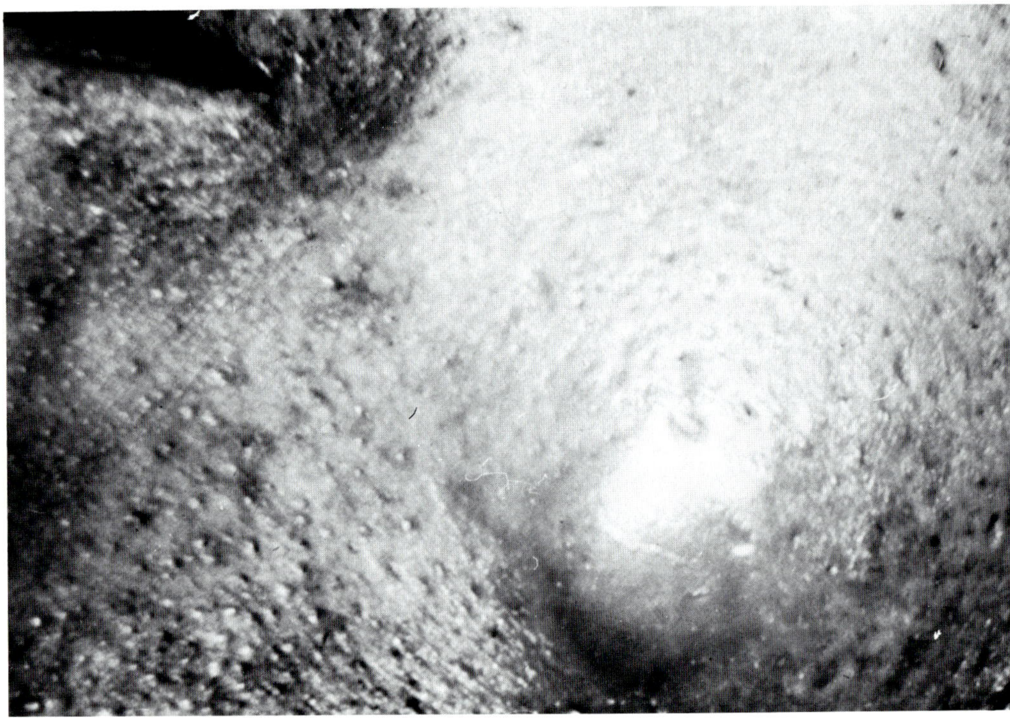

Figure 5.23. Facial abscess near corner of mouth about to drain or be drained. This abscess generated from an abscessed tooth.

loma appears as a radiolucency, usually clearly demarcated, about the apical portion of the involved tooth (Figs. 5.24 and 5.25). Treatment consists of root canal therapy or extraction. After therapy the localized area of destruction heals and new bone forms to obliterate the defect on a radiograph.

The periapical or radicular (root end) cyst is as common as the dental granuloma

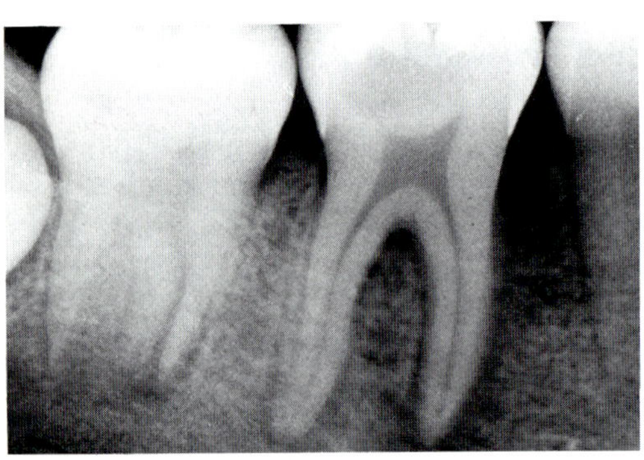

Figure 5.24. Radiograph of an 11-year-old female. First molar has extensive occlusal caries, periapical inflammation of both roots.

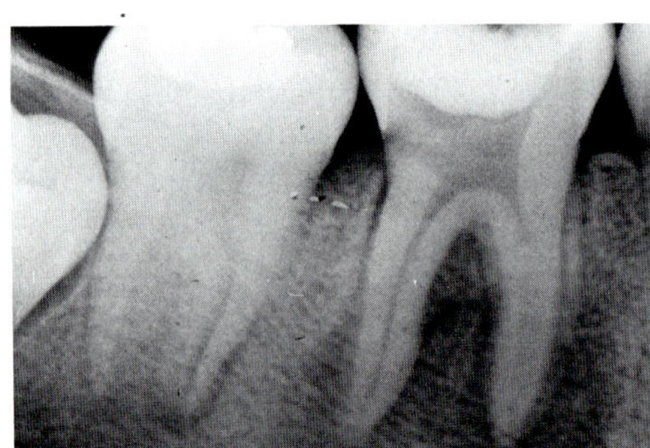

Figure 5.25. Radiograph of same patient as in Figure 5.24, 6 months later, showing progressive involvement of bone and enlarged and more prominent radiolucencies about the roots. The lesion was a dental granuloma with abscess, and the patient had an enlarged jaw (see Fig. 5.32).

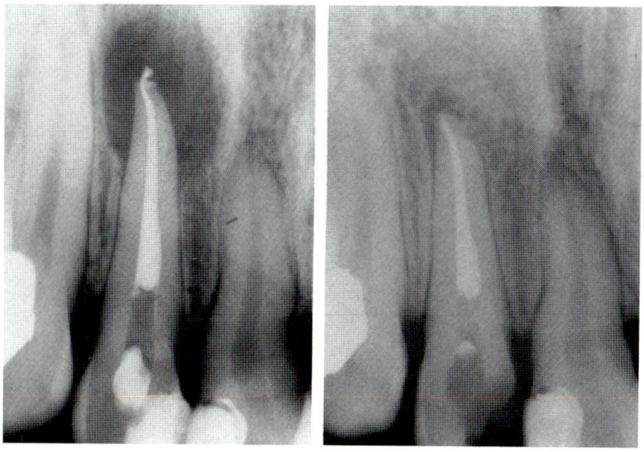

Figure 5.26. Periapical inflammatory lesion, a granuloma, cyst, or abscess. Sequential photos show *A*, root canal therapy completed and *B*, subsequent healing of periapical area by regeneration of bone.

from which it is derived. Clinically, these cysts are asymptomatic. The involved teeth are usually necrotic. Radiographically, the radicular cyst resembles the dental granuloma and chronic abscess with an area of radiolucent bone loss (Fig. 5.26). The radiograph cannot be used to distinguish the nature of the lesion. (A radiograph merely shows shadows, which is not a diagnosis. Therefore, a periapical radiolucency is consistent most often with a granuloma, a cyst, or an abscess.) The cyst is diagnosed because of its microscopic features.

By definition a cyst is a sac of fibrous tissue containing fluid or semisolid material, like cells, in a lumen that is lined by epithelium. The radicular cyst is derived from the epithelial rests of Malassez, which are within the periodontal membrane surrounding a tooth (Fig. 5.27). In the presence

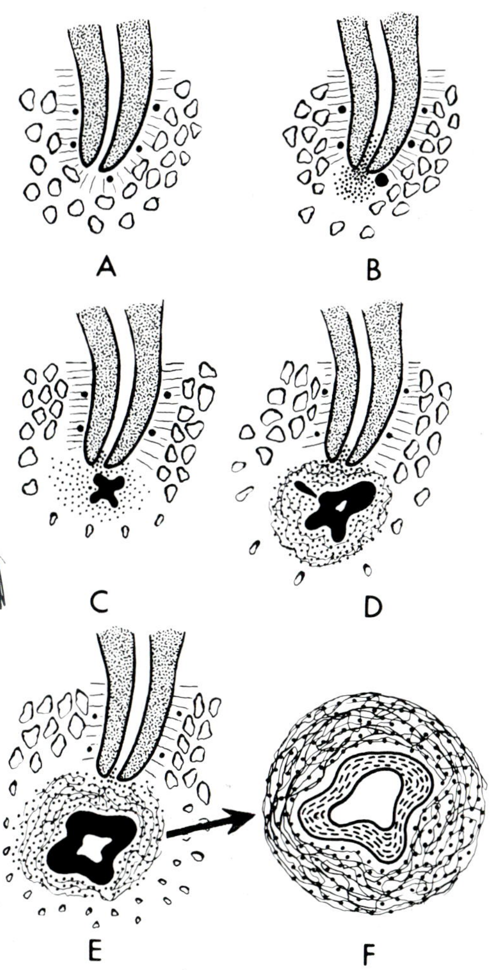

Figure 5.27. Schematic diagram depicting the development of a periapical cyst. *A*, normal root apex with adjacent periodontal ligament containing epithelial rests of Malassez (*black dots*) and clear areas surrounding root representing alveolar bone; *B*, inflammation from pulp extends into periapical area (granuloma) where bone is resorbed, and epithelial rest near the inflammation has begun to proliferate and is larger; *C*, continued growth of granuloma and rest epithelium; *D*, early liquefaction necrosis in center of epithelial mass; *E*, cyst with central lumen; and *F*, expanded view, lumen in center has fluid, surrounded by stratified squamous epithelium contained with inflamed connective tissue.

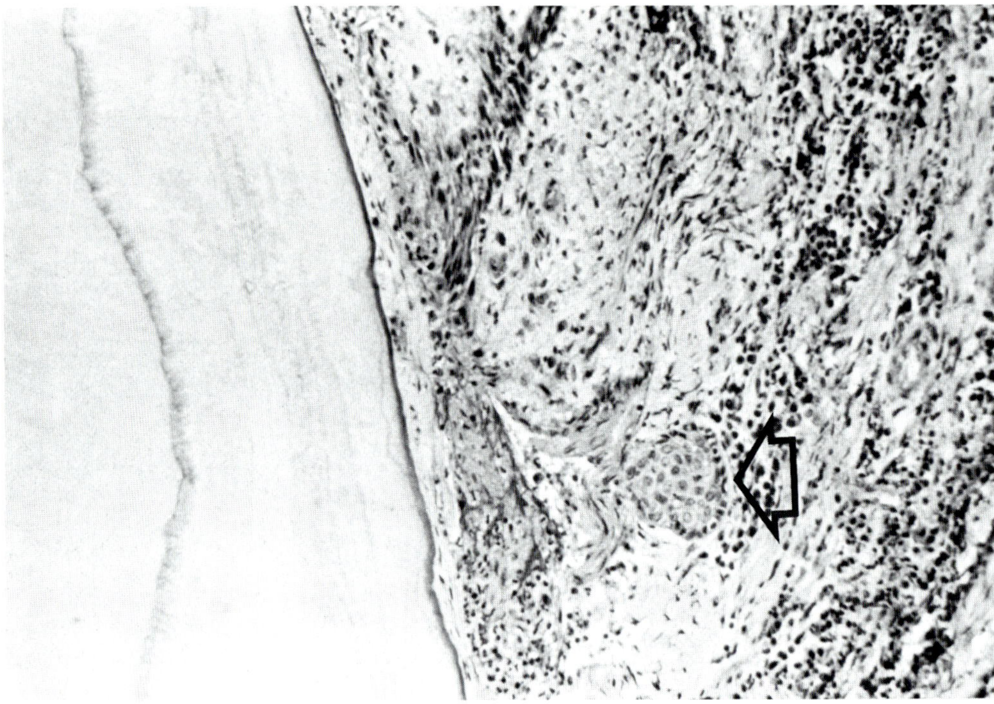

Figure 5.28. Proliferating epithelium (*arrow*) within granuloma at root end of tooth (*left*).

of chronic inflammation of the granuloma, the epithelial rests proliferate (Fig. 5.28). Sometimes, the growing ball of epithelial cells enlarges to such a degree that the nutrients to the central core of cells are too far removed from the connective tissue that contains the blood supply. Those central cells undergo necrosis and liquefy (liquefaction necrosis). This forms a small cavity or lumen with fluid and/or cells lined by epithelium (cyst). This inflammatory cyst can continue to enlarge and replace the apical alveolar bone. They may become several centimeters in size (Figs. 5.29 and 5.30). Following treatment the bone usually regenerates. Sometimes it may not, and scar tissue repair persists (apical scar), leaving a radiolucent, asymptomatic lesion that does not enlarge. Both the cystic cavity and the cyst wall account for the radiolucent radiographic appearance. The treatment for radicular cyst is root canal therapy or extraction and surgical removal of the cyst.

Besides periapical granuloma, cyst, and abscess, there are other sequelae of pulpitis. There may be an infection of the jaw bone (osteomyelitis) caused by various organ-

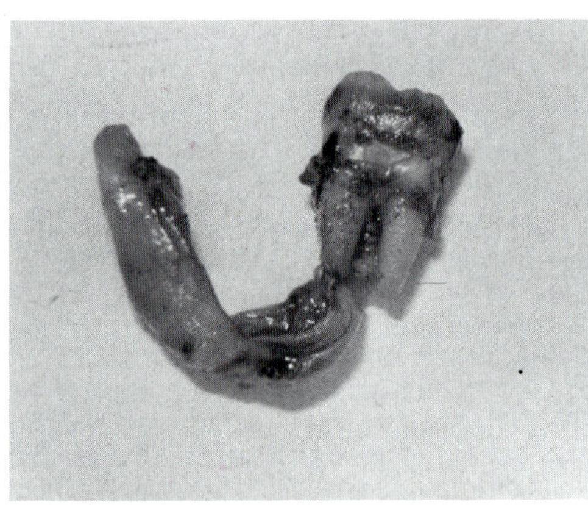

Figure 5.29. Large periapical cyst attached to the root of a molar. The sac was originally filled with fluid. The bone defect extended from second molar to first bicuspid.

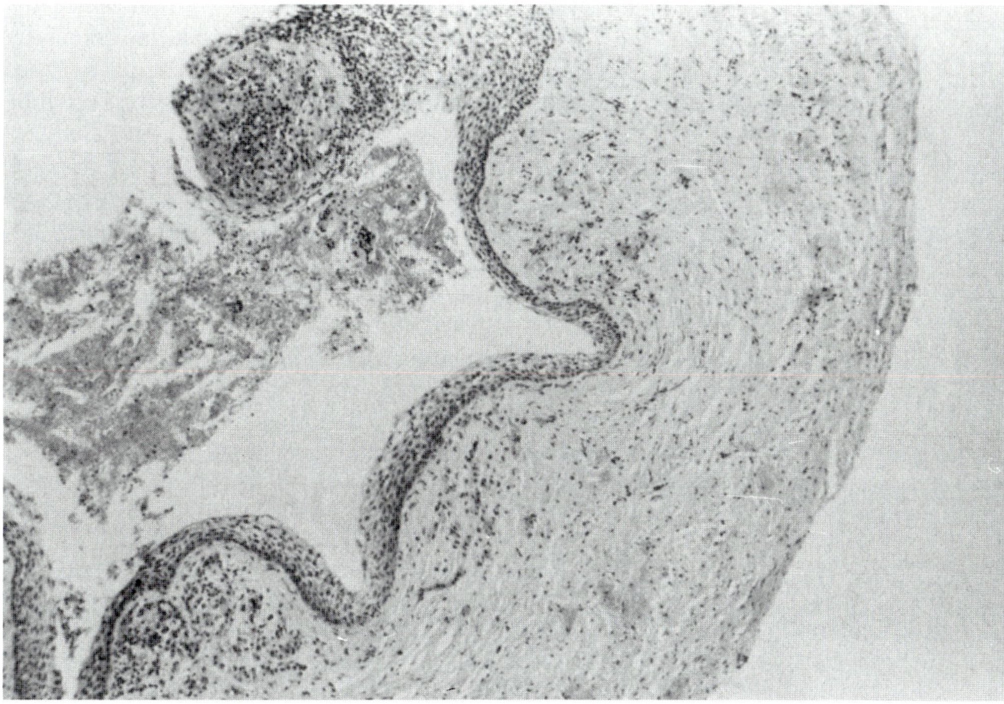

Figure 5.30. Cyst wall. Lumen (*left*) with fluid and debris, epithelial lining, and connective tissue wall.

isms. It is characterized by pain and sometimes by the death of the bone (a sequestrum), which must be removed. Two that involve exaggerated spread of the inflammation are Ludwig's angina and cavernous sinus thrombosis. Though both are rare, they are life threatening. Ludwig's angina is a painful purulent inflammation spreading in the submandibular spaces and ultimately the pharynx, which can choke the patient (Fig. 5.31). In cavernous sinus thrombosis, the inflammation spreads rapidly from the face to the brain, and a thrombus affects vital parts. Infections other than from pulpitis may cause these. Both conditions require hospitalization and high dosages of antibiotics.

Two other sequelae are characterized by the proliferation of bone. In Garrè's osteomyelitis, there usually is a painful swelling of the mandible similar to a cellulitis and secondary to an infected radicular granuloma or cyst. But the swelling is firm because there is extra bone formed on the outer (periosteal) surface of the mandible (Fig. 5.32). After the tooth is treated by

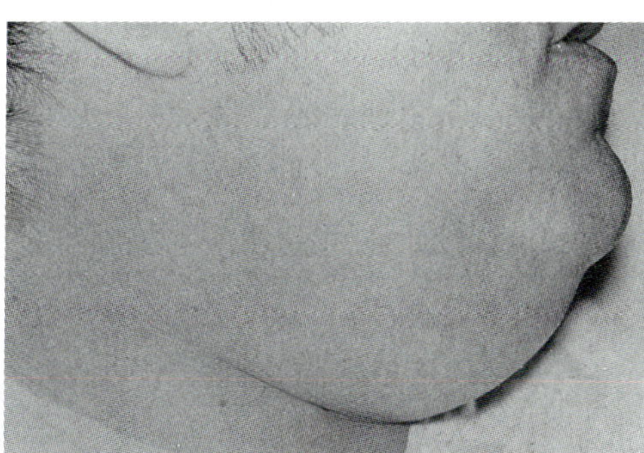

Figure 5.31. Ludwig's angina. Severe cellulitis from infected lower anterior teeth results in swelling of submandibular and lateral pharyngeal spaces and causes compromised breathing. Hospitalization and massive doses of antibiotics are required.

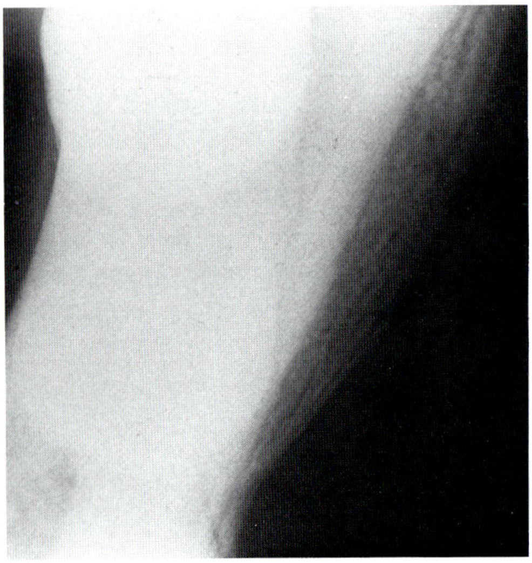

Figure 5.32. Proliferation of periosteal bone causing swelling of mandible in a young patient with an abscessed tooth (Garrè's osteomyelitis).

endodontics or extraction, the bone remodels and the swelling subsides.

Condensing osteitis (focal sclerosing osteitis) is a common sequela of low-grade pulpitis. It is usually seen as a radiopaque lesion associated with the roots of the mandibular molar teeth, usually the mesial root of the first molar. It occurs in younger people on a tooth with caries or a large restoration. Instead of the apical bone resorbing, the low-grade inflammation induces extra dense bone to form. There is mild inflammation. Unless the tooth is symptomatic, no treatment is required. In theory, the opacity should decrease after endodontic therapy. However, it may persist in the bone after extraction of the tooth; then it is called a bone scar, an area of osteosclerosis.

Cysts other than radicular cysts do occur in the head and neck, but their frequency is far less than the radicular cyst. Like the radicular cyst, the cyst is an abnormal sac or fibrous tissue, containing fluid or cells or more solid material. Lining the lumen is epithelium from which the cyst was derived. Unlike the radicular cyst, the cause of the development of the other cysts is unknown. Epithelial remnants or rests proliferate but not due to inflammation. Thus, there may be no inflammation associated with these other cysts unless there is secondary infection or irritation. In other words, they are noninflammatory cysts. They are expansile, usually asymptomatic, lesions occurring in soft tissue but mostly in bone. In either case they may be discovered routinely by noticing a swelling or a radiolucent area on radiographs. The area of destruction is always greater than that outlined on the radiograph. The radiographic appearance and site may suggest the presence of a cyst. However, cysts, abscesses, benign and malignant neoplasms, metabolic diseases, trauma, surgically removed tissue, and normal structures can all produce radiolucent areas on radiographs. Therefore, the final diagnosis can be made only after considering the radiographic image, an adequate history, other clinical features, and microscopic analysis.

Table 5.2.
Developmental cysts

- I. Odontogenic: dental origin
  - A. Periodontal: rests of Malassez in periodontal ligament
    1. Periapical: most common
    2. Residual: no tooth present
    3. Lateral periodontal
  - B. Follicular: dental lamina, dental follicle, enamel organ
    1. Primordial: no tooth present
    2. Dentigerous: common
    3. Eruption
    4. Gingival: soft tissue
  - C. Globulomaxillary: between lateral and canine
  - D. Odontogenic keratocyst: recurrence
- II. Nonodontogenic: Nondental origin
  - A. Bony (fissural): rests in areas of fusion of developing processes
    1. Nasopalatine (incisive canal): common; midline
    2. Median palatine: midline
    3. Median mandibular: very rare
  - B. Soft tissue
    1. Nasolabial (nasoalveolar)
    2. Lymphoepithelial
       Lateral neck (branchial cleft)
       Floor of mouth, etc.: oral tonsils
    3. Dermoid: floor, mouth, neck; midline
    4. Thyroglossal duct: midline

Cysts are derived from embryonic epithelium that in development remains as a small cluster of cells entrapped in bone or soft tissue. For convenience cysts are classified as odontogenic if they are derived from epithelium related to tooth development, or as nonodontogenic. The following classification is offered with additional comments relevant to frequency and location of developmental cysts of the head and neck (Table 5.2; Fig. 5.33).

Periodontal cysts arise from the epithelial rests of Malassez remaining in the periodontal ligament. The periapical cyst is the most common of all the cysts and has been covered in detail. It occurs in both the maxilla and mandible in relation to inflammation proceeding from the pulp. The residual cyst is a periapical cyst that persists after the removal of the involved tooth. The cyst is not curetted effectively at surgery, fails to heal, and remains (Fig. 5.34). The lateral periodontal cyst occurs at the middle third of the root of a tooth that usually tests vital. This cyst is associated with periodontal disease or trauma.

The follicular cysts arise from epithelium associated with tooth development. The primordial cyst arises from a tooth germ that fails to form. Therefore, there is a history of a missing tooth, most commonly the mandibular third molar. This cyst must be distinguished from the residual cyst by an accurate history. The dentigerous cyst is the most common follicular cyst (Fig. 5.35). It is always associated with a tooth that is

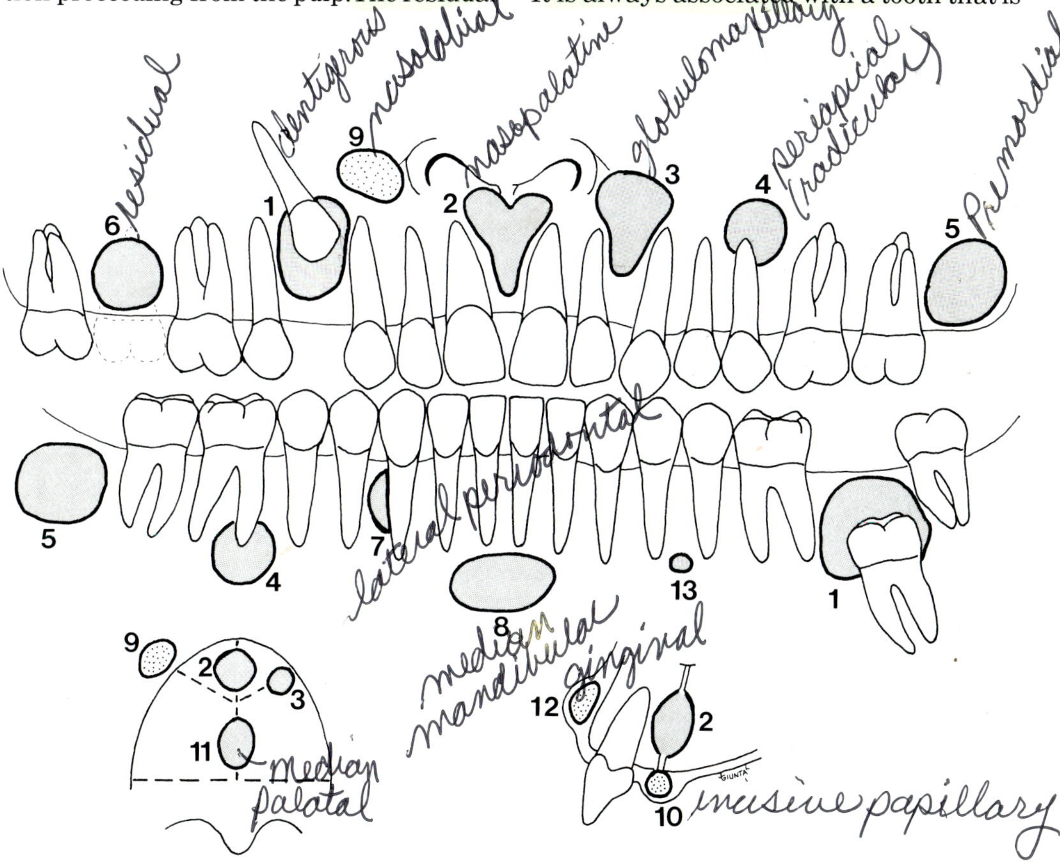

Figure 5.33. Various developmental cysts. Shaded cysts would be radiolucencies within bone. Stippled cysts would be in soft tissue, causing no radiolucency unless there is pressure atrophy of bone. 1, dentigerous; 2, nasopalatine (incisive canal); 3, globulomaxillary; 4, periapical (radicular); 5, primordial; 6, residual; 7, lateral periodontal; 8, median mandibular; 9, nasolabial (nasoalveolar); 10, incisive papillary; 11, median palatal; 12, gingival; and 13, mental foramen (not a cyst). The odontogenic keratocyst has specific histology and radiographically could appear like 1, 3, 5, 7, or even 4.

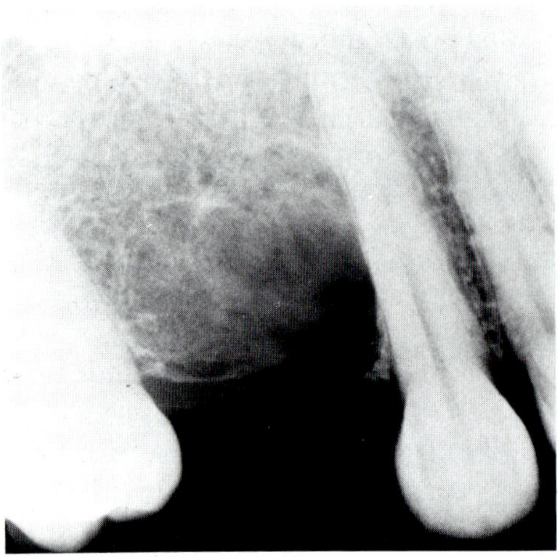

Figure 5.34. Residual cyst. This represents a periapical cyst which surrounded a tooth that was extracted.

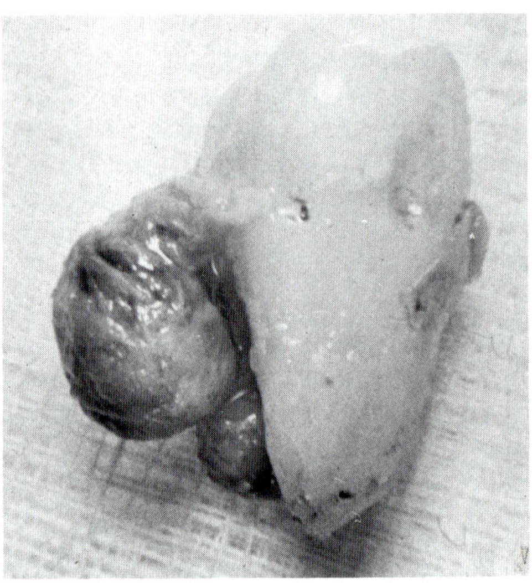

Figure 5.35. Dentigerous cyst or lateral periodontal cyst. Saclike structure contained fluid.

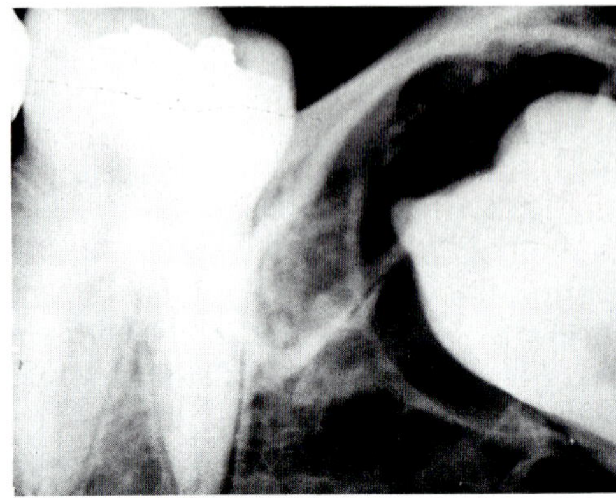

Figure 5.36. Radiolucency about crown of impacted third molar. Consistent with dentigerous cyst.

part of the wall of the cyst. It occurs particularly about impacted mandibular third molars and maxillary cuspids and is responsible for considerable bone destruction and possible swelling (Fig. 5.36). Rarely, tumors, such as ameloblastoma or carcinoma, may arise in the wall of a dentigerous cyst. Moreover, there are several odontogenic tumors that can have the same radiographic pattern as a dentigerous cyst. The eruption cyst occurs over erupting teeth and thus is seen mainly in children. It is seen clinically as a blue-purple mucosal swelling over the erupting tooth and resembles a blood blister (Fig. 5.37). The cyst usually disappears spontaneously with further eruption of the tooth into the oral cavity, or it may be surgically removed. The gingival cyst is derived from epithelium of the dental lamina, and there are two types, both in soft tissue. Gingival cysts of the newborn (Epstein's pearls) occur in most infants (see Fig. 6.98). They are pearl-like keratin-filled cysts on the gum pads. They disappear quickly and spontaneously as the cysts open into the oral cavity.

The gingival cyst of the adult is rare. The counterpart of the lateral periodontal cyst, it occurs labially on the attached or unattached gingiva and appears similar to a mucocele. With pressure atrophy of the bone, there can be a radiolucency. Treatment is surgical removal.

The globulomaxillary cyst, in the past considered to be a fissural cyst, is probably a lateral periodontal cyst, a primordial, or a lateral dentigerous cyst derived from the respective odontogenic epithelium. It is characterized by its specific location, be-

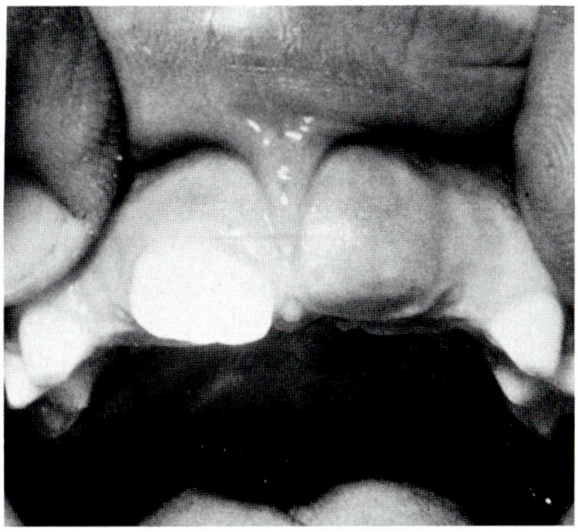

Figure 5.37. Eruption cyst overlying erupting left maxillary central incisor. Mucosa was bluish-purple.

tween the maxillary lateral and canine teeth. Usually it appears as an inverted pear-shaped radiolucency causing divergence of those roots. The teeth are usually vital, although a radicular granuloma or cyst of either tooth could look similar radiographically. Treatment is surgical enucleation.

The odontogenic keratocyst, most likely derived from dental lamina, is an unusual cyst that has an aggressive behavior in that it can recur following surgical excision. The name is derived from the histologic pattern, which is specific and unique. One of the features is keratin formation. They may appear in several locations, commonly the posterior mandible in the form of a primordial cyst. Many of the other odontogenic cysts already covered may be keratocysts. Because of their behavior they are called by their histologic name rather than by their location in the jaw. They may cause extensive bone destruction and may recur several times. Rarely, they occur in patients with the basal cell nevus syndrome.

The nonodontogenic cysts include fissural cysts and other cysts that occur in specific locations in soft tissue. The fissural cysts are developmental, arising from epithelial remnants of embryonic processes that fused in embryogenesis. The midline of the palate is the common location.

The nasopalatine or incisive canal cyst arises from epithelium of the nasopalatine duct. Most common of the fissural cysts, it occurs posterior to and between the roots of the maxillary central incisors. In a periapical film the radiolucency may be heart-shaped (Fig. 5.38). They can become so enlarged as to cause a swelling of the palate. If they arise in the soft tissue, they can cause an enlargement of the incisive papilla and are called incisive papilla cysts. The median palatine cyst occurs in the midline of the hard palate. It may or may not appear as a radiolucency mistaken for another cyst until an occlusal radiograph shows the midline radiolucency. As with all of the fissural cysts, the teeth test vital. The median mandibular cyst is a rare cyst occurring in the midline of the mandible below the apices of the incisors, which test vital.

The nonodontogenic cysts of soft tissue

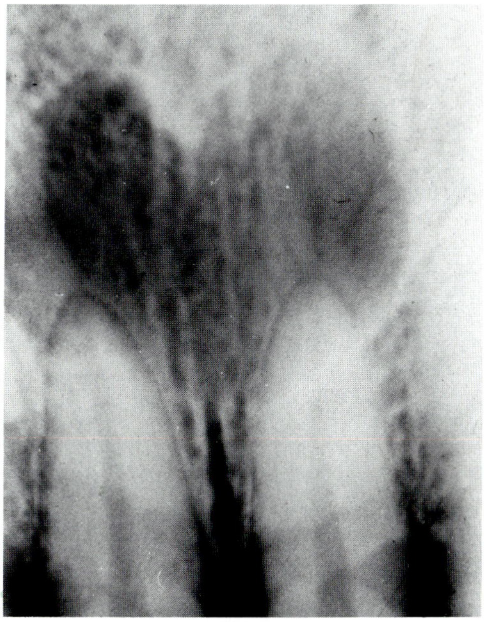

Figure 5.38. Heart-shaped radiolucency characteristic of a nasopalatine cyst.

are all rare lesions. The nasolabial (nasoalveolar) cyst occurs at the nasolabial fold region as a swelling that obliterates the fold and can appear in the mucolabial fold intraorally. Arising probably from nasolacrimal duct epithelium, its location is the soft tissue counterpart of the globulomaxillary cyst.

Lymphoepithelial cysts occur in the lateral neck (branchial cleft cyst) or in the floor of the mouth. They are derived from epithelium proliferating in lymph node tissue, yielding a distinctive pattern and the name. In the neck they may be large and fluctuant swellings, mimicking tumors. In the mouth they are small, yellowish lesions resembling pseudocysts and arising in the oral tonsillar tissue (Fig. 5.39). Dermoid cysts occur in the midline and histologically contain keratin, and the wall may resemble skin. They may appear above the mylohyoid muscle within the tongue or in the floor of the mouth, where they may enlarge and raise up the tongue. Or they may occur below the mylohyoid muscle and appear as a swelling in the submental area. In this area they may resemble the thyroglossal duct cyst, another midline cyst found in the neck (Fig. 5.40) or at the base of the tongue. Thyroid tissue may be in the wall of these cysts.

The treatment for developmental cysts is local surgical removal or interruption of the cyst wall with ultimate filling in with granulation tissue and restitution of the original tissue.

There are several cystlike lesions that occur in the jaws, some of which are mentioned here. The traumatic bone "cyst" is an asymptomatic, radiolucent lesion, usually of the mandible in the premolar region in a young person (Fig. 5.41). The teeth test vital. When the lesion is surgically explored, an empty, sometimes hemorrhagic, cavity is found. The lesion heals after the surgery. A history of trauma may or may not be elicited. The lingual mandibular bone concavity (Stafne's bone defect or "cyst") is an anatomical depression on the medial man-

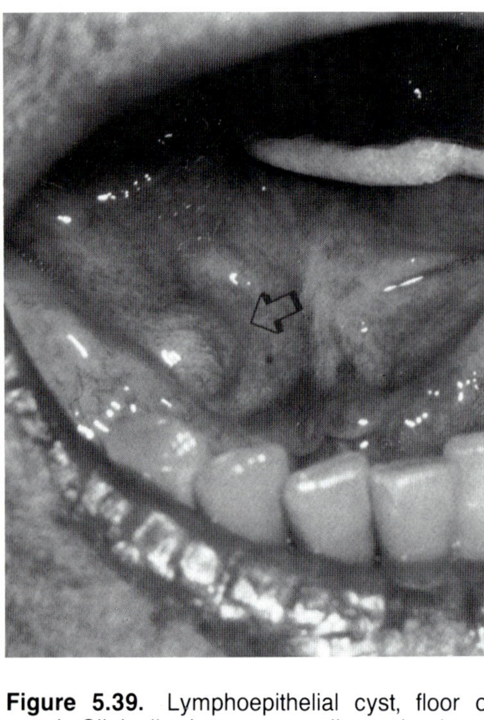

Figure 5.39. Lymphoepithelial cyst, floor of mouth. Clinically, there was a yellow color due to the keratinized cells within the cyst, which was arising in an oral tonsil.

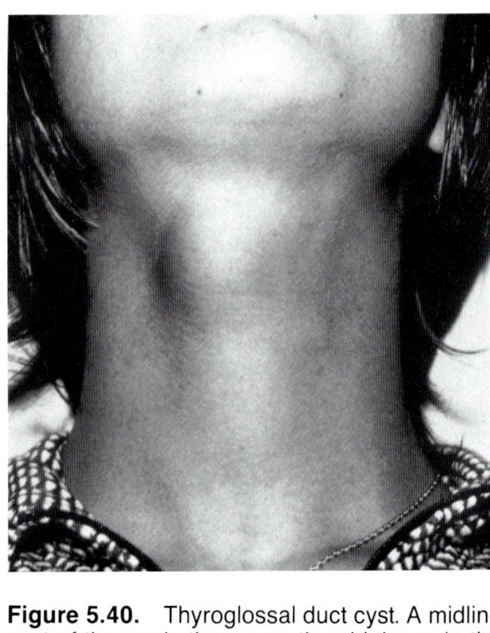

Figure 5.40. Thyroglossal duct cyst. A midline cyst of the neck, there was thyroid tissue in the wall.

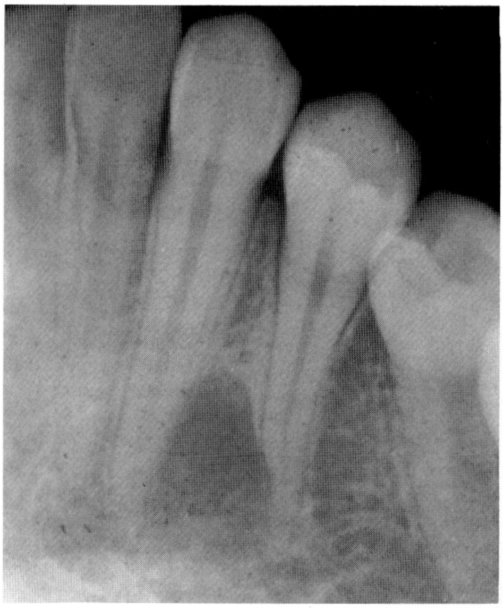

Figure 5.41. Traumatic bone "cyst" in a young person. The teeth were vital. On surgical exploration, there was an empty cavity.

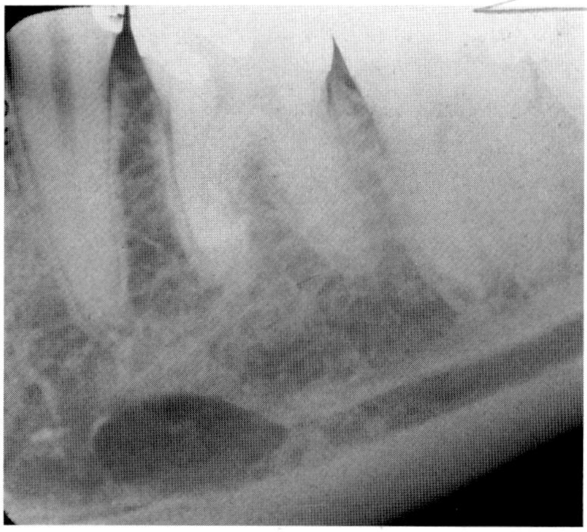

Figure 5.42. Lingual mandibular bone concavity (Stafne's bone defect or "cyst"). The depression, corresponding to the radiolucency, could be palpated on the lingual side of the mandible.

dibular bone usually posterior and inferior to the mandibular canal, appearing as a cystic radiolucency (Fig. 5.42). Frequently it occurs anteriorly below the roots of teeth and resembles a cyst. In the anterior locations the depression may be felt, to confirm the diagnosis. A similar condition occurs on the labial side of the maxilla and mandible and is therefore called a labial bone concavity. An example is the cupped-out area of the canine fossa in the maxilla. If exaggerated, it may resemble a cyst. The osteoporotic marrow defect of bone is a cystlike radiolucency, usually in the mandible of middle-aged women, in whom there is red marrow replacing mandibular bone. The diagnosis is made after surgical exploration and biopsy of the suspected "cyst."

Periapical cemental dysplasia (cementoma) is a condition in which the bone is replaced by fibrous tissue in which bone or bonelike material can form. Before the bone forms, the lesion appears cystic. There is a radiolucency near the apices usually of the mandibular anterior teeth that mimics a periapical inflammatory lesion (Fig. 5.43). However, the teeth test vital, and endodontic therapy need not be performed. Instead, the lesion(s) are followed radiographically, and eventually opacities corresponding to bone are noted within the lesion.

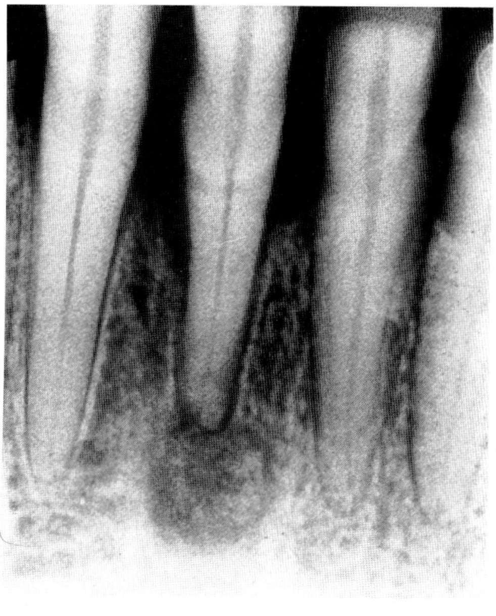

Figure 5.43. Periapical cemental dysplasia, cementoma, at apex of mandibular incisor. Tooth tested vital. Note opacities within radiolucency. No treatment is needed.

Chapter 6

ORAL MUCOUS MEMBRANE PATHOLOGY

Review of Normal Skin and Oral Mucosa

Because the face and oral cavity are constantly under observation by the dental team, some knowledge of the normal histology of the skin and oral mucosa is required to appreciate the changes that can and do occur.

The skin is composed of surface epithelium (epidermis), skin appendages (hair, hair follicles, sweat and sebaceous glands), and the underlying connective tissue (dermis). The epithelium is basically composed of four layers: the stratum basalis or germinal layer, the stratum spinosum or prickle cell layer, the stratum granulosum or granular cell layer, and the corneal or surface layer composed of keratin. Beneath the basal layer is a basement membrane area that connects the epithelium to the connective tissue, which is composed of collagen fibers.

Normal mucosa is similar to skin in that it also is composed of surface stratified squamous epithelium overlying connective tissue. However, there are several differences between skin and oral mucosa. Whereas skin is always keratinized, the mucosa is mostly parakeratinized. There are essentially three layers of cells in the epithelium (Fig. 6.1). The basal cell layer next to the connective tissue is a single cell layer with the capacity for cell division. Only the basal layer is responsible for the addition of new cells. When cell division does occur, daughter cells cause lateral pressure and "squeeze" other, older basal cells toward the surface. These cells are then called prickle cells or spinous cells because of the spiny projections seen under the light microscope connecting one cell to the other. This stratum spinosum is several cell layers in thickness. Actually, it is much wider than the spinous cell layer of skin and accounts for the fact that the epithelium of oral mucosa is more than two times thicker than the epithelium of skin. In most cases the surface or corneal layer of mucosa contains parakeratin, not keratin. This means that the thin layer of cells at the surface resembles keratin but still retains the nuclei of the cells. Keratin is the tough end product of the squamous epithelial cell. No nuclei are seen in a keratinized layer. In the oral cavity, the attached gingivae, the dorsum of the tongue (papillae), and the hard palate are keratinized. The remaining mucosa is parakeratinized. Keratin tends to give a whiter color to the mucosa, because keratin is white clinically. In addition to being mostly parakeratinized and having a thicker epithelium, the mucosa does not have skin appendages. It does, however, contain clusters of accessory salivary glands that secrete mainly mucus on the surface of the mucosa to keep it moist. The major salivary glands—the parotid, the submandibular, and the sublingual—also add to the moist atmosphere of the mucosa. The underlying connective tissue of mucosa is fibrous, usually with dense bundles of collagen. There may be some inflammatory cells in the connective tissue, but they are not seen in large numbers. These cells are mainly plasma cells and lymphocytes and indicate that the oral mucosa is constantly warding off foreign agents and bacteria because these cells are responsible for antigen–antibody types of reactions. The gingival cuff region, in particular, always contains these cells.

The epithelial cells reproduce in the basal

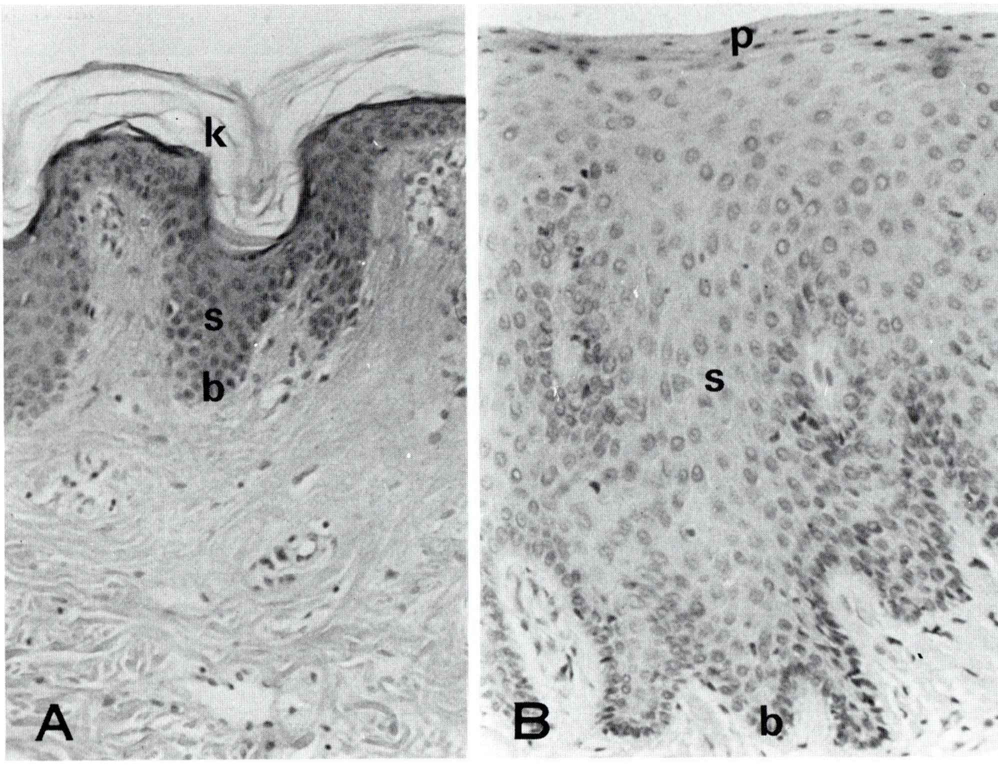

Figure 6.1 *A*, normal skin, and *B*, normal oral mucosa at approximately ×200 magnification. Epithelial cell layers are: *b*, basal; *s*, spinous; *k*, keratin; and *p*, parakeratin.

cell layers and move toward the surface in a process of maturation by which they become spinous cells and finally keratin or parakeratin. The transit time from the basal cell layer to the time of desquamation is approximately 10 to 12 days. Thus the mucosa could rebuild itself in about 2 weeks.

The oral mucosa has a great capacity for healing. Coupled with the rapid regeneration time is the fact that it is bathed constantly in saliva. The saliva has antibacterial properties including antibodies, and the moisture it produces results in rapid healing. Therefore, lesions that do not heal in a 2-week period should be suspicious until a proper diagnosis can be made. When the mucosa does heal, it generally does so by regeneration and rarely by scarring. Scars, however, can be seen following deep-seated chronic inflammation, accidents, gingivectomies, and apicoectomies.

Biopsy

The removal and examination of tissue from the living body is called a biopsy. For many diseases a biopsy is not required for diagnosis. The clinical features may be so characteristic that removal of all or part of the lesion is not necessary. On the other hand, there are times that microscopic examination of tissue gives greater knowledge of a disease and in many instances allows a definite diagnosis. Biopsy is required whenever a lesion is suspected of being a cancer. A biopsy can confirm or rule out malignancy and is a highly reliable and accurate procedure for this purpose. When additional information is needed to distinguish conditions with similar clinical features, the biopsy is most useful in aiding the diagnosis and approach to treatment. In addition, in cases in which the treatment for a known lesion is surgical removal, the surgical specimen should be submitted routinely to confirm the diagnosis. In some cases it may reveal an unsuspected diagnosis.

Biopsy may be either excisional or incisional. Excisional biopsy refers to the surgical removal of the entire lesion plus a surrounding rim of normal tissue. Small lesions are usually removed in this manner (Figs. 6.2 to 6.4). Incisional biopsy is the removal of only a small portion of the lesion. The site of removal is either sutured or closed or left open to heal. The specimen is placed in a fixative solution, usually 10 percent neutral buffered formalin, and is submitted along with adequate history and features of the clinical lesion to a diagnostic laboratory. At the laboratory, microscopic slides are prepared for examination by a pathologist.

Oral Cytology

Oral exfoliative cytology refers to the scraping of the surface of soft tissue lesions and examination of these cells under a microscope. It is not a substitute for biopsy. It may, however, be useful as an adjunct in diagnosing lesions due to cancer, viruses, fungi, and other diseases. If cytology is used, one must bear in mind that it is not as accurate a test as the biopsy. A significant percentage of false negatives occurs in cases relating to cancer detection. If a smear is reported as positive for abnormal cells, a biopsy is mandatory.

The technique for cytology, like the biopsy, is simple and painless. A wooden tongue blade or metal spatula is used to collect the cells from the surface. The tongue blade should be wet with water or saliva. Then the lesion is stroked firmly. The collected cells are smeared on a glass slide with the name of the patient and location of the lesion indicated on the frosted end of the slide. The smeared cells are immediately fixed with spraycyte. After drying, the slides and history form are forwarded to a diagnostic laboratory. The slides are stained by the Papanicolaou method and then read as (a) normal cells present—negative for cancer or (b) abnormal cells present (Fig. 6.5). If the latter is true, then a biopsy is mandatory so that adequate treatment can be instituted.

Microscopic Changes of the Oral Mucosa

The microscopic changes seen in the oral mucous membrane consequent to pathologic conditions can be divided into those of the epithelium and those of the connective tissue, for convenience. In reality, changes occur in both at the same time; however, the change may be more striking in the epithe-

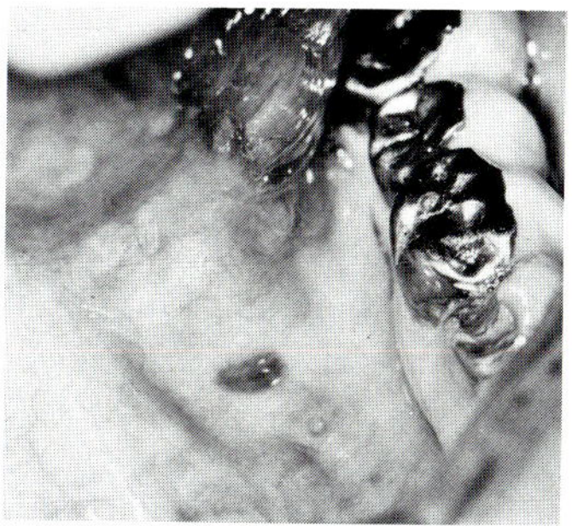

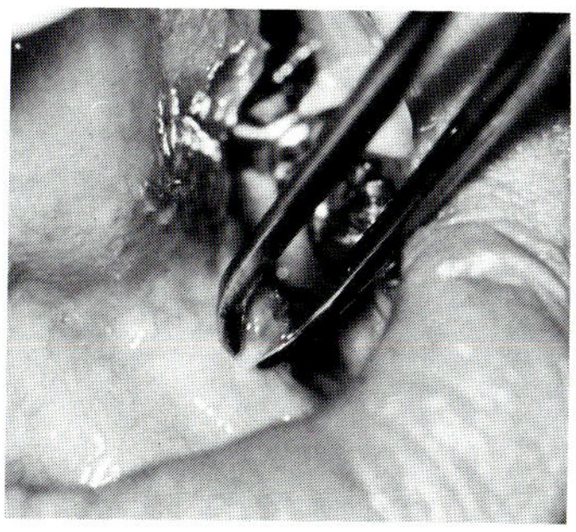

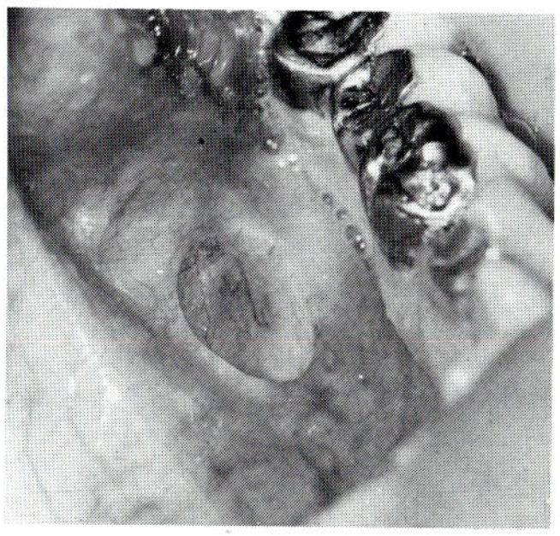

Figure 6.2. *Left*, biopsy of pigmented lesion (amalgam tattoo) from the floor of the mouth.
Figure 6.3. *Middle*, biopsy procedure. Forceps grasp black lesion and some normal tissue. Tissue is cut below forceps.
Figure 6.4. *Right*, biopsy procedure. Black lesion has been removed and placed in formalin fixative. Defect will heal without a suture in this case.

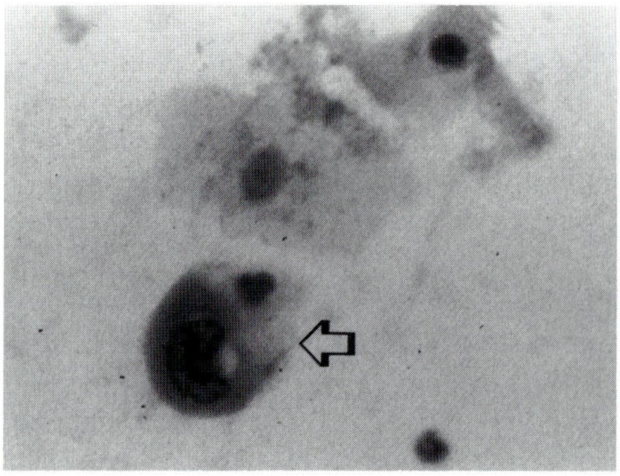

Figure 6.5. Oral cytologic smear of a proven oral cancer. Note positive cancer cell with enlarged nucleus, multiple nucleoli, and reversed ratio of nucleus to cytoplasm, in contrast to normal squamous cells above.

lium, in the connective tissue, or even in both. The following terms refer to these changes.

Epithelial Changes

Hyperkeratosis refers to an increase or widening in the stratum corneum (Fig. 6.6). This results in excess keratin (hyperorthokeratosis) or parakeratin (hyperparakeratosis) at the surface and yields a white appearance clinically. If the white surface is in the form of a patch, it is called leukoplakia (white patch).

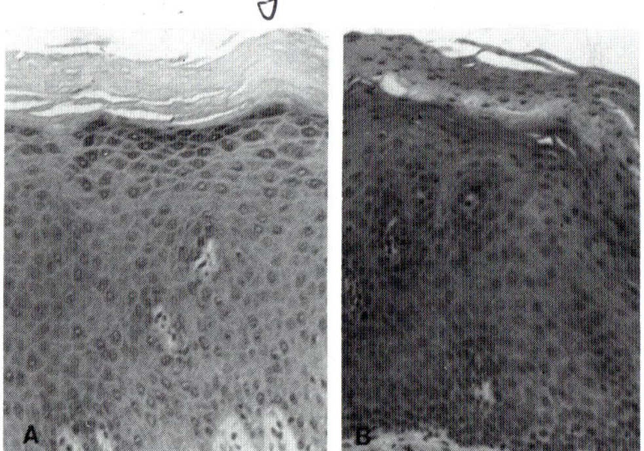

Figure 6.6. *A*, hyperorthokeratosis. Increased thickness of cornified layer with true keratin above granular cell layer. *B*, hyperparakeratosis. Increased thickness of cornified layer with parakeratin (note retained nuclei versus no nuclei in keratin).

Hyperplasia of the epithelium occurs with the widening or increase in the number of cells in the stratum spinosum (acanthosis). This thickening also results in a white lesion. Another form of hyperplasia is the extension of rete pegs with their penetration into the connective tissue (Fig. 6.7).

Epithelial dysplasia (dyskeratosis) refers to the abnormal growth pattern or disorientation of the normal layers of epithelium (Fig. 6.8). It generally indicates premalignant changes. The changes can be so severe that they resemble cancer, in which case the term carcinoma in situ is used because all the cellular characteristics of cancer are present but are confined to the epithelium with no invasion into the connective tissue. This also can be a white or red lesion.

Vesicles can be of two types. Subepithelial vesicles are more common. The accumulation of fluid is beneath the stratum basalis, so all the layers of epithelium are raised (Fig. 6.9). Intraepithelial vesicles are those in which the fluid collects within the epithelial layers, usually the stratum spinosum. The basal layer remains attached to the connective tissue. A rarer type of vesicle, it is important because it can signify the presence of a serious disease, pemphigus. Vesicles rarely are found intact. When they break, an ulcer is formed.

An ulcer is a break in the continuity of epithelium. The peripheral epithelium is slightly hyperplastic and clinically shows a rolled margin. The central depressed area without epithelium is covered with a necrotic plug or scab covering granulation tissue. Most often this central portion appears white and the margins are red.

Spongiosis refers to the accumulation of fluid within the cells of the stratum spinosum. This reflects a degeneration of these cells, and the microscopic picture resembles a sponge (Fig. 6.10). Clinically, the lesion appears white and is most commonly seen on the buccal mucosa as leukoedema.

Text continues on page 97

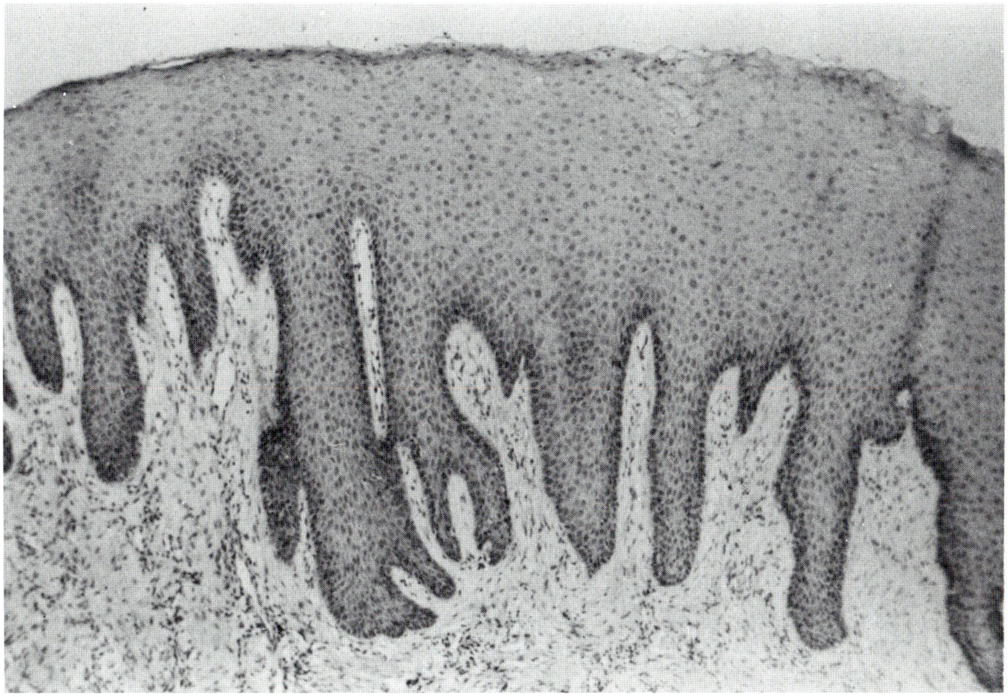

Figure 6.7. Epithelial hyperplasia, an increase in the spinous cell layer, and extension of rete pegs; epithelium extends like fingers into connective tissue.

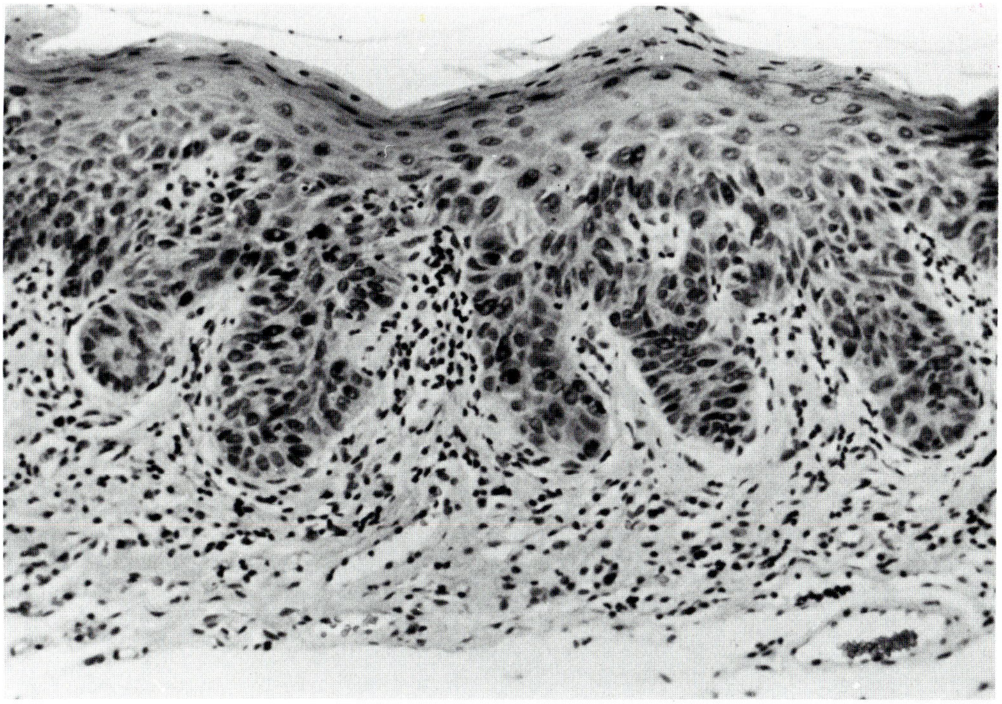

Figure 6.8. Epithelial dysplasia of oral epithelium. Note the haphazard arrangement of cells, particularly in and about the basal cells and drop-shaped rete ridges. The surface shows hyperparakeratosis. This is a premalignant change showing cancer cell changes within the epithelium (magnification ×200).

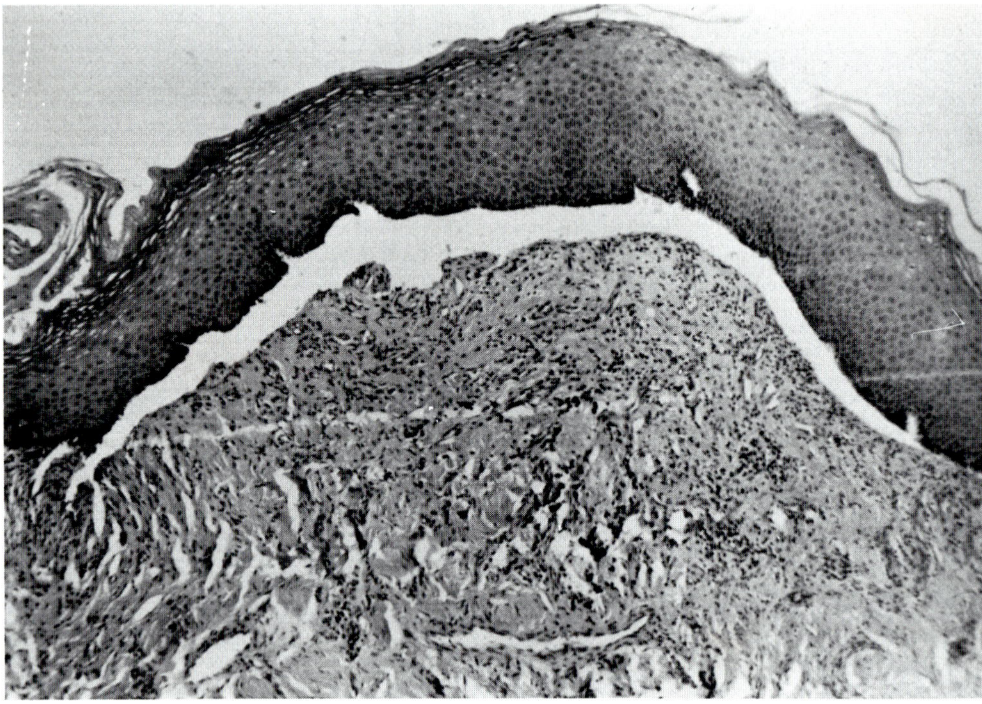

Figure 6.9. Subepithelial vesicle. Space beneath epithelium contained fluid. All layers of epithelium are raised away from connective tissue (magnification ×80).

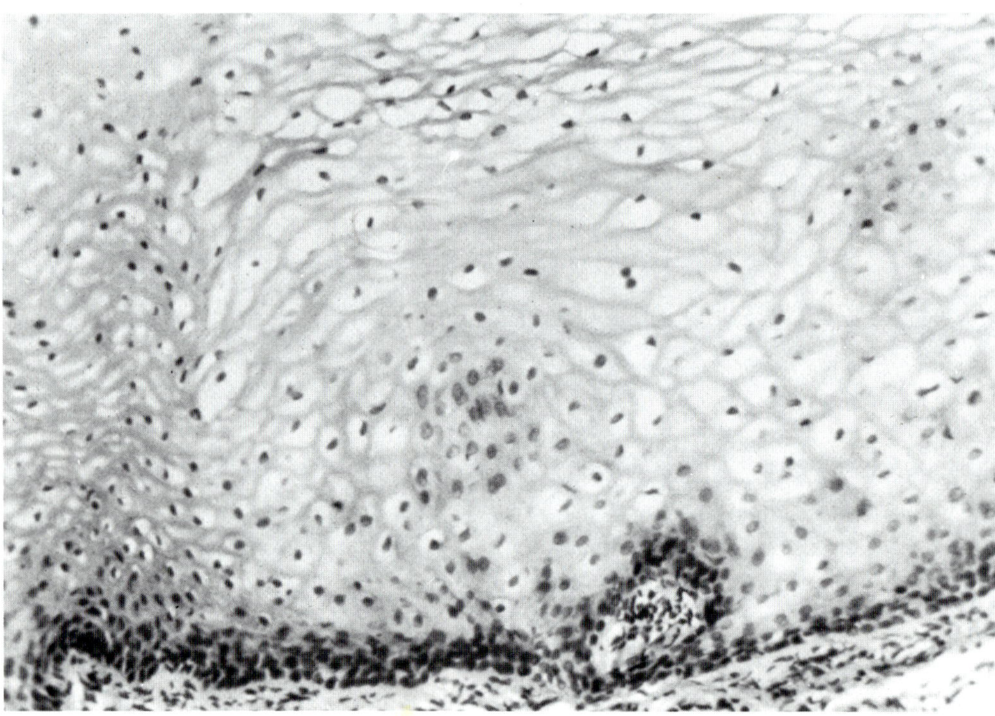

Figure 6.10. Spongiosis of epithelium. Fluid within epithelial cells gives them the appearance of a sponge (magnification ×200).

Connective Tissue Changes

Inflammatory infiltrates are common. Most often chronic inflammatory cells are present (Fig. 6.11). A prime example is gingivitis.

Hyperplasia of connective tissues refers to an increase in the amount of collagen fibers.

Glandular and ductal distention can be seen in the many accessory mucous glands due to pressure and obstruction.

Clinical Changes in the Oral Mucosa

Despite the numerous diseases that can affect the oral mucosa, there are only a limited number of gross lesions that can be seen clinically. A lesion is any wound or pathologic alteration of tissue. Oral mucosal diseases are characterized by one or more lesions that can be categorized into these basic types: macule, papule, plaque, vesicle, bulla, ulcer, erosion, nodule, tumor, atrophic area, scar, and crust (Fig. 6.12; see also Figs. 6.18 and 6.23). The recognition of these lesions is of prime importance, because unless these are noted, oral disease will be overlooked.

A *macule* or macula is a flat spot, stain, or blemish on the mucosa (Fig. 6.13). It varies in size and color and may be red, blue, black, or another color. Examples are the common amalgam tattoo (see Fig. 6.2), melanin pigmentation of a nevus, the rash of secondary syphilis, or a small area of hemorrhage, a petechia.

A *papule* or papula is a small, rounded, pimplelike, variably colored elevation. They usually appear in clumps and are commonly seen in lichen planus in which they appear as white elevations with variable patterns (Fig. 6.14).

A *plaque* is a small or large, demarcated patch that can be smooth or fissured (Fig. 6.15). Leukoplakia refers to a white patch or plaque. The leukoplakia may represent simple hyperkeratosis, dysplasia, or cancer. Erythroplakia is a red patch. It tends to

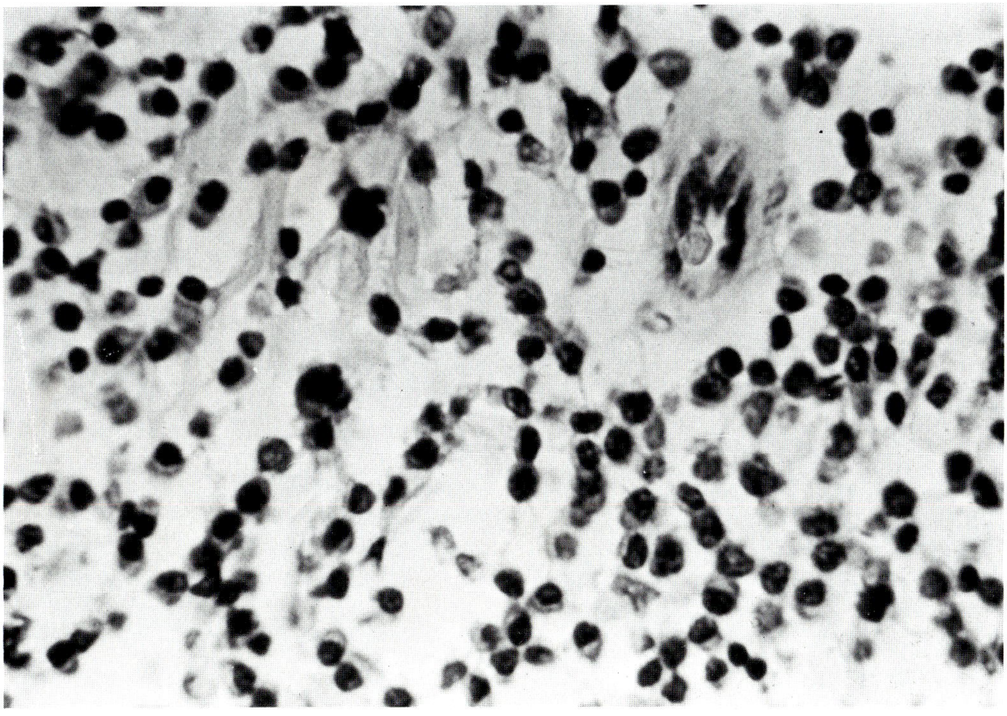

Figure 6.11. Chronic inflammatory cells, mostly lymphocytes and plasma cells (magnification ×400).

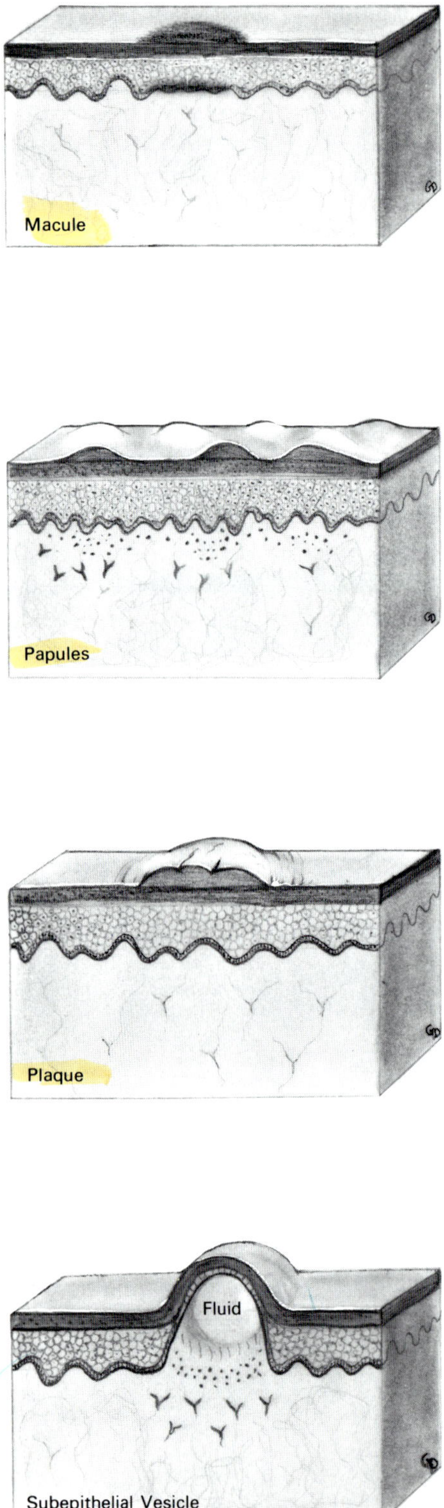

Figure 6.12. Diagrams of oral mucosal changes.

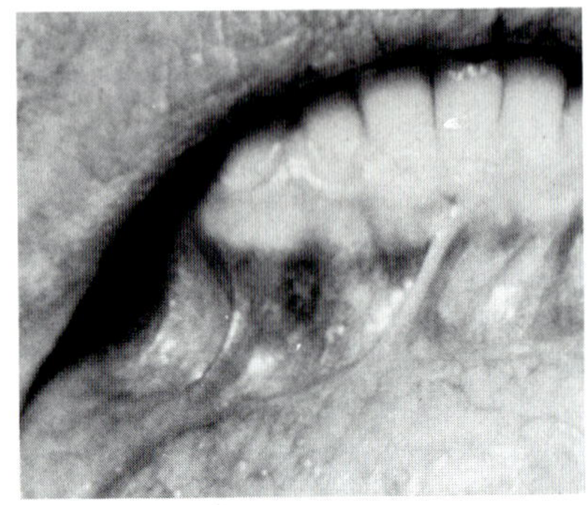

Figure 6.13. Black macule, unattached gingiva. Carbon tattoo from a pencil.

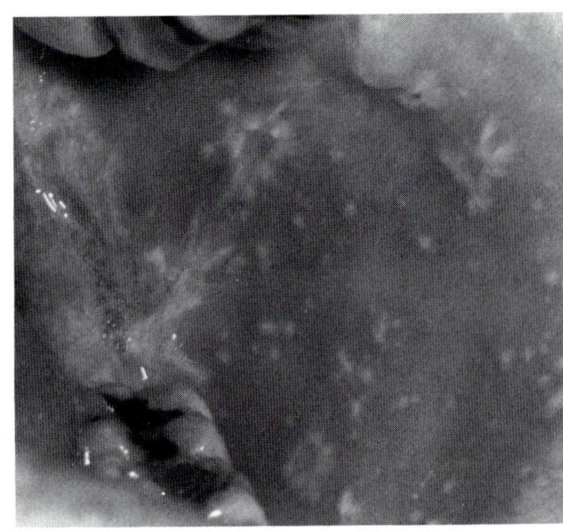

Figure 6.14. Lichen planus. There are white, keratotic, nonremovable papules, some of which form patterns.

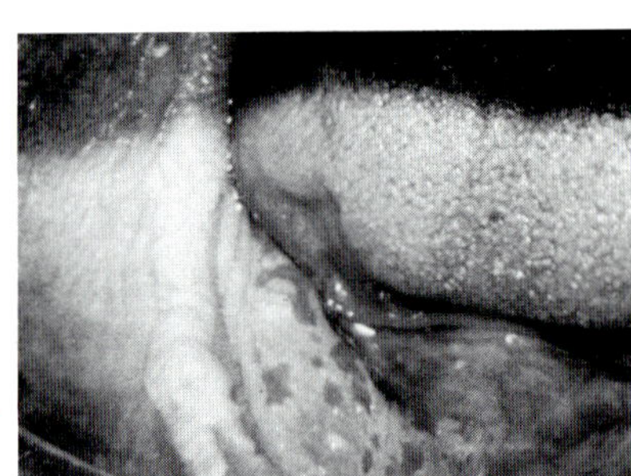

Figure 6.15. Leukoplakia (white patch), buccal mucosa, alveolar ridge, and floor of mouth.

be flat rather than raised and is usually malignant or premalignant unless it is associated with another known disease. It must be differentiated from a rash.

A *vesicle* is a small bleb or blister representing accumulation of fluid beneath or within the epithelium (Fig. 6.16). Clinically, the subepithelial type cannot be distinguished from the intraepithelial type. Viral diseases cause vesicles to form. Intact vesicles are commonly seen in herpes labialis of the lips. However, within the oral cavity intact vesicles are rarely seen because they are traumatized readily. Once a vesicle is traumatized or the membrane is ruptured spontaneously, an ulcer is formed.

A *bulla* is merely a large vesicle or blister (Fig. 6.17). It may form when several vesicles coalesce. Pemphigus and drug reactions are characterized by bullae. The bulla may appear white due to the necrosis of the overlying degenerating epithelium (Figs. 6.18 and 6.19).

An *ulcer* is a sore characterized by the loss of epithelium yielding a punched out shallow or deep area. The central zone of necrosis appears as a white or yellowish membrane and is surrounded by a red halo (Fig. 6.20). They may be large or small and the border may be hard and raised. Traumatic ulcers are the most common. Ulcers are also seen in aphthous stomatitis, cancer, and tuberculosis.

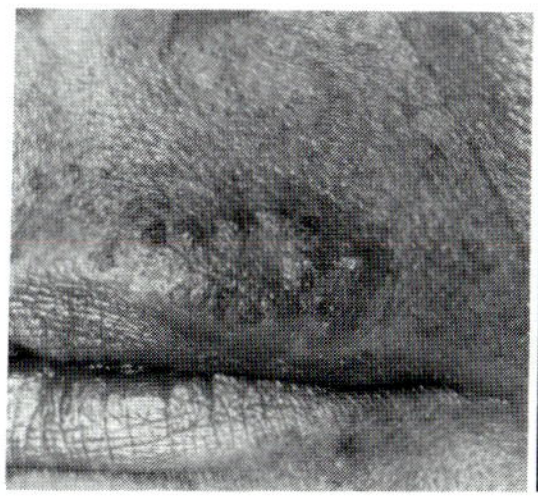

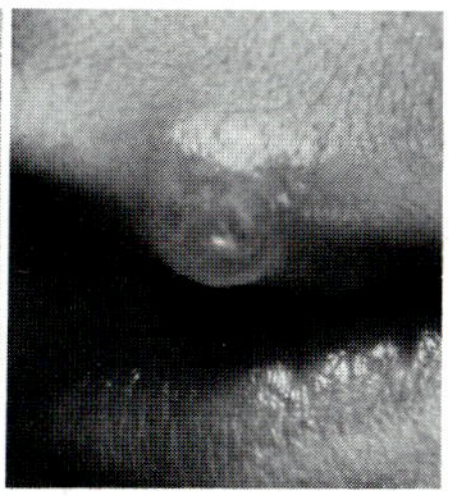

Figure 6.16. *Left*, numerous small vesicles on the skin of the upper lip (herpes labialis).
Figure 6.17. *Right*, several vesicles have coalesced to form a large vesicle or bulla on the upper lip (herpes labialis).

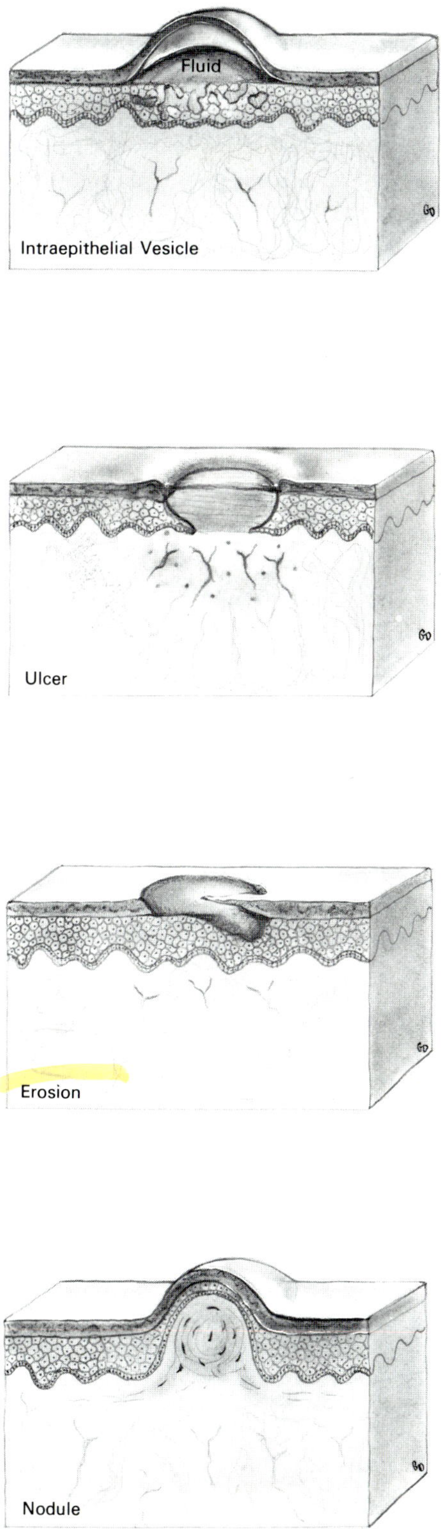

Figure 6.18. Diagrams of oral mucosal changes.

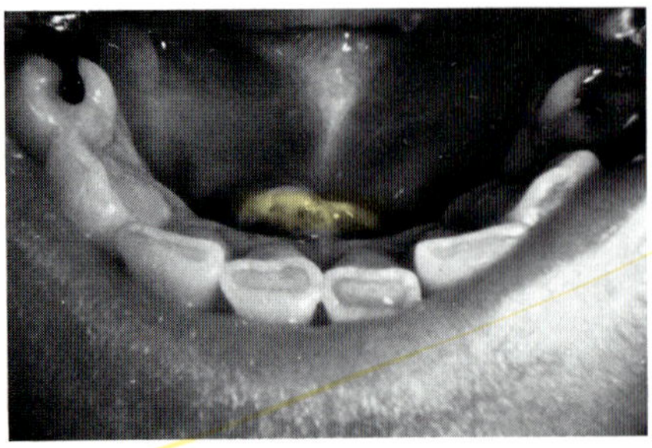

Figure 6.19. Bulla, floor of the mouth. Surface is degenerative and appears white (pemphigus).

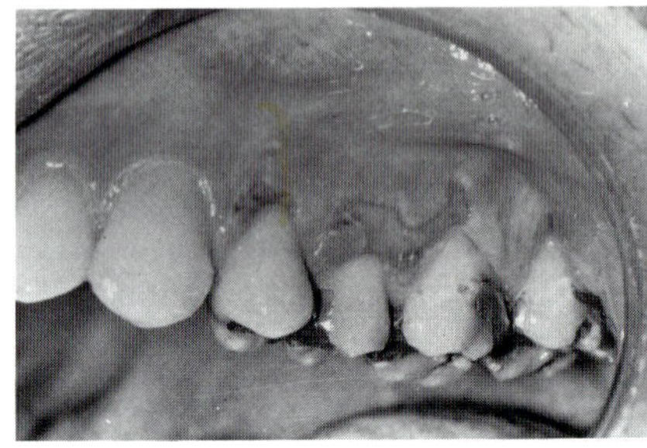

Figure 6.21. Erosion and ulcer of traumatic origin (toothbrush). Erosion is red area on gingiva over the first bicuspid.

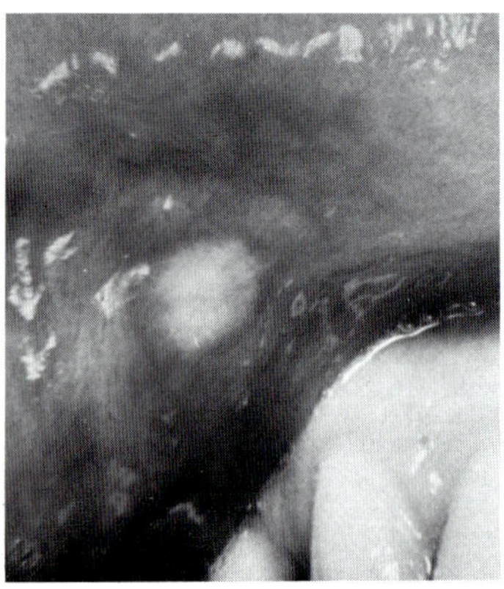

Figure 6.20. Ulcer, inner aspect upper lip (aphthous stomatitis).

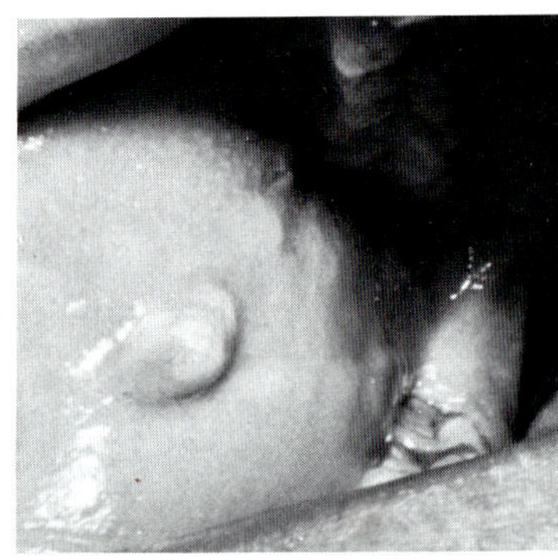

Figure 6.22. Nodule on buccal mucosa (fibroma).

An *erosion* of the mucosa refers to the partial loss of the upper layers of the epithelium. These lesions appear red because the blood supply in the connective tissue can be seen more easily in the area where there is less epithelium. Examples of mucosal erosions are traumatic erosion caused by toothbrushing (Fig. 6.21) and a form of lichen planus called erosive lichen planus. These lesions appear as red, raw denuded areas.

A *nodule* is a localized swelling or protuberance. It is usually solid, raised, and firm and can measure from millimeters to centimeters. It usually represents a growth from the connective tissue. A common example is the fibroma (Fig. 6.22). Mucosal cysts and cystlike masses are specialized nodules in that they are not firm. A mucocele of the lip presents as a nodular mass.

A *tumor* is a swelling of a part (Fig. 6.23). It could be inflammatory but often is considered as a developmental or neoplastic solid growth projecting outward and arising from the mucosa. A hemangioma is a benign tumor (Fig. 6.24). Carcinoma or cancer is a malignant tumor (Fig. 6.25).

Atrophy refers to reddened areas of the mucosa where the epithelium is thin and the blood supply of the connective tissue is seen (Fig. 6.26). It differs from erosion in that there are fewer cells in the epithelium because of atrophy of the epithelium, not because of trauma. Examples of atrophy are seen in geographic tongue where the filiform papillae are lost, as well as in vitamin deficiency states, anemias, and tertiary syphilis.

A *scar* is a white depressed mark, line, or

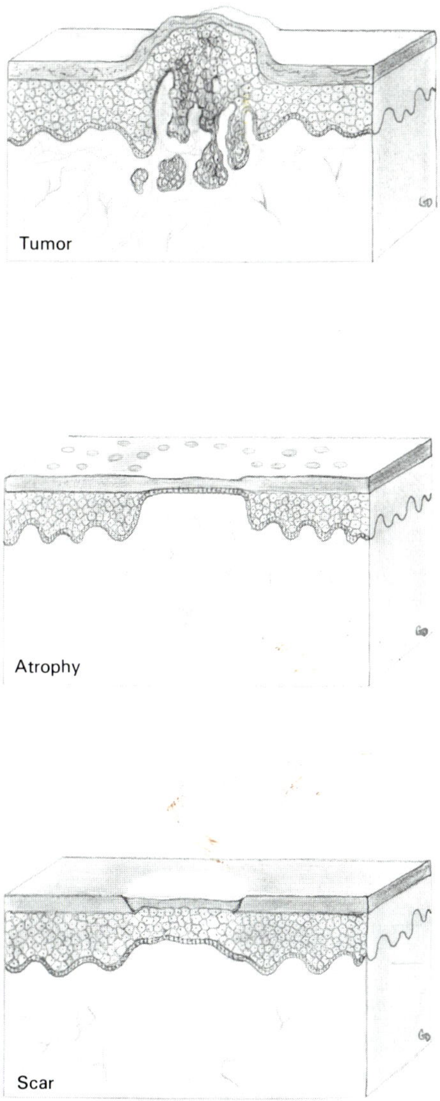

Figure 6.23. Further diagrams of oral mucosal changes.

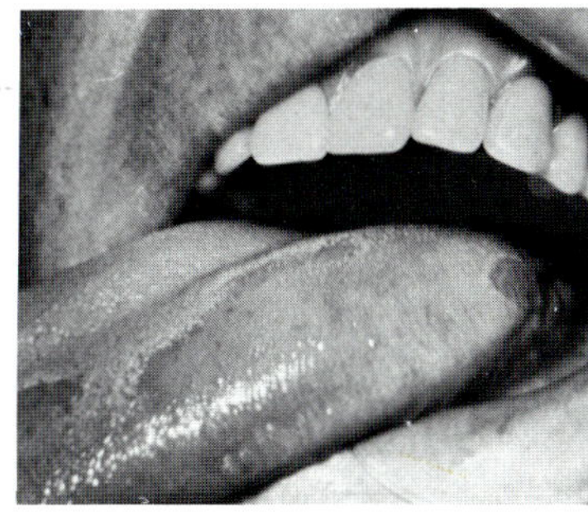

Figure 6.26. Atrophy of filiform papillae due to denture trauma caused large red denuded area on left lateral border of tongue. A lesion of geographic tongue appears at posterior lateral border.

area that represents healing after injury. It is rare in the oral cavity, but is seen following gingivectomies, apicoectomies, and deep inflammation. Scars are frequently seen on the lips (Fig. 6.27), mucosa, and skin surface as reminders of previous trauma.

A *crust* is a scab or dry outer layer. It is usually seen with brown pigmentation of the skin or outer surface of the lips (Fig. 6.28). A scab in the mouth is white and is represented by the central white necrotic area of an ulcer.

Viral Infections of the Oral Cavity

Viruses are the smallest of microorganisms that can produce infection. Infection

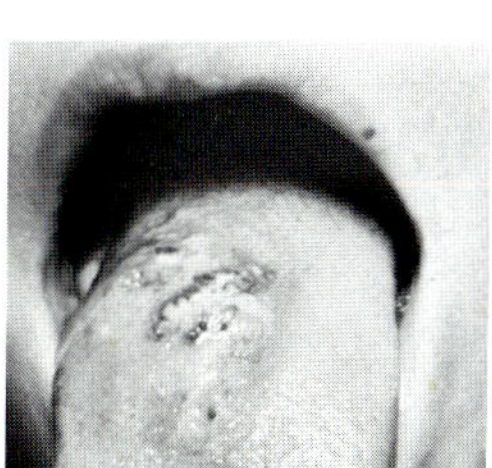

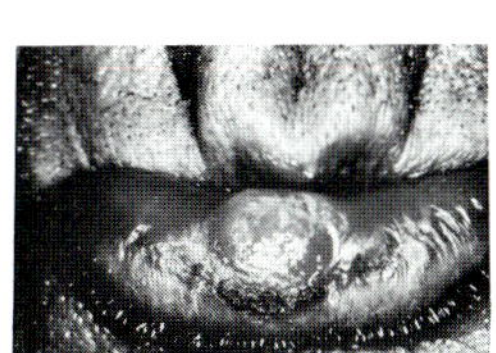

Figure 6.24. *Left*, benign tumor involving over half the tongue (hemangioma).
Figure 6.25. *Right*, malignant tumor of the lower lip (carcinoma).

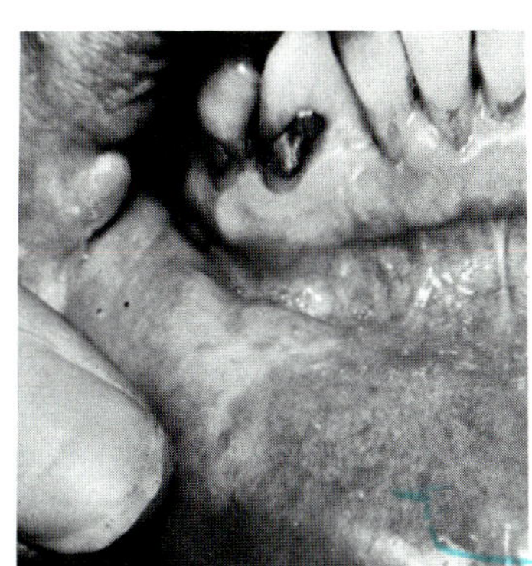

Figure 6.27. Scars, inner aspect lower lip (healed deep aphthous ulcers).

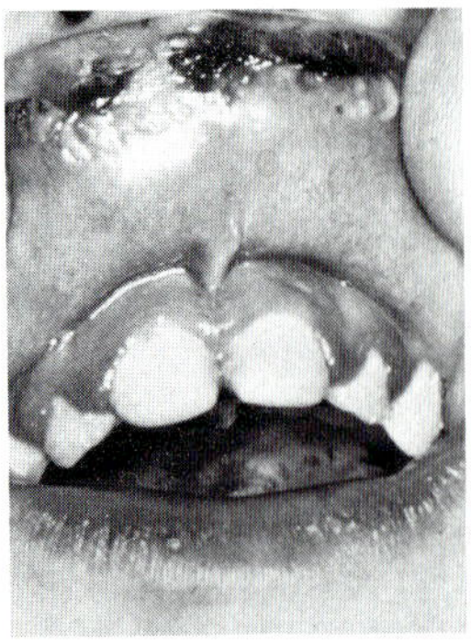

Figure 6.28. Crusts on upper lip (herpetic stomatitis).

is the invasion of tissue by pathologic microorganisms with resulting damage to the tissue, inflammation, and systemic involvement. Viruses are smaller than bacteria; they can be isolated by special technique and observed by electron microscopy. They are composed of an outer protein coating surrounding an inner core of either ribonucleic acid (RNA) or deoxyribonucleic acid (DNA). Found everywhere, they infect animals, plants, and bacteria. They live within cells and utilize the cell's metabolic machinery for their own reproduction. Characteristically, they choose specific cells of the body. This tendency to turn to, to choose, or to have an affinity for certain cells and not others is called tropism. Viruses, then, can be categorized according to the tissue that is mainly involved or infected.

Dermotropic viruses select the skin and mucous membranes. Included in this group are the viruses that cause chickenpox, smallpox, measles, and the herpes simplex virus that involves mainly the mouth.

Pneumotropic viruses affect the respiratory system and are responsible for the common cold and influenza.

Neurotropic viruses involve nerve tissue. Herpes zoster, encephalitis, rabies, and poliomyelitis are diseases caused by these viruses.

Glandulotropic viruses infect glands. Mumps of the parotid gland is an example.

Oral involvement by viruses is very common. The disease may affect only the mouth, or the oral mucosa may be involved concurrent with spread of infection from other parts that are infected. Those infections confined to the mouth are herpetic stomatitis (*stomato*—mouth), herpes labialis, and herpangina. Those that include both the skin and the mouth are chickenpox, measles, mumps, and herpes zoster.

Usually, once an individual is infected with a virus, the defense system of the body reacts. Lymphocytes recognize the virus as foreign and plasma cells produce neutralizing antibodies against it to overcome the infection. Characteristically, for most viruses, the immunity to further infection is long-lasting. However, important exceptions to this are the common cold virus, the herpes simplex virus, and the chickenpox virus.

Humans are the natural host of six of about 100 herpesviruses. Sharing morphologic characteristics, these human herpesviruses are important in several diseases of the oral cavity. They include: herpes simplex virus type 1 and 2 (HSV1 and HSV2), cytomegalovirus (CMV), Epstein-Barr virus (EBV), varicella-zoster virus (VZV), and the recently described human B-cell lymphotropic virus (HBLV). All of them have an inner DNA structure, surrounded by a capsid and an outer protein skin. Replicating in the nucleus of the host's cells, they produce a primary infection that is followed by a latent period, after which they may be reactivated despite circulating antibody to them in the host. The primary infection may be subclinical, having no signs or symptoms, but causing the formation of antibodies; or it may be clinical, characterized by disease manifestations. Following the development of antibodies, the virus remains latent or hidden in a specific site in the body, not producing disease. Later, in some patients, the virus may be reactivated, producing a secondary disease that is not similar to the primary disease.

Primary Herpetic Stomatitis (Acute Herpetic Gingivostomatitis)

Herpetic stomatitis occurs in 10 percent of the cases, following primary contact with the HSV1. (HSV2 is responsible for the genital herpetic infections. However, type 2 herpes has been isolated from the oral cavity and type 1 from the genital area, probably from orogenital transmission from active lesions or from viruses shed in the saliva. Type 1 and 2 lesions cannot be distinguished clinically.) Maternal antibodies offer protection until about 6 months of age, after which the virus may be infective on exposure. Usually children between 3 and 10 years are affected. However, primary herpes is also seen in teenagers, adults in the third and fourth decades, and immunecompromised patients. Following exposure from the saliva or from a vesicle from a patient with active early disease, there is an incubation period of about 1 week during which the virus resides in the patient but does not produce any manifestations. Then there are two possibilities. In most infected individuals there is no clinical disease and the immune mechanism begins to develop antibodies to the virus at about the sixth day following the incubation period. In about 10 percent the virus produces clinical disease, the most common being primary gingivostomatitis. Other areas that can be affected are the skin, conjunctiva, and the meninges, which could be fatal.

During the incubation period, the virus is establishing itself in the tissues it prefers; in this in case the oral epithelial cells near the surface. As the virus replicates itself in the nuclei of the epithelial cells, the nuclei swell and become greatly distorted and swollen. Eventually the nucleus degenerates, and viral particles are released. Lymphocytes respond, and fluid accumulates. The patient experiences a prodromal period because of the cellular changes and the reaction of the body to them. The patient feels ill and runs a high fever, 104+ °F in children, 101+ °F in others. Swelling and pain appear in the mouth, and vesicles develop from the inflammatory response pursuant to the degeneration and necrosis of the epithelial cells. Occurring anywhere in the oral cavity (stomatitis) and on the gingiva (gingivitis), the vesicles may be few and scattered or many. Some may coalesce and form a bulla. The vesicles or blisters quickly rupture to form ulcers with a red halo (Figs. 6.29 and 6.30). The vesicles continue to develop for a week and then begin to fade as the immune response develops antibodies starting at day 6 of the active disease. By about 2 weeks the lesions disappear, and the mucosa heals without scarring and appears normal.

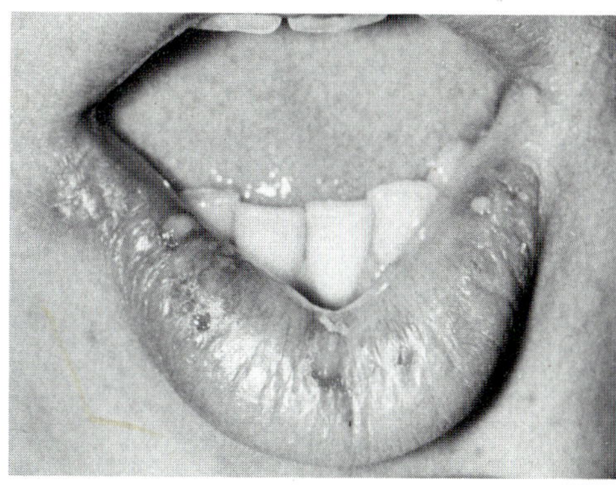

Figure 6.29. Herpetic stomatitis, 24-year-old female. Many vesicles have ruptures leaving discrete ulcers with halos on lower lip.

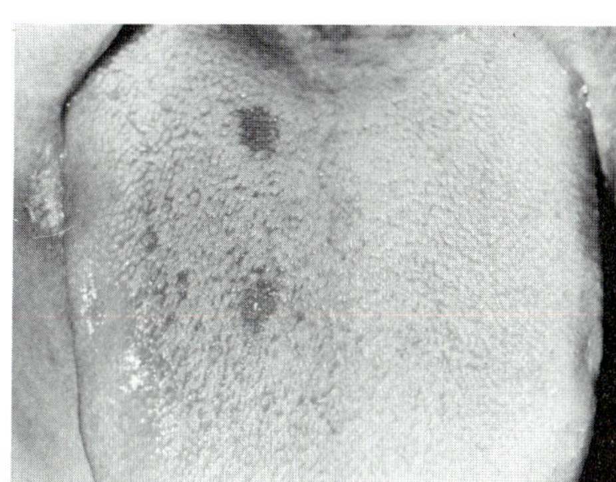

Figure 6.30. Herpetic stomatitis, same patient as in Figure 6.29. Note intact small vesicle below, and atrophic area of ruptured vesicle, above. Tongue is uniformly coated and whitened.

Besides the vesicular eruptions, typically the gingivae are intensely inflamed, appearing fiery red on the marginal attached and unattached gingivae, such that the mucogingival line is obliterated (Fig. 6.31). The tongue is usually coated, appearing white, because fever causes the delayed desquamation of the filiform papillae (Fig. 6.32). The fungiform papillae may be prominent because of the edema. The lips may swell, and as vesicles break there can be pseudomembranous white lesions on the mucous membrane and crusts on the dry skin surface. Lymph nodes on both sides of the neck are usually swollen and tender (see Fig. 1.8).

The treatment is generally to alleviate the symptoms, because the disease naturally resolves itself. A soothing anesthetic mouth rinse is used for the sore mouth, aspirin or aspirin substitutes for the fever, plus bed rest and nutritional supplements. In immunocompromised patients, acyclovir, which inhibits replication of the virus, is used and is effective. However, it does not prevent the virus from remaining in the body. Antibiotics are ineffective against viruses, but sometimes they are used against secondary bacterial infections.

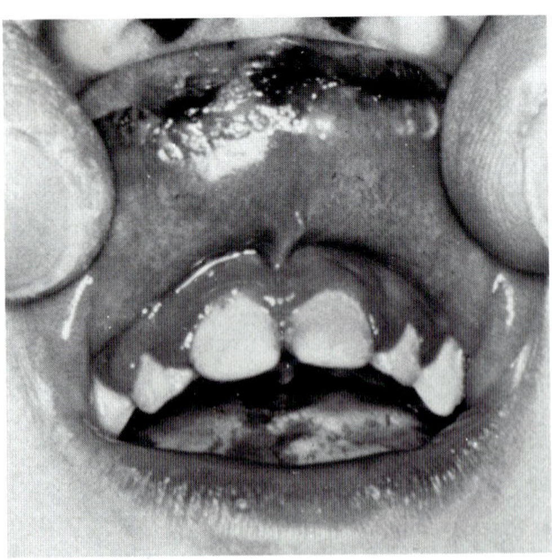

Figure 6.31. Primary herpetic gingivostomatitis, 9-year-old male. Gingivae uniformly reddened. Lips are crusted.

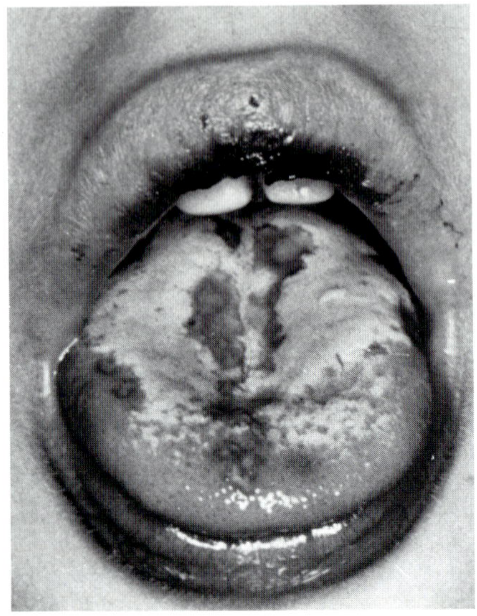

Figure 6.32. Primary herpetic gingivostomatitis, same as Figure 6.31. Note many ulcers on white-coated tongue.

Following the primary infection, clinical or subclinical, the virus lies dormant or latent in the trigeminal ganglion. Because of this, despite neutralizing antibodies and antiviral medications, the virus may be reactivated, establishing itself in the tissues and causing a secondary disease either in the mouth or on the lips. By an unknown triggering mechanism, the virus is reactivated and spreads along the nerve pathway, producing disease at a peripheral site. Triggering factors are: trauma, emotions, fever, infections, menstruation, and allergy.

Recurrent Intraoral Herpes Simplex

These are called recurrent herpetic ulcers because the vesicles are rarely seen intact. The manifestations of these recurrent episodes are in no way as dramatic as the primary disease. Usually, there is a prodromal symptom of tingling or slight pain, followed by the eruption of a vesicle that soon ruptures. The resulting ulcers are small but may be large if several vesicles coalesce. Characteristically, they occur on bound-down or firmly attached mucosa, such as the hard palate and attached gin-

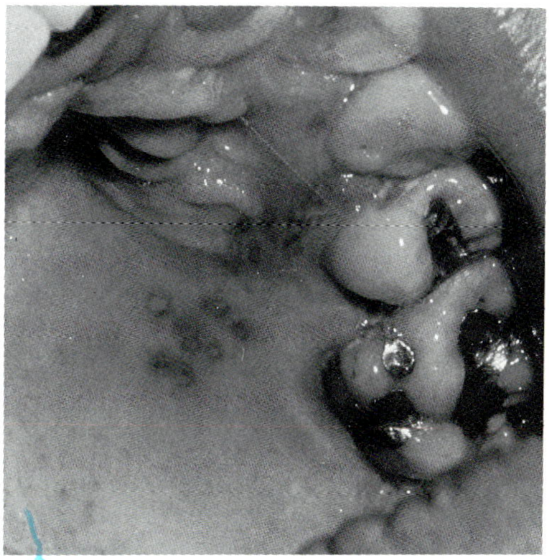

Figure 6.33. Recurrent intraoral herpes of hard palate. Note small, punctate, clustered ulcers. The patient felt a burning sensation before the outbreak of vesicles.

givae, and not on movable mucosa (Fig. 6.33). (This is important in distinguishing the recurrent herpetic ulcer from recurrent aphthous ulcerations.) A cytologic smear in the early phases often shows swollen, distorted nuclei of affected epithelial cells. The ulcers heal in about 7 days. Treatment should be toward reducing the pain. Topical anesthetic solutions are helpful, along with topical corticosteroids or other adherent medications.

Recurrent Herpes Labialis

Herpes labialis (cold sores) is the more common of the recurrent herpetic infections. Some of the precipitating factors are the common cold, febrile diseases, and exposure to direct sunlight, which have led to the names in common usage of cold sores, fever blisters, and sun blisters, respectively.

The disease starts with prodromal symptoms such as a tingling or burning sensation in the lip at the future site of the vesicles (Figs. 6.34 to 6.38). Within 24 hours small vesicles appear in clusters, usually

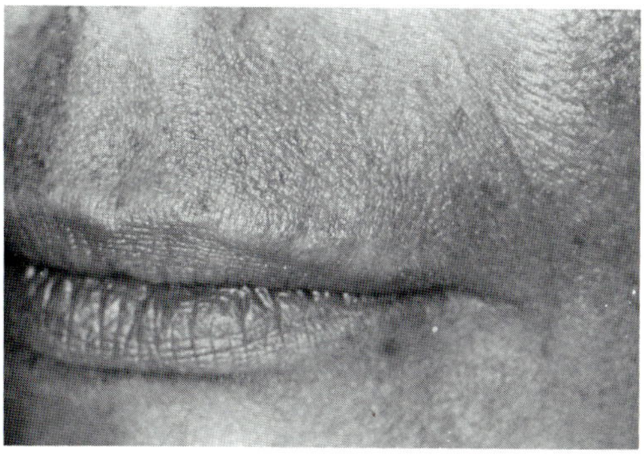

Figure 6.34. Herpes labialis, upper lip, day 1: prodromal stage, tingling, following exposure to sun.

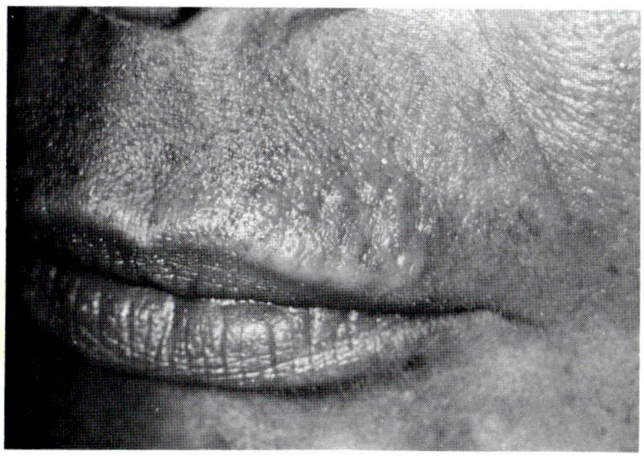

Figure 6.35. Same patient as in Figure 6.34. Herpes labialis, day 2: vesicles at site of tingling.

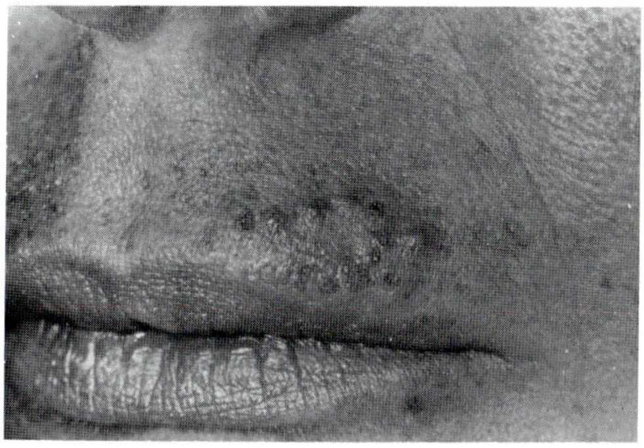

Figure 6.36. Same patient as in Figure 6.35. Herpes labialis, day 3: vesicles have begun to weep and ulcerate.

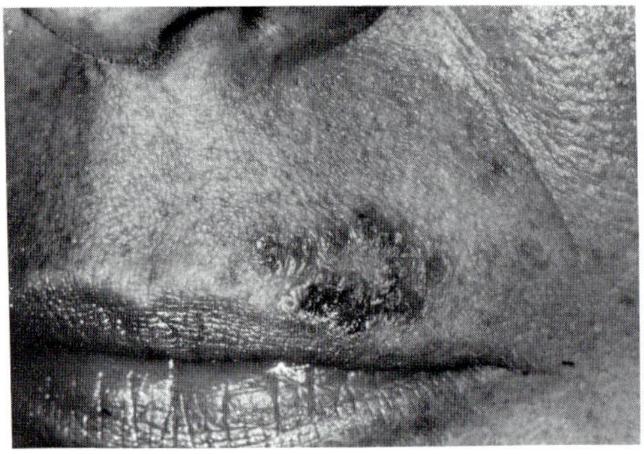

Figure 6.37. Same patient as in Figure 6.36. Herpes labialis, day 5: ulcers have crusted.

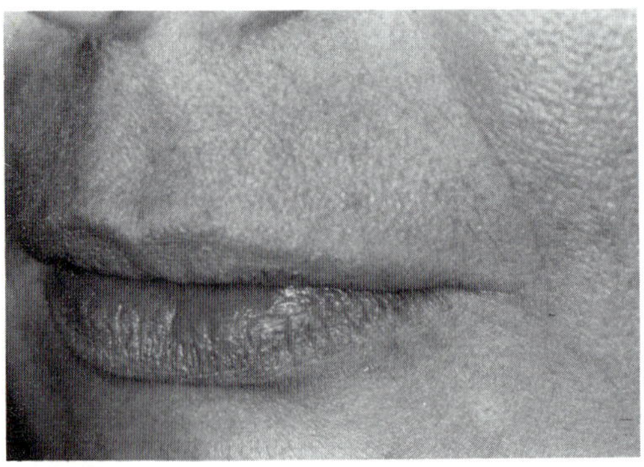

Figure 6.38. Same patient as in Figure 6.37. Herpes labialis, day 7: skin healed, normal.

on the skin surface of the upper or lower lips. There may be a few or many vesicles (Fig. 6.39). Some may coalesce to form a bulla (Fig. 6.40). The vesicles rupture leaving ulcers that crust on the skin surface and appear brown. There may be extensive edema, with redness and swelling (Fig. 6.41). Scratching can spread the infection. The lesions usually heal naturally in 5 to 7 days without scarring but may last as long as 2 weeks.

If the disease is treated in the prodromal stage, it may be aborted. However, after the first 24 hours, treatments only shorten the course of the disease but do not abort it. Topical applications such as 70 percent alcohol, ether, and antiviral medication such as acyclovir can be effective.

For the dental team, precautions should be taken. If the patient has vesicles at an appointment, and unless there is an emergency, it would be prudent to reschedule the patient. Gloves should be worn for infection control anyway, keeping in mind that the herpesvirus is shed in the saliva even without active disease. Moreover, the virus can be inoculated directly into the finger, creating an infection called herpetic whitlow, even if the dental member has antibodies against the virus (Fig. 6.42).

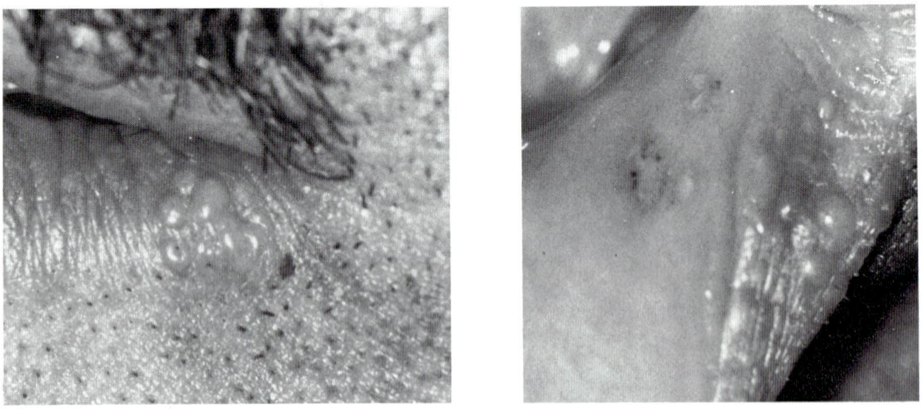

Figure 6.39. Recurrent herpes labialis due to the trauma of a lip bite. *A*, multiple vesicles on skin side of lower lip; and *B*, corresponding ulcer on inner lip.

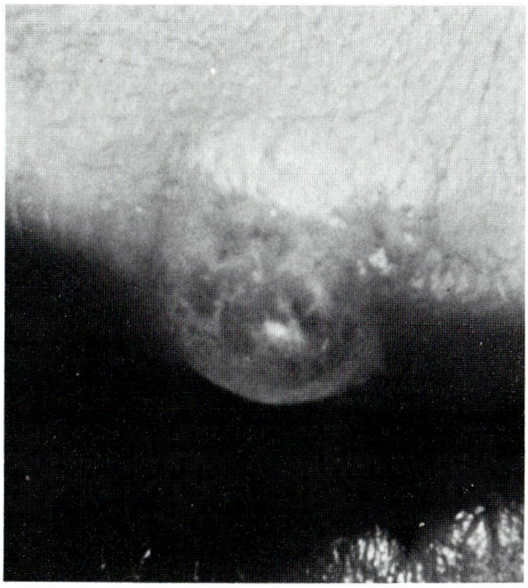

Figure 6.40. Herpes labialis, upper lip. Several vesicles have coalesced to form a large blister.

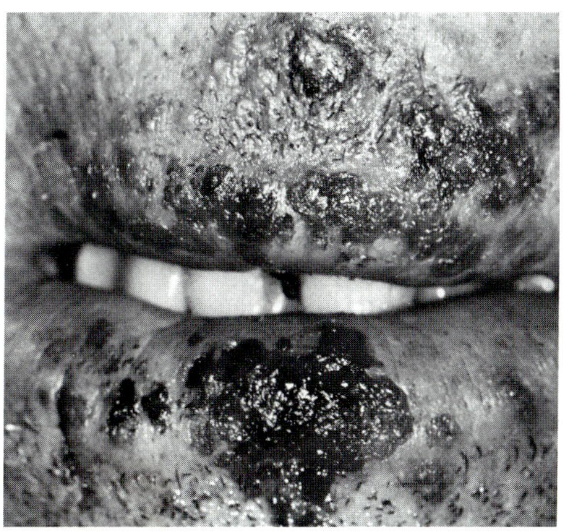

Figure 6.41. Herpes labialis, upper and lower lips, after only one exposure to sun. There are several vesicles, ulcers, crusts, and extensive swelling and edema.

Herpangina

Herpangina, caused by various strains of the coxsackievirus (not a herpesvirus, despite the name), affects the posterior part of the mouth (Fig. 6.43). There is a prodromal period of fever and ill feeling. Following

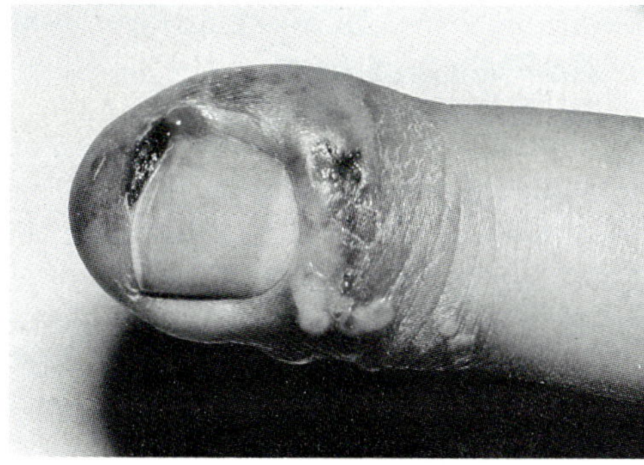

Figure 6.42. Herpetic whitlow, showing some intact herpetic blisters and open ulcers with severe swelling of tip of finger.

this, groups of vesicles appear mainly on the soft palate and tonsillar areas. The vesicles then rupture. Patients complain of a severe sore throat that may be confused with a "strep throat." The disease runs its course in 7 to 10 days. Only symptomatic treatment is required.

Herpes Zoster

Herpes zoster (shingles) is caused by the chickenpox (varicella) virus (a herpesvirus) that becomes reactivated. It may also occur following exogenous exposure to someone with chickenpox. Occurring in older or immunosuppressed individuals, the disease erupts along peripheral sensory nerves lead-

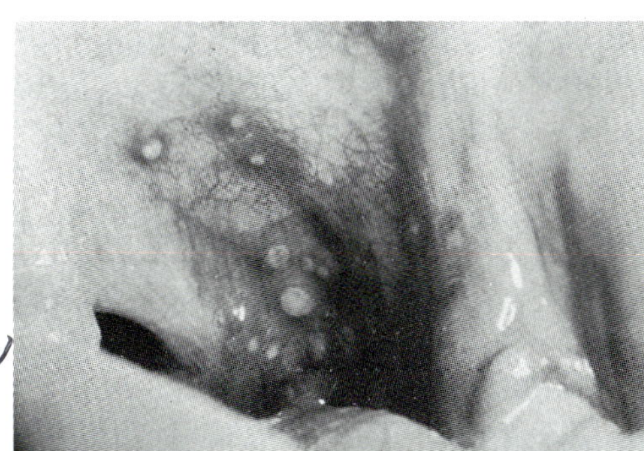

Figure 6.43. Herpangina; multiple vesicular and ulcerative lesions on the red base in the posterior part of the mouth.

ing from the dorsal root ganglion where the virus was lying dormant. Starting as pain along the nerve, this is followed by painful eruptions of vesicles on the skin, usually on the trunk under the axilla from the vertebra to the midline on one side. The oral cavity may be affected when the trigeminal nerve is involved. Strikingly, the eruptions are *unilateral*, appearing on the skin on one side of the face and on one side of the mouth (palate, tongue), following the distribution of the particular nerves involved (Figs. 6.44 and 6.45). The disease runs a course of weeks and months without treatment, and pain may linger after lesions heal.

Other viruses affecting the skin also may have vesicular eruptions in the mouth, but the oral eruptions are secondary features. Chickenpox (varicella) and measles (rubeola) are exanthematous viral diseases of childhood, usually characterized by vesicles and fever. Some vesicles may appear in the mouth. The Koplik spots of measles are supposed to appear on the buccal mucosa 24 hours before the outbreak of the disease. Clinicians, however, are hard pressed to find and prove the existence of these spots.

Occasionally, on examination, one may find a single vesicle on the soft palate. Follow-up of these cases shows that the patient has a cold or is about to get one. The vesicle represents an attack by a pneumotropic virus.

Mumps is a glandular viral disease usually affecting the parotid gland. High fever is followed by a painful swelling behind the ear. The papilla to the parotid (Stensen's) duct may be swollen, and the secretions of the parotid are lessened so the mouth may be dry. The pain subsides, but the swelling persists for about 5 days and then abates. The submandibular and sublingual glands may also be affected. The facial swelling can mimic a cellulitis (Fig. 6.46).

Infectious mononucleosis, caused by the herpesvirus Epstein-Barr virus, manifests

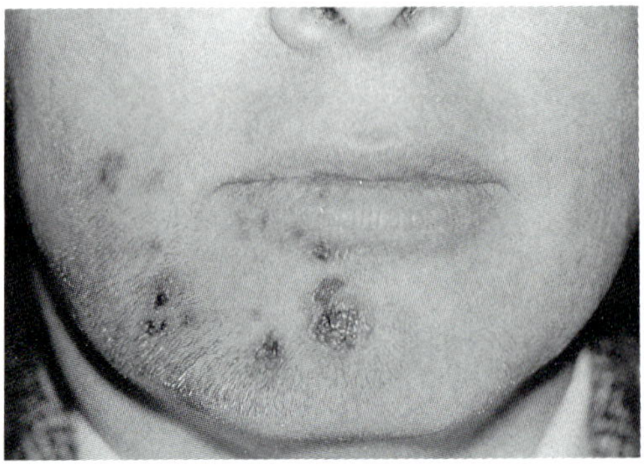

Figure 6.44. Herpes zoster; painful unilateral vesicular ulcers on right side of face along mandibular branch of trigeminal nerve.

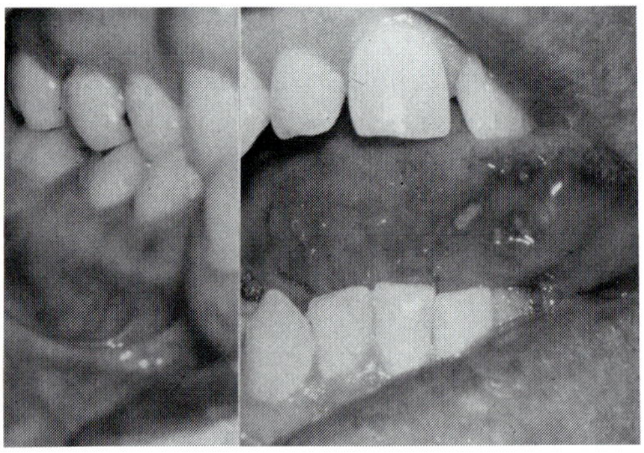

Figure 6.45. Herpes zoster; painful unilateral ulcers on right side of gingiva and tongue in same patient as Figure 6.44. This episode started as a toothache in tooth #30 with no other lesions present at the initial appointment.

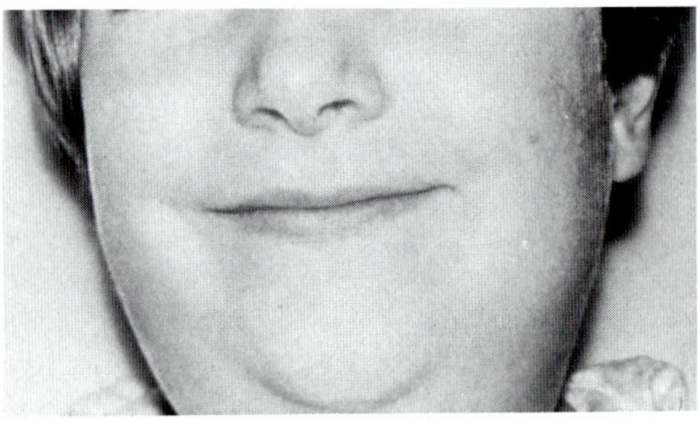

Figure 6.46. Facial swelling in a 7-year-old female who had mumps for 4 days when this photo was taken.

with swollen neck nodes, a sore throat, and abnormal blood monocytes. The palatine tonsils are frequently involved and in the early stages may resemble "strep throat" (Fig. 6.47). The tonsils become greatly enlarged and necrotic. Petechiae of the palate may be noted. There is no effective treatment. The disease may last for months and involve the liver.

It is to be noted that viral diseases manifest themselves mainly with the eruption of vesicles when they involve the oral cavity. However, other conditions may cause vesicular eruptions. Among these are drug reactions, allergies, and several dermatologic-oral diseases. In addition, because the vesicles rupture and leave ulcers, it may be difficult at times to label them as viral ulcers. Other ulcerative conditions must then be considered.

Recurrent Aphthous Stomatitis (Canker Sores)

Aphtha means small ulcer or white spot. The common disease of aphthous stomatitis is characterized by one or more, usually small, painful ulcers affecting the movable or mucous gland-bearing mucosa. The small ulcers often resemble those formed by the rupture of a herpetic vesicle, showing as a white spot with a red halo. Thus the two diseases may be confused. However, aphthous stomatitis is not a viral disease. The aphthae do not arise from vesicles. They start as pain followed by a red macule in the painful area. The center of the macule becomes ischemic and an ulcer forms (Fig. 6.48). There are etiologic as well as precipitating factors.

A streptococcal organism, *Streptococcus sanguis*, of the normal oral flora has been isolated as a possible etiologic agent. There appears to be a localized altered immune response against this organism, as well as to the oral epithelium of the host. The ensuing inflammatory response causes localized damage to the host in the form of degeneration and necrosis. The overlying epithelium loses its blood supply, and

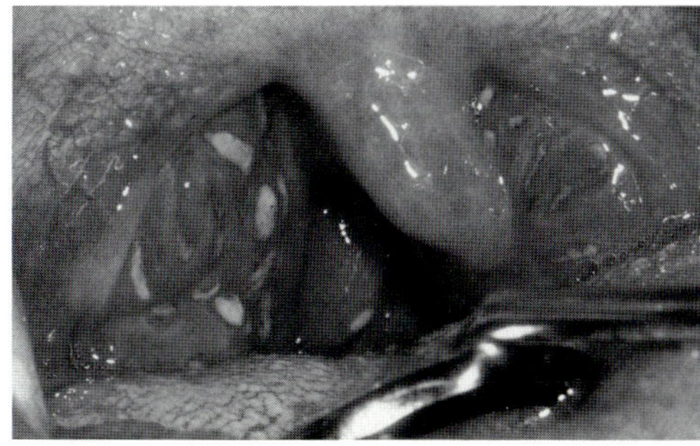

Figure 6.47. Infectious mononucleosis, early phase. Positive serologic tests. Swollen palatine tonsils with necrotic material in crypts in an 18-year-old with sore throat and posterior neck adenopathy. A "strep throat" would look similar.

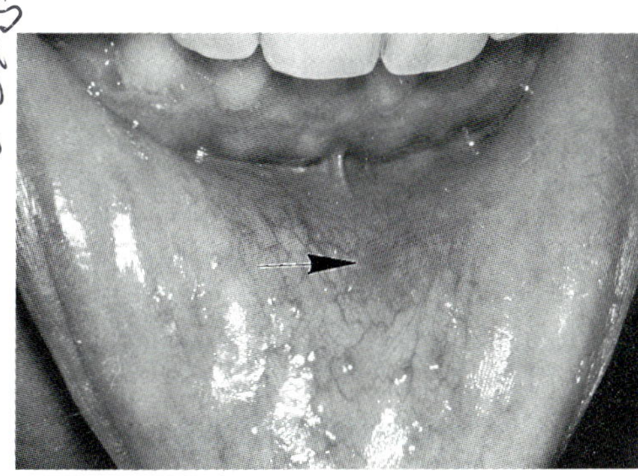

Figure 6.48. Beginning aphthous stomatitis; red macule (*arrow*).

an ulcer is formed. Invariably in patients with aphthous stomatitis, there is an associated, emotionally stressful event antecedent to the formation of the ulcer. For this reason, aphthous stomatitis is considered one of the psychosomatic diseases. Other precipitating factors are trauma, hormonal changes such as menses, and allergy to foods. Some nutritional deficiencies manifest with cankerlike ulcers.

Patients give a history of some sensation such as tingling at the site of the future ulcer. Then a red macule appears. This is followed by a breakdown of the epithelium (ulceration). The ulcers are characteristic with a central white or yellow area surrounded by a halo of erythema (Fig. 6.49). They appear punched out, usually oval or round, but may be linear. The ulcers may be singular or multiple (Fig. 6.50). They can occur anywhere in the mouth and lips. In contrast to recurrent intraoral herpetic ulcers, aphthous ulcers occur on the unattached and movable mucosa. Small ulcers are called minor aphthae. Large, longstanding ones are major aphthae and heal by scarring. Some ulcers may coexist with genital ulcers (Behçet's syndrome). Some patients may have only one episode, whereas others may have recurrent attacks. The intervals vary from years to months. Some individuals are never free of the ulcers, with a new one appearing as the older ones heal. Thus, a history of recurrence is significant for diagnosis. All age groups can be affected, but the incidence is highest in young adults. The ulcers are extremely painful so the patient often seeks aid.

Treatment varies with the severity of the lesions and the attitude of the patients. Tetracycline mouth rinses, topical corticosteroids, and anesthetic mouth rinses are effective. Wiping off the scab and using hydrogen peroxide work well. Sometimes, systemic corticosteroids are used. However, there are no curative measures to date. The small ulcers heal unaided in 5 to 14 days; a very large ulcer can take months. Minor aphthae usually heal without scarring, but major aphthae with deep inflammation heal with scars (Figs. 6.51 and 6.52).

The clinical appearance of ulcers in aphthous stomatitis is sufficiently characteristic that the term aphthous ulcer is often used. An ulcer with the typical aphthous characteristics coupled with a history of

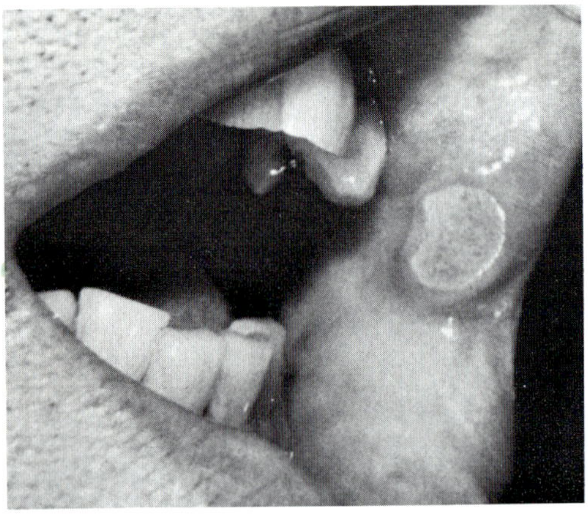

Figure 6.49. Aphthous stomatitis, buccal mucosa near commissure. A large ulcer with oval white central area surrounded by a wide zone of erythema. This was extremely painful.

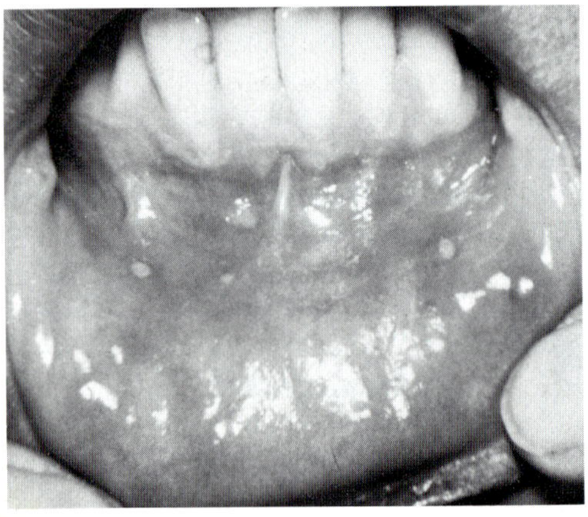

Figure 6.50. Aphthous stomatitis. Multiple discrete small ulcers on labial mucosa. They resemble herpetic ulcers; however, note gingivae are not involved.

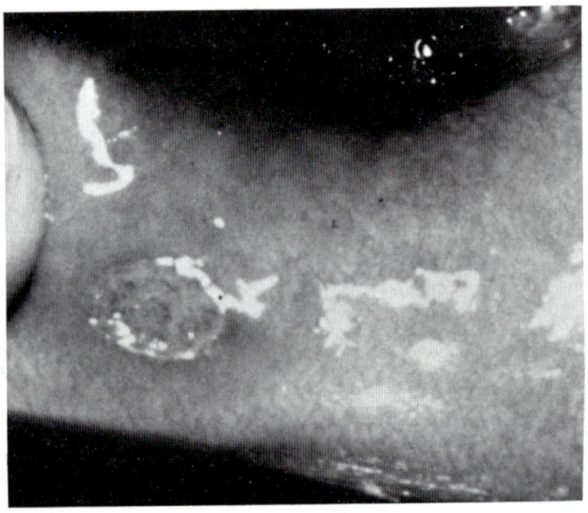

Figure 6.51. Aphthous stomatitis. Healing ulcer. Necrotic area is being replaced by new epithelial surface.

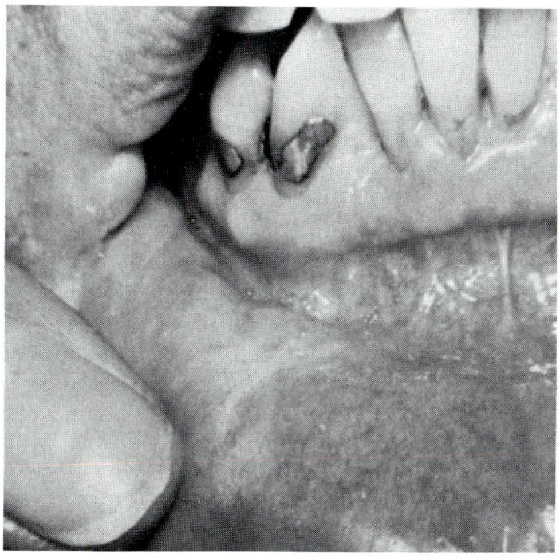

Figure 6.52. Aphthous stomatitis. Deep, long-standing ulcers have healed by scarring of the labial mucosa.

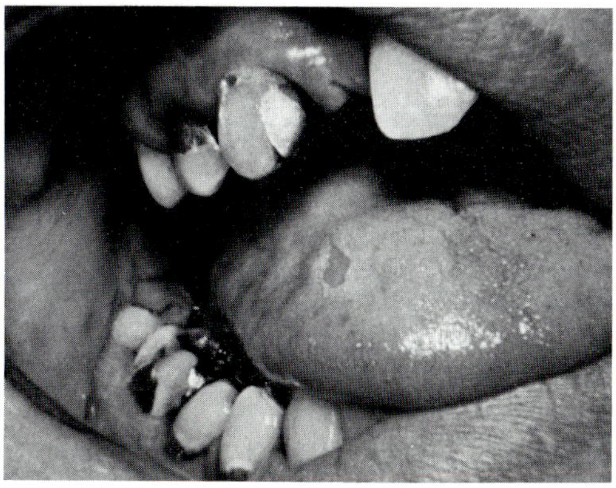

Figure 6.53. Traumatic ulcer on tongue. Patient rubbed tongue over sharp edges of buccal surface of decayed molar.

pain and recurrence probably represents aphthous stomatitis. However, there are many other conditions with ulcerations that must be considered possibilities before a final diagnosis is made.

Besides ulcerations of viral, drug, or allergic source, there are the common ulcers produced by trauma. These traumatic ulcers become infected secondarily by oral bacteria and therefore can be considered bacterial infections. Traumatic ulcers and traumatic lesions of the oral mucosa are extremely common, and trauma should be considered first when ulcers, erosions, and atrophic areas are noted.

The trauma may be mechanical, chemical, thermal, or electrical, the most common being mechanical. This includes lacerations and abrasions by many objects, such as teeth, restorations, dental procedures, and foreign objects. A badly decayed tooth often has sharp edges of enamel that tear the mucosa (Fig. 6.53). Dental protheses and worn restorations may have sharp edges. Orthodontic appliances frequently cause ulcerations. Accidental biting of the mucosa causes painful sores. Any sharp object introduced into the mouth by the patient, hygienist, or dentist can create trauma. Trauma may be induced by the patient (factitial trauma), in which case a careful inquiry elicits that history. Ill-fitting dentures are a common source of traumatic lesions, one of which is the traumatic ulcer.

Traumatic ulcers vary according to the nature of the cause, the duration of the infliction, and the amount of secondary bacterial invasion. Generally, they are discrete ulcers, with a punched-out appearance. The shape can vary, and often the borders are jagged. Like other ulcers, the central necrotic zone is white and there is a variable red halo surrounding it. They can be painful, but pain is not always a prominent feature as it is with aphthous ulcers. They heal within 7 to 10 days, usually depending on the size and the removal of the source of the problem. The cause is usually apparent, either through history or through examination. For example, toothbrush abrasion with erosions and ulcerations is frequently seen because patients are overzealous about brushing prior to appointments (Fig. 6.54). A newly placed denture often results in ulcerations. When the denture is relined, the ulcers heal uneventfully. Conversely, an ill-fitting denture moves and cuts into the mucosa. Relin-

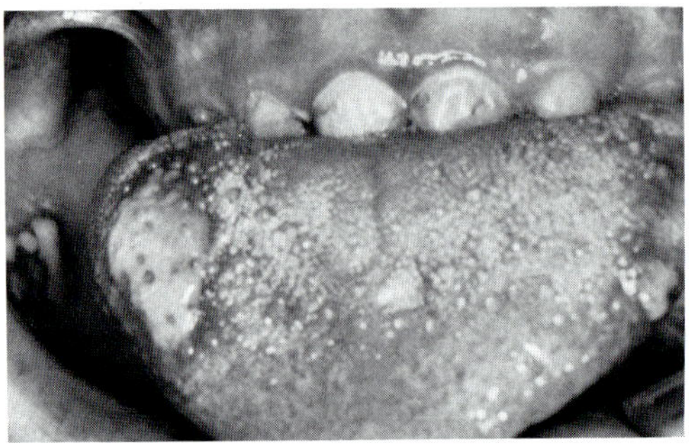

Figure 6.54. Traumatic ulcers of tongue and buccal mucosa, caused by overzealous toothbrushing in a youngster. Ulcers have a thick white necrotic pseudomembrane.

ing or remaking the denture is required to alleviate the problem. Thus, therapy for the traumatic ulcer depends on the symptoms and on finding and removing the cause. If an ulcer fails to heal within 2 weeks, it should be suspected of being cancer until proven otherwise (Fig. 6.55).

There are other traumatic lesions produced by dentures. A traumatic glossitis-appearing geographic tongue may be seen on the lateral border of the tongue. The lingual surface is devoid of filiform papillae, is atrophic, and appears red, swollen, and shiny. The cause is the abrasion of the tongue against the lingual surfaces of the denture teeth either by neurotic habit or poor alignment of the teeth. The atrophic areas do not change as they do with geographic tongue.

Denture sore mouth is another condition related to dentures. The palate and maxillary and mandibular ridges in particular appear bright red, swollen, and often are burning and painful. The cause appears to be poorly adapted dentures. This condition is treated with soft tissue-relining material until healing occurs; then new dentures are constructed. Sometimes a fungal infection, candidiasis, is associated with denture sore mouth.

Chemical trauma is caused by the application of drugs or burning chemical to the mucosa. An aspirin burn can be caused by placing aspirins against a painful tooth, a practice that should be discouraged. The aspirin, being acid, burns the mucosa and leaves a white pseudomembrane representing the necrotic epithelium (Fig. 6.56). The white membrane can be removed leaving a raw ulcer. Other chemicals include household items such a lye that can cause severe burns. Mouthwashes, if used full strength over a sufficient period of time, can cause chemical erosion and burns. Some tooth-

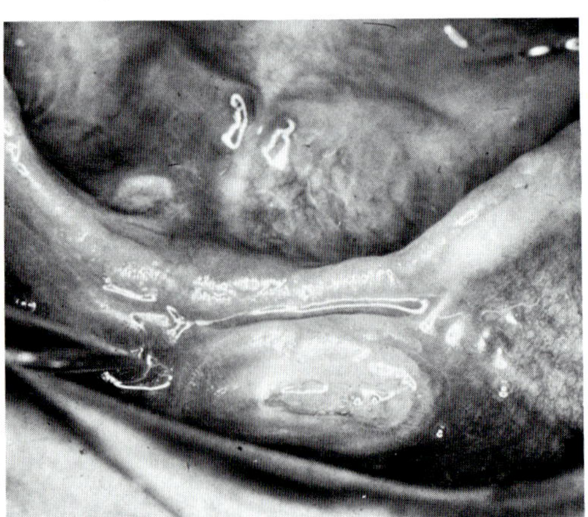

Figure 6.55. Two ulcers associated with denture trauma. When denture was withheld from patient, the large ulcer on the labial sulcus healed, but the smaller ulcer on the lingual sulcus did not. Biopsy proved it to be a squamous cell carcinoma.

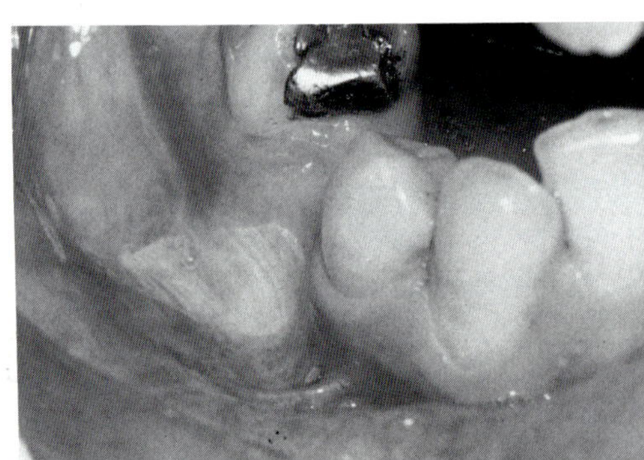

Figure 6.56. Aspirin burn, right buccal vestibule. The acid has coagulated the epithelium causing a white lesion.

pastes, because of their preservatives, also have this capability. Silver nitrate, a cauterizing and disinfecting agent, burns and necrotizes mucosa when it is applied.

Thermal injury can also cause severe damage to the mucosa. The most common examples are those caused by hot food or liquids taken into the mouth (Fig. 6.57). Soups frequently cause burns on the lips, and the mucosa appears white and may form a vesicle. Hot cheese, as in grilled sandwiches and pizza, is a common offender. The pizza burn usually occurs on the palate. The lesion is a striking, irregular, white-yellow slough with underlying ulceration. The pain may be severe. Ointments may help alleviate the discomfort and aid healing, which takes about 10 days to 2 weeks.

Factitial trauma (that produced by the patient unintentionally or subconsciously) is responsible for many lesions, usually ulcerations. However, the diagnosis may be elusive at first, so the practitioner must persist if factitial trauma is suspected. Often, a biting habit that produces whitened lesions is not realized by the patient. An example of factitial trauma is noted in Figure 6.58. The treatment is to get the patient to realize the self-inflicted trauma and to stop it. Topical corticosteroids can hasten healing.

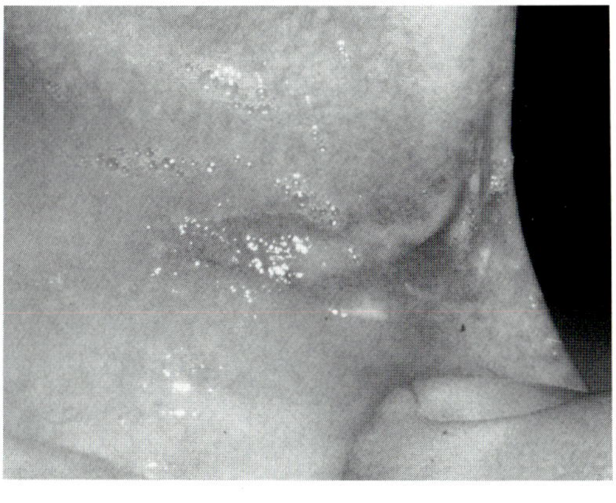

Figure 6.57. Thermal burn, left buccal mucosa, caused by hot fork. Necrotic epithelium and scab appear white.

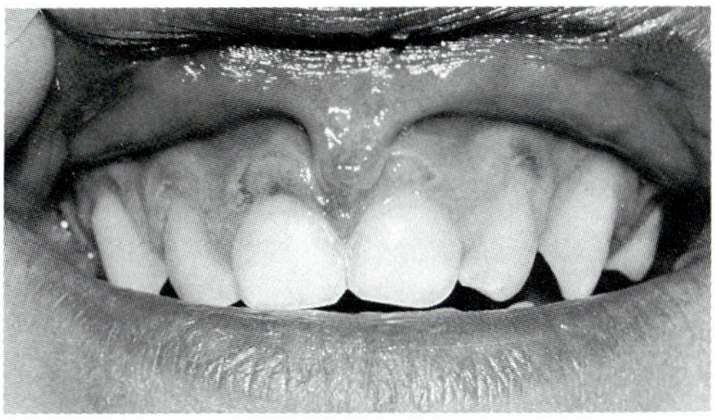

Figure 6.58. Factitial trauma; this 18-month-old patient has scraped away the marginal gingivae with his sharp fingernails.

Electrical burns are rare, with the exception of those purposefully done as part of therapy utilizing electrosurgery or electrocautery. A child biting into an electrical cord may get a severe irregular burn, with white slough on the lip. Treatment in this case would include plastic surgery.

There are other common lesions of the mucosa related to irritation and trauma that can also be considered as nonspecific bacterial infections. The oral flora is that group of bacteria that are normally present in the mouth and usually are nonpathogenic. These flora may exaggerate traumatic lesions, ulcers, and other conditions. The lesions listed below are at one time or another involved with these bacteria. Because there are many bacteria and no single microbial agent responsible, these infections are called nonspecific. In addition, because of their clinical appearance these same lesions can be considered tumorlike, because they are essentially swellings and resemble some tumors. In fact, however, they are inflammatory responses to irritation. The inflammation is longstanding, though, and so the component of hyperplasia is present and responsible for the tumorlike appearance.

Most of the time these inflammatory hyperplastic overgrowths occur on the gingivae. Therefore, they have been called epulides. An epulis is a swelling of the gingiva. Although most are caused by local irritation and may look alike, they have different names, depending on the microscopic diagnosis. Thus, an epulis may be: a pyogenic granuloma, a peripheral fibroma, a peripheral ossifying fibroma, a peripheral giant cell granuloma, a hemangioma, or granulation tissue, depending on the microscopic pattern.

The pyogenic granuloma is a common lesion that usually occurs on the labial gingiva, although it can occur anywhere in the mouth. Clinically, it is a nodular, raised, rounded mass with a red to purple hue, often with scattered white masses representing ulcerative zones. Bacteria are involved with these surface ulcerations and originally were thought to be the causative agent. (Pyogenic refers to pus-producing organisms.) The growth is, in fact, an overgrowth of granulation tissue, accounting for the red color and for the ease of bleeding. The treatment is surgical removal; sometimes the lesions recur (Fig. 6.59).

Pregnancy tumors are pyogenic granulomas that occur on the gingiva of pregnant women. They have the same clinical appearance and undoubtedly are responses to local irritation. The gingiva in pregnant women can have an exaggerated response to irritants such as calculus. Unless the lesions are particularly bothersome, they are effectively removed following delivery. They are not true tumors and are not premalignant.

Following the extraction of teeth, there may be an exuberant inflammatory response in the socket site. Frequently a lesion similar to the pyogenic granuloma is seen protruding from the socket like a raspberry. These are called epulis granulomatosa or granulation tissue, and often foreign bodies are noted within them. They bleed readily. Simple surgical removal is the treatment.

Peripheral giant cell granuloma or giant cell epulis is a red, blue, raised firm swelling occurring only on the gingiva (Fig. 6.60). It resembles the pyogenic granuloma and differs only histologically in that numerous giant cells are found scattered throughout the granulation tissue. It appears suddenly and rapidly increases in size. Treatment is surgical removal. They also may recur. The term peripheral is used because there is a similar histologic lesion that can occur within the jaw, in which instance it is termed central giant cell granuloma. When it occurs in the bone there is a cystic appearance on the radiograph.

Besides the denture ulcer, an ill-fitting

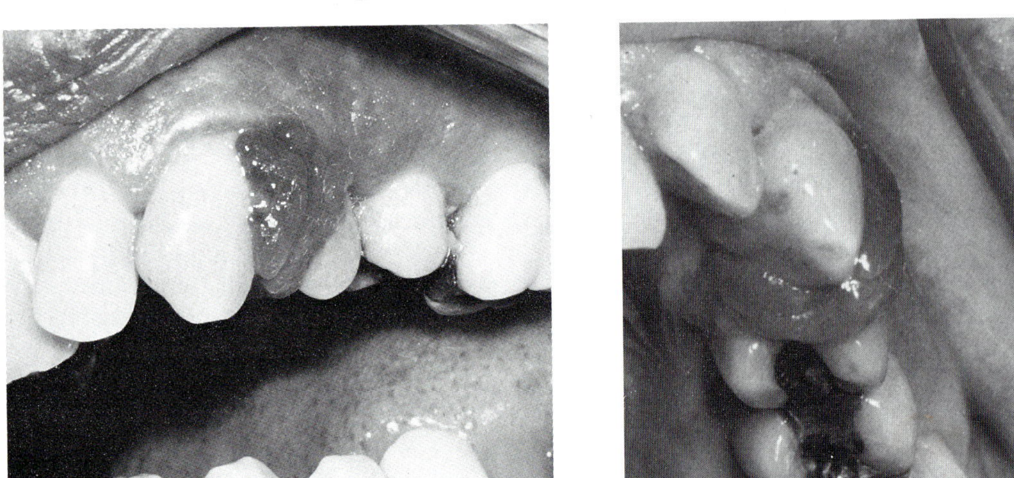

Figure 6.59. Epulis. Microscopically, a pyogenic granuloma. This red lesion grew rapidly and bled easily (two views of same patient).

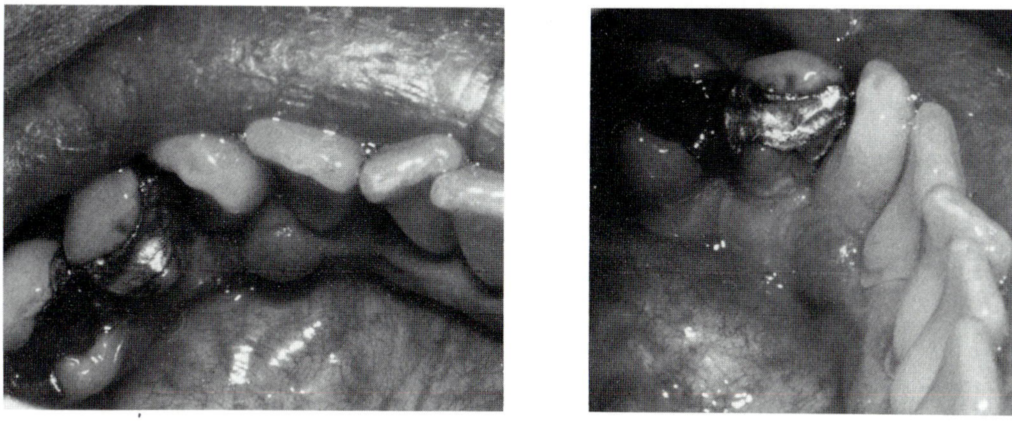

Figure 6.60. Epulis, gingiva lingual to mandibular canine and lateral incisor. A peripheral giant cell granuloma, this was blue-purple like a hemangioma (two views of same patient).

denture is responsible for two common hyperplastic and tumorlike lesions. Epulis fissuratum or denture hyperplasia represents the reaction of the tissue at the flanges or peripheral borders of a loose denture (Figs. 6.61 to 6.63). The tissue appears as red, flabby, grooved folds, running along the margins of the denture. Often the patients give a history of not having had an adjustment of the denture when it was first inserted. It is also often seen when the patient has a maxillary denture and mandibular anterior teeth but no posterior teeth. Then every time the patient bites, the mandibular anterior teeth cause the maxillary denture to move in the anterior area, thus producing the hyperplastic tissue. With an overextended margin, an ulcer develops. If the denture is not

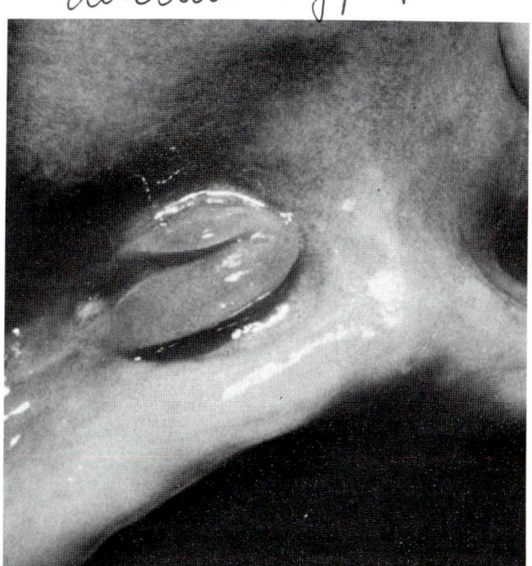

Figure 6.61. Epulis fissuratum, denture hyperplasia. Growth of tissue in labial sulcus corresponding to position of denture flange that caused the trauma.

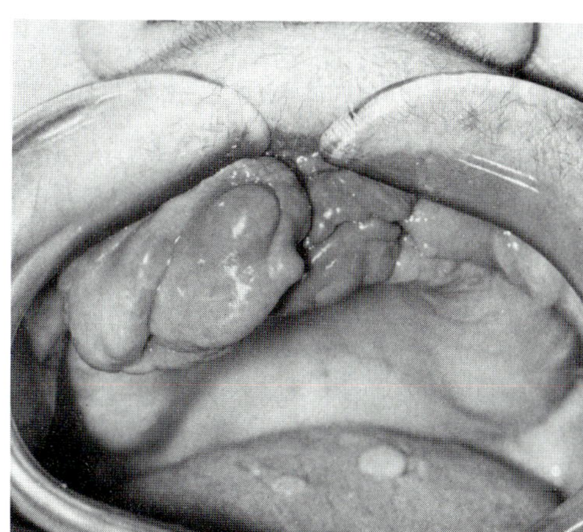

Figure 6.62. Epulis fissuratum, extensive overgrowth of flabby tissue related to poorly fitting denture.

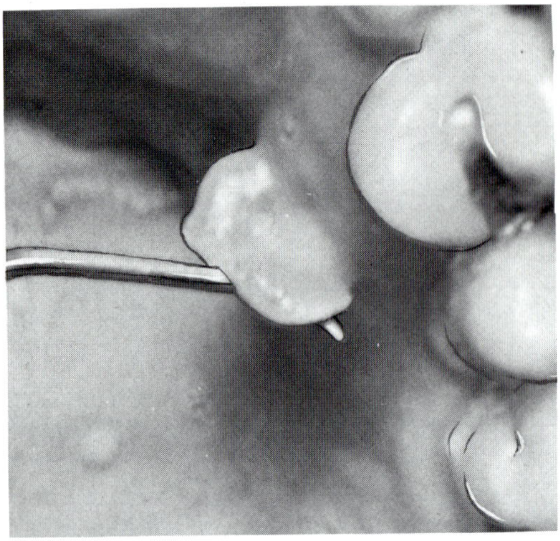

Figure 6.63. Denture hyperplasia. Inflammatory growth associated with a temporary acrylic appliance used to replace missing anterior incisors.

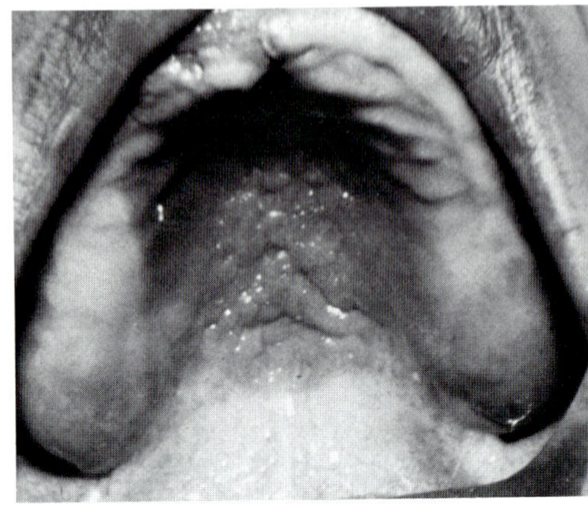

Figure 6.64. Inflammatory papillary hyperplasia, palate. Space between tissue and poorly adapted denture was filled in by this inflammatory growth.

corrected, the longstanding inflammation and continued trauma lead to the excess of tissue. The overgrowth is of both the epithelium and connective tissue, which is usually quite vascular, accounting for the red color. The treatment is surgical removal of the redundant folds and fabrication of a new, properly fitting denture.

Inflammatory papillary hyperplasia or papillary hyperplasia of the palate refers to a reddened palate with numerous small pebblelike projections or nodules, much like a raspberry (Fig. 6.64). It occurs mainly on the palate and is usually related to ill-fitting dentures and also to poor hygiene. Besides bacteria, fungal organisms (*Candida albicans*) may be found associated with the lesion. The growths are individual masses similar histologically to epulis fissuratum. Treatment consists of removal of the denture, after which the condition may subside and new dentures can be made. If the lesions do not subside, surgical excision is followed by the making of new dentures.

Pericoronitis is a common bacterial infection of the gingival tissue overlying the occlusal of an erupting or partially impacted tooth, usually a third molar. A pocket is created by the flap of tissue (operculum) over the tooth and around the crown (pericoronal) (Fig. 6.65). Food debris can lodge and set up an infection. The ensuing inflammation causes swelling. Often the opposing tooth compounds the problem by adding trauma to the tissue, and a cycle of irritation is set into motion. Young adults are mainly affected. There is swelling, extreme pain, some necrosis of marginal gingiva,

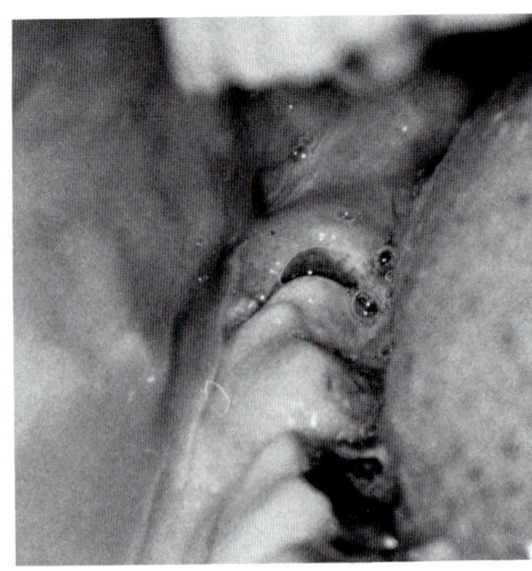

Figure 6.65. Pericoronitis. Note pocket and inflamed tissue distal to a newly erupted third molar.

and foul odor. Depending on host resistance, there can be fever, lymphadenopathy, spread of the infection, and pain referred to the ear from the mandibular tooth. Treatment consists of irrigation of the pocket area and frequent rinses with peroxide and water. Antibiotics may be necessary. A gingivectomy or extraction may eventually have to be done, because the condition tends to recur.

Specific bacterial infections of the oral cavity are rare. In these instances, the causative organisms are known specifically. The infections in the mouth may be due to bacteria acting locally to produce specific clinical lesions or acting systemically and yielding oral manifestations.

Acute necrotizing ulcerative gingivitis (ANUG) (i.e., necrotizing ulcerative gingivitis [NUG], ulceromembranous gingivitis, Vincent's infection, trench mouth) is a relatively common bacterial infection caused by anaerobic opportunistic pathogens. Not contagious, it is seen frequently in younger individuals such as students and armed forces personnel who share a common environment with many physical and emotional stresses. Besides life stress, other risk factors include smoking, poor nutrition, ascorbic acid deficiency, debilitating diseases such as cancer, and immune dysfunctions. ANUG may be familial; it is seen primarily in whites, but seldom in blacks despite the risk factors. With the tissue defense mechanism being lowered, as by stress, there is a likely reduction in blood flow to the gingivae and the interdental papillae in particular. This ischemia may change the local nutrient environment of the plaque. Specific organisms, normally in the plaque in smaller numbers, are nourished by the ischemic by-products, begin to proliferate, and contribute to the necrosis of the gingivae. The anaerobic bacteria are the fusospirochetal complex of *Fusobacterium* species and *Treponema* species, as well as *Bacteroides melaninogenicus intermedius* and *Actinomyces odontolyticus*.

Clinically, the manifestations are characteristic (Fig. 6.66). With a rapid or acute onset, the gingivae develop severely painful lesions characterized by necrosis of the interdental papillae that appear cut off with a white pseudomembrane at the apex and red and swollen at the base. Most often ANUG affects the labial surfaces of the lower incisors, but it may appear at any site and can spread to the marginal gingivae and other areas. In the palate, it can resemble a herpetic infection (Fig. 6.67). Because of the extensive necrosis, there is a

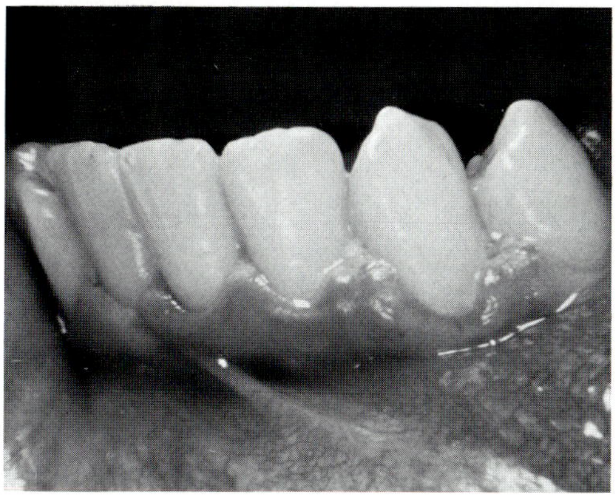

Figure 6.66. Acute necrotizing ulcerative gingivostomatitis (ANUG). Note a progression in severity of involvement from left to right. The interdental papillae become necrotic and disappear. A white pseudomembrane covers the ulcerated gingivae.

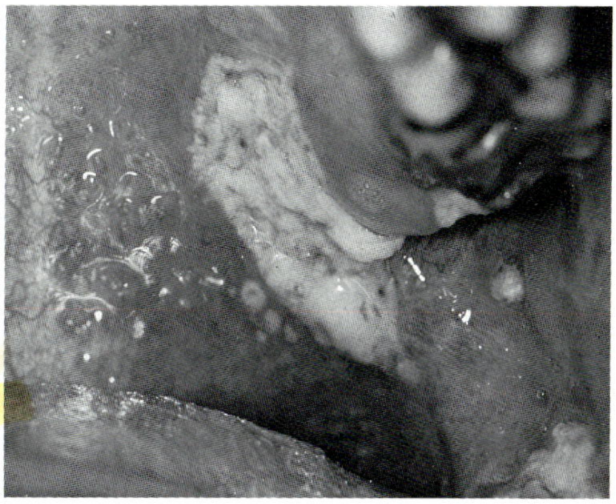

Figure 6.67. ANUG spread from gingivae to palate; note white pseudomembrane of necrotic tissue and erythema of palate, and not pericoronitis of upper and lower molars.

fetid odor and there may be a metallic taste. The teeth feel "wedged," and the gingivae bleed readily on probing. There can be a fever and lymphadenopathy with tenderness in the neck.

Treatment consists of several phases. First, the acute phase requires gross, superficial scaling and debridement with lavage, peroxide mouth rises, and aspirin or aspirin substitutes for control of the fever. The antibiotic metronidazole effectively controls the anaerobic organisms and resolves the infection. Following mechanical debridement, there must be further appointments for more scaling, along with advice on proper rest, oral hygiene, and diet until healing ensues. The interdental papillae usually regenerate, unless the condition was ignored and had become chronic. With repeated episodes there can be severe gingival destruction with no regeneration of the papillae and possible periodontal involvement.

Gangrenous stomatitis or noma is a severe complication of necrotizing stomatitis. Occurring in severely debilitated individuals with protein deficiency or in those being treated with chemotherapy, it is a fulminating infection starting in the mouth and necrotizing through to the facial surfaces. The major problem is malnutrition and debilitation.

Scarlet fever (scarlatina) is a streptococcal disease characterized by a skin rash and a stomatitis. The oral involvement consists of a severe sore throat with a fiery red pharynx and tonsils. The tongue is swollen, red, and coated because of the fever in this disease. The fungiform papillae, also swollen, appear red against the white background, resulting in the name "strawberry tongue." This appearance is not specific to scarlet fever, which is now infrequent since the arrival of penicillin. Scarlet fever is caused by a β-hemolytic streptococcus. Oral and throat infections by such bacteria are important to know about, because there can be serious postdisease complications. In some individuals there is a sensitization toward the organisms and, after the disease, the body reacts with an immune response that damages its own tissue. Rheumatic fever, kidney disease, meningitis, and subacute bacterial endocarditis may also follow a streptococcal infection.

Syphilis (Lues)

Syphilis is a systemic communicable disease that may have oral lesions. A bacterial infection, it is caused by a spirochete (*Treponema pallidum*—meaning a pale, twisting thread). A sexually transmitted or venereal disease (VD), the spirochetes are transmitted from one person to another by intimate sexual contact or by close body contact involving the sex organs, mouth, or rectum. The organisms are fragile and cannot live long in light and air; they require warm moist areas for survival. To enter the body, the spirochetes must penetrate mucosa or skin, usually through a wound or area that is not intact. The disease that may ensue has a natural course of three stages with two periods of remission if preventive measures are not taken (Table 6.1).

The primary stage is characterized by the appearance of a chancre (pronounced *shank*-er). This primary chancre develops at the site of initial inoculation about 2 weeks following intimate contact. Of the lesions, 90 percent occur on the genitalia and 10 percent occur in or about the mouth, on the lips, tongue, or palate. The chancre is a hard ulcer that clinically is nonspecific and resembles a traumatic ulcer (Fig. 6.68). However, it does contain organisms. Because of the hard ulcer, cancer is suspected rather than oral syphilis. The ulcer is usually painless and heals spontaneously in weeks. The bacteria spread throughout the bloodstream, and antibody titers begin to rise. A blood test may be either positive or negative at this time. With the disappearance of the chancre, there is a remission period of months during which time there are no signs or symptoms of disease, except that the organisms are in the blood and blood tests are positive. Besides the serologic tests, there are antibody tests, such as

Table 6.1.
Natural course of syphilis by stage with indications of oral, systemic, and serologic manifestations

Stages	Incubation Period	Primary Stage	Latent Period	Secondary Stage	Latent Period	Tertiary Stage
Time	3 weeks, (9-90 days)	3 weeks	3-6 weeks	6 weeks	Months-years	Years
Oral		Chancre (painless), lip, tongue, tonsil		Mucous patch, papule, rash, condyloma lata		Gumma, atrophic glossitis
Systemic		Adenopathy (painless) ? malaise		Adenopathy malaise syndromes (protean signs)		Cardiovascular disease; central nervous system discasc; other
Serology		−+	++	++++	+++	+−

the *Treponema* immobilization test, that are helpful in diagnosing syphilis.

The secondary stage follows the intermission and is characterized by a skin rash, fever, and illness. The skin rash is not distinct and is composed of numerous red macules and papules. These eruptions can occur in the mouth, usually on the palate (Figs. 6.69 and 6.70). The mucous patch is the other oral lesion of secondary syphilis. This is a silvery-white necrotic slough that is highly contagious. It mimics cancer, which is what is usually suspected. The lesions of this stage heal without treatment in several weeks. The blood tests at this stage are definitely positive. With the disappearance of the lesions there is a second period of remission; however, the disease persists. During this time, which can last from many months to several years, the

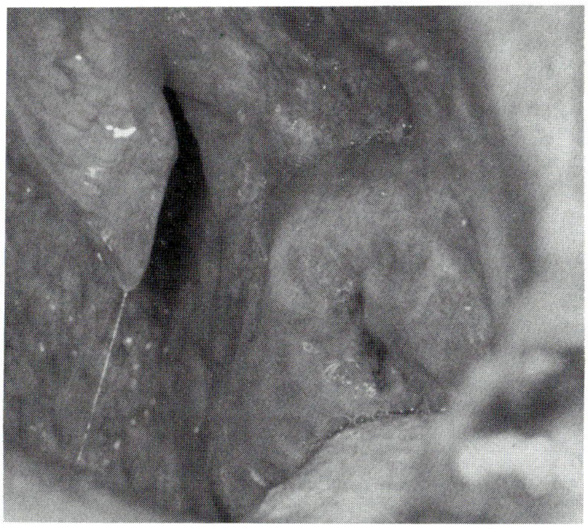

Figure 6.68. Primary syphilitic chancre of left palatine tonsil. The tonsil was very hard, painless, and ulcerated.

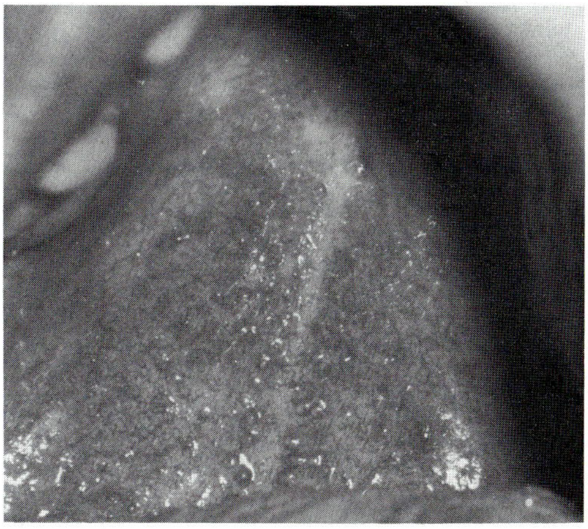

Figure 6.69. Secondary syphilis, oral rash of soft palate similar to herpangina. There was a maculopapular skin rash (see Fig. 2.65) including palmar and plantar lesions. Serology was positive.

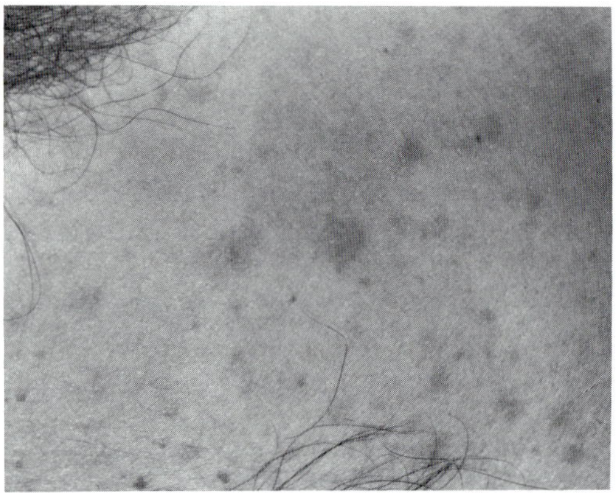

Figure 6.70. Macular skin rash, secondary syphilis.

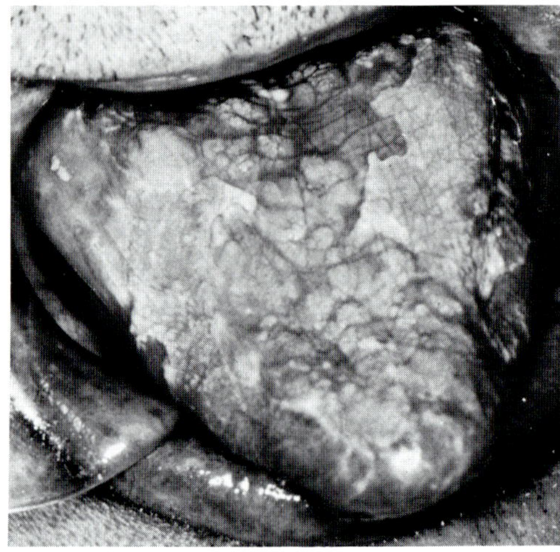

Figure 6.71. Atrophic glossitis of syphilis with leukoplakia.

spirochetes settle in various areas of the body and elicit a reaction that in one-third of the patients eventually results in severe damage. Because the oral lesions of primary and secondary syphilis are infectious and contagious, dental personnel should take precautions, such as wearing gloves.

The third stage of syphilis manifests itself primarily with changes in the nervous system and the heart. There is tissue destruction without regeneration, and patients suffer from insanity, lose motor control, and loss of balance. The aorta of the heart in some patients is damaged and causes heart disease. Besides these major findings, there can be oral lesions at this stage. One is atrophic glossitis. The tongue appears smooth, shiny, and bald owing to loss or atrophy of the papillae. A characteristic microscopic picture of syphilis is a perivascular endarteritis. The end arteries become damaged, undergo inflammation, and fail to regenerate, causing a loss of the epithelial specialized structures, the papillae. With the normal protection of the papillae being lost, the surface is prone to irritation, and white lesions develop (Fig. 6.71). Some of these areas may become cancerous.

The gumma is the other lesion of tertiary syphilis that can involve the oral cavity. They are most frequently seen on the palate. They begin as a nonhealing ulcer that usually is suspected for cancer. There is progressive and extensive replacement of tissue, and the destruction may cause a perforation through the soft tissue and bone of the hard palate, leaving a permanent opening from the mouth to the floor of the nose (Fig. 6.72).

In the tertiary stage the blood level of antibody usually decreases so that blood tests can be negative despite the presence of disease. The lesions are not contagious at this stage.

Syphilis can be treated effectively with penicillin. This antibiotic kills the spirochetes at any stage and stops the disease.

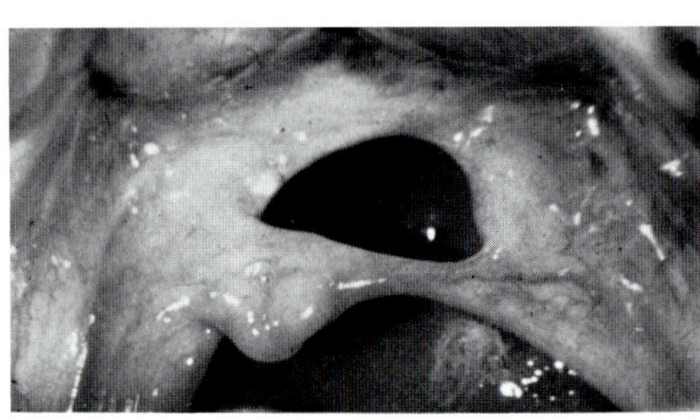

Figure 6.72. Gumma of soft palate, syphilis.

However, once the third stage is reached, the damage to nerve, heart, and other tissue continues on course despite treatment.

Syphilis can be prevented not only by antibiotics and other prophylactic measures but also by conscientious measures and adequate education at all age levels. Syphilis is not simply a bacterial disease. More so, it is a social disease. With better education and responsible social conscience, syphilis could be eliminated.

Congenital or prenatal syphilis is not venereal but is passed on to the fetus by an infected pregnant woman. If the woman is treated within the first 3 months of pregnancy, the fetus is not affected. After the first trimester the spirochetes pass the placental barrier and infect the fetus. If untreated, most often the disease is fulminating and causes death of the fetus with spontaneous abortion. In other cases, particularly in those fetuses infected later in pregnancy, the baby survives and is born with disease in its secondary or tertiary stages. Numerous organs and tissues can be affected during their development. Visible malformations of having had the disease linger for the life of the child and are called the stigmata of congenital syphilis. These occur in a large percentage, but certainly not in all, of those afflicted with the disease.

Some of these stigmata have been covered under enamel hypoplasia. There can be severe hypoplasia of the primary teeth. In the permanent teeth, Hutchinson's incisors, peg laterals, and mulberry molars can be seen. All are characterized by a decrease in the mesiodistal dimension or a narrowing at the biting surface. Besides these oral lesions, the lesions of tertiary syphilis may ultimately become noted. Sometimes puckering and folds due to scars around the mouth (rhagades) are visible. Bone defects are those manifested by a saddle-shaped nose (depression) and by frontal bossae or bone depressions of the forehead. As a sign of brain damage, the children may be mentally deficient.

Gonorrhea is one of the leading communicable diseases in the United States. Also a venereal disease, the gonococcus organism produces infection with pus. It can be responsible for sterility in women. Women can harbor the disease without signs. During birth the disease can be transmitted to the eyes of the newborn. For this reason silver nitrate drops are applied to the eyes of the newborn for prophylaxis. Gonorrhea is treated with antibiotics, but some strains are resistant. However, a vaccination will be available.

The oral lesions of gonorrhea are rare. They are so nonspecific that the suspicion of the disease must be raised by the patient. There may be irregular ulcerations and pharyngitis. Cultures can prove the diagnosis. The oral lesions disappear after antibiotic therapy for the urethral disease. Because the gonococci are anaerobic, there is little chance of transmission of the disease from oral lesions to the dental personnel.

Genital herpes, caused by herpes simplex type 2, is another common sexually transmitted disease. Its pathogenesis is similar to oral herpes (herpes simplex type 1), in that there may be primary disease and secondary disease caused by reactivation of the dormant virus despite the presence of antibodies. The genital lesions may be transmitted to the oral cavity where vesicles would rupture and a herpetiform ulcer would appear. Likewise, oral herpes may be transmitted to the genitalia.

Tuberculosis

Tuberculosis is an ancient disease caused by the tubercle bacillus, *Mycobacterium tuberculosis*. Whereas in the past it was feared (in 1900, it was the major cause of death) and a disease of social stigma, today it is well controlled because of antibiotics and the centers that were originally established primarily to treat tuberculosis are treating other diseases. Tuberculosis is primarily a disease affecting the lungs; however, it can involve many other organs. The oral lesions are rare and, except when the disease is contracted from unpasteurized milk, the oral lesions are secondary to lesions in the lung.

Three strains that can infect humans are the human, the bovine (cattle), and the avian (bird). With the advent of pasteurization, it is primarily the human strain that involves people. The bacteria are passed by air through dirt, dust, or continued close contact. They settle in the lung, and the body usually reacts with an inflammatory response that effectively seals off the affected area with fibrosis. This can be seen on a chest radiograph and is a sign of primary contact with the organism. Skin testing may reveal a positive response in many individuals, particularly those living in crowded areas of the city. If the defenses of the body are inadequate on primary contact or with secondary infection, because of an increased sensitivity to the organism, severe damage can take place. The disease can spread in the lung and to the lymph nodes. The organisms are rods with a waxy capsule. By special stain, they appear red or acid-fast. The normal inflammatory response is ineffective, and the bacilli cause death of the host cells. Microscopically, granulomas are formed. These are areas of central necrosis in which host tissue is destroyed. Macrophages attempt to ingest the bacteria and form a wall around it. Some of them group together to form giant cells called Langhans' giant cells because the nuclei are placed at the periphery of the cell. Special stains may indicate the tubercle bacillus in the cytoplasm of these cells. Also in the granuloma are lymphocytes signifying an immune response and fibroblasts to lay down collagen in an attempt to wall off the response. It presents a specialized picture of chronic inflammation, so that microscopic sections can often suggest the presence of tuberculosis. If the host resistance is good, the damage is localized; otherwise it spreads. The necrosis of tissue is called caseation necrosis, because clinically it looks like a white cheese. This eventually leaves a cavity in the lung tissue. If it breaks through blood vessels and a bronchus, there is a spitting of blood and coughing up of organisms for further spread.

The oral lesions are usually ulcers but may be granulomatous, bumpy, nodular masses. They are nonhealing, persistent ulcers and cancer is usually suspected (Fig. 6.73). A biopsy reveals that it is not cancer but a granulomatous disease with Langhans' giant cells. If tuberculosis was not known to occur in the patient, further laboratory studies would undoubtedly reveal pulmonary tuberculosis. Tuberculosis may affect lateral neck lymph nodes draining from the oral cavity or a possible jaw lesion. Tuberculosis of a cervical lymph node is called scrofula and presents as a swollen gland by the lower border of the mandible (Fig. 6.74).

Tuberculosis is treated by some isolation, prolonged rest, and the use of appropriate antibiotics combining to effectively reduce the morbidity and mortality of this once major disease.

There are several other granulomatous diseases, some caused by specific organisms, others by foreign materials. Except for foreign body reactions, the other diseases are rare in the oral cavity (histoplasmosis, blastomycosis, sarcoidosis). When they do manifest, there are longstanding

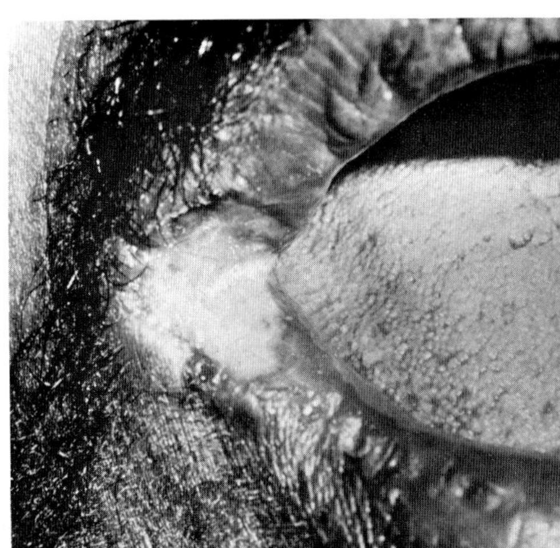

Figure 6.73. A nonhealing ulcer at the commissure of the lips that on biopsy was a tuberculous ulcer. The patient was then found to have active tuberculosis of the lungs.

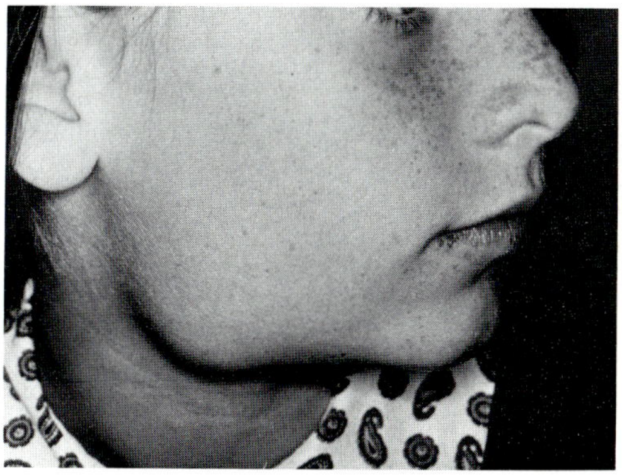

Figure 6.74. Swelling at angle of mandible, firm, movable. On investigation it proved to be a tuberculous lymph node, scrofula.

lumps, fissures, pebbly or erythematous areas. There is suspicion of cancer and the biopsy shows chronic granulomatous disease. Further testing helps to make a definitive diagnosis. The foreign body reaction is the most common granulomatous disease process of the oral cavity.

Mucocele

Mucoceles (mucous retention phenomenon) are nodular tumorlike masses caused by some traumatic incident to the mucosa and the minor salivary glands in particular. The oral cavity has numerous clusters of mucous glands with ducts that normally excrete the mucus onto the surface, maintaining a moist atmosphere, accounting for the term mucous membrane. In addition, the oral cavity is the site of frequent trauma, which is the leading etiologic factor in many lesions of the mouth. Whereas other lesions created by trauma may have a bacterial component due to secondary infection, mucoceles do not unless surface ulceration occurs.

Mucoceles are common lesions and are diagnosed usually by their clinical appearance. They consist of a soft fluctuant bluish or translucent swelling that can vary in size from a few millimeters to several centimeters. They occur most frequently on the lower lip but may be seen on the buccal mucosa, floor of the mouth, palate, upper lip, and tongue (Figs. 6.75 and 6.76). All age groups are affected, but mucoceles are seen most frequently in children and young adults. The cause is some traumatic injury with the severance of a duct or ducts. The mucus pours into and collects in the adjacent connective tissue rather than the surface of the mucosa. The mucus is foreign to the connective tissue, and the body mounts an inflammatory response with granulation tissue to wall it off. A cystlike space filled with mucus is formed, but a

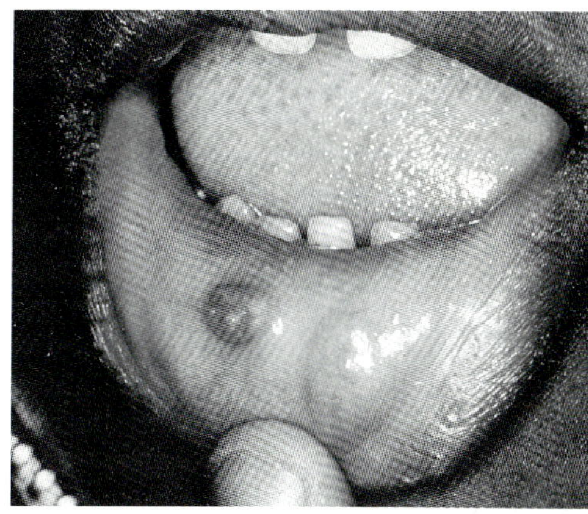

Figure 6.75. Mucocele, inner aspect of lip in a child; the lesion had swelled up and subsided and contained fluid.

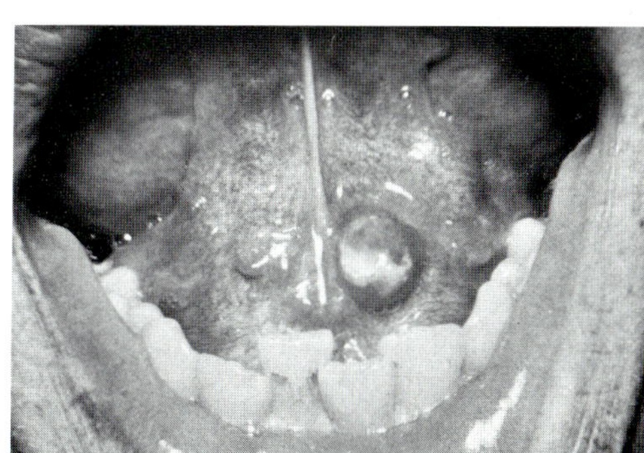

Figure 6.76. Mucocele, floor of mouth at Wharton's duct. Trauma has caused a white lesion on the surface of the soft fluctuant swelling.

mucocele is not a cyst because there is no epithelial lining. Clinically, the fluctuant (fluid motion in a cavity) swelling appears clear like a vesicle if the fluid accumulation is close to the surface epithelium. If the mucus collects deeper in the connective tissue, the swelling appears bluish and may resemble a hemangioma or other blue-black lesion. Often there is a history of swelling, spontaneous rupture, and subsequent swelling. The treatment is adequate surgical removal that should include the associated glands.

A *ranula* is a large mucocele in the lateral aspect of the floor of the mouth arising from a blocked sublingual gland duct (Fig. 6.77). It is called a ranula because of a clinical resemblance to the belly of a frog. The ranula can push the tongue up toward the palate or can dissect through the mylohyoid muscle into the neck (Fig. 6.78). It is treated surgically either by total or partial removal (marsupialization—removal of cystic contents and healing by secondary intention).

A swelling similar to a mucocele in the floor of the mouth (see Fig. 6.76) may be due to a stone within Wharton's duct (sialolithiasis). The patient may complain of pain (not a symptom of mucoceles) and a history that the gland and swelling enlarge while eating. An occlusal radiograph may reveal a round-to-oval opaque mass with concentric laminations (Fig. 6.79). If raised above the surface, it will be a yellow nodule beneath the stretched mucosa. Along with the blockage, there is a retrograde bacterial infection in the gland that undergoes pressure atrophy and fibrosis unless treated. The stone should be surgically removed and the infection treated with antibiotics. Sometimes, the gland has to be removed. Although the submandibular gland and duct are more commonly affected, any gland may be involved, major or minor.

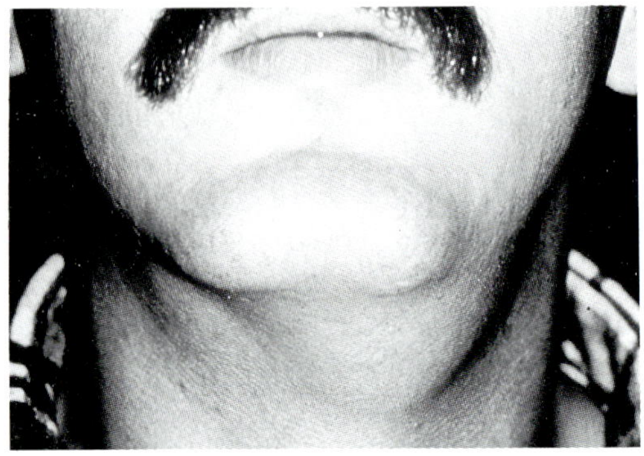

Figure 6.78. Mucocele presenting in lateral neck; dissected through the mylohyoid muscle from floor of mouth.

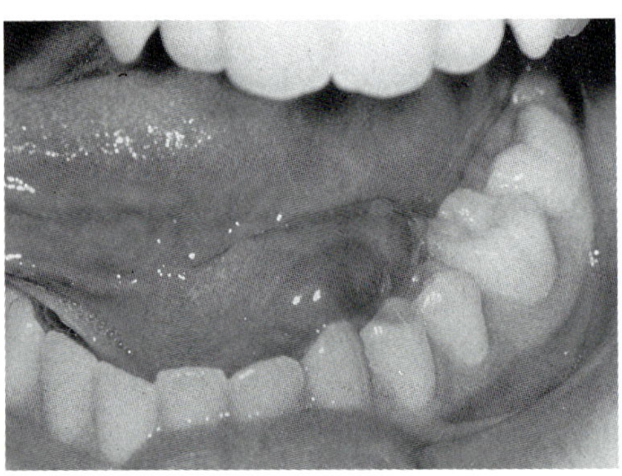

Figure 6.77. Ranula; mucocele, floor of mouth from severed duct of sublingual gland.

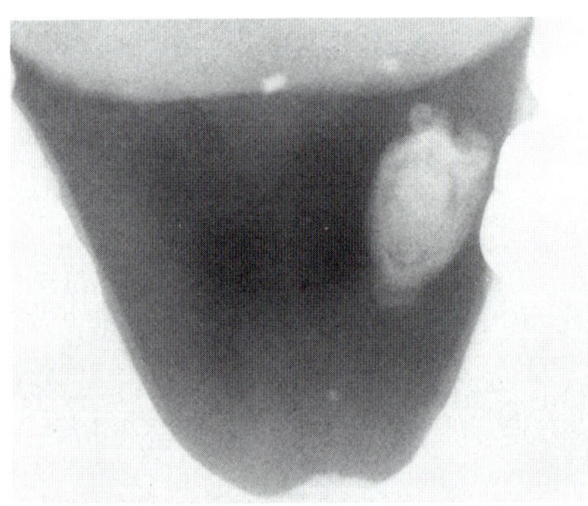

Figure 6.79. Sialolith, floor of mouth, blocking Wharton's duct, radiograph. Submandibular gland was painful and swollen.

Mycotic (Fungal) Infections

Fungi are small plants lacking chlorophyll. They are much larger than bacteria and vary in size and shape from round-to-oval cellular masses to long, slender, rodlike hyphae. They are found in plants and animals and generally live a symbiotic parasitic relationship. Fungi occur normally in the oral flora of humans. With a lowered resistance or change of the normal floral environment, these fungi can infect humans and cause disease. Other fungi, not normally present, may at times also be pathogenic.

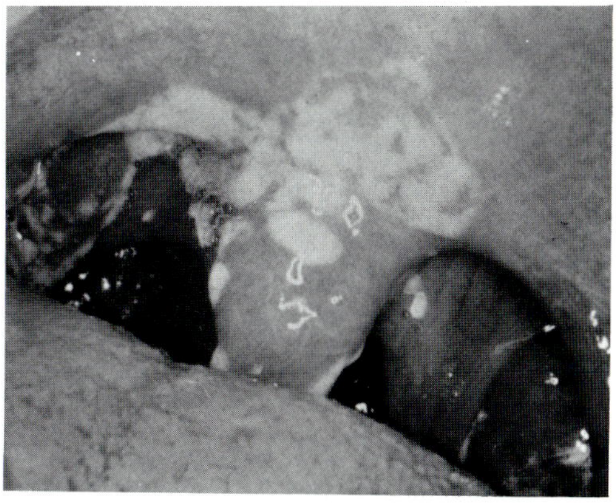

Figure 6.80. Candidiasis, thrush, soft palate and uvula. The white organisms resemble milk curds.

Candidiasis (Moniliasis; Thrush)

Candidiasis is a surface infection caused by a yeastlike fungus, *Candida albicans*. The name refers to the appearance of the growth being a glowing white, a characteristic that also places this infection in the category with "white lesions" (see below). The disease occurs essentially in three groups of people. In newborns and babies it is called thrush. The baby presumably contracts the fungus from the vaginal canal during birth. Perhaps the *Candida* flourishes because the oral flora is not well established in newborns, and proper balances among organisms have not been achieved as yet. The *Candida* flourishes, appearing as curds of milk on the membrane (Fig. 6.80). Young adults receiving antibiotics or with a lowered resistance are susceptible to candidiasis. The antibiotic presumably alters the content of the flora, and the fungus grows in excess. Other circumstances besides the antibiotic must also be responsible, because the incidence of the disease related to the administration of antibiotics is not high. Factors similar to those seen in necrotizing gingivitis are frequently present in cases of candidiasis in young adults. The last groups of individuals affected are debilitated adult patients, most commonly terminal cancer patients, but also those with longstanding disease. With a lowered resistance, the usually nonpathogenic *Candida* becomes infectious. Of note, it is common in diabetic patients. The organism flourishes with a lowered immune response, as in immunotherapy and the disease of AIDS. Where macrophages and T cells are affected, candidiasis occurs early and, as in AIDS, may be the first sign of the disease. It is the most common oral infection seen in patients with AIDS. Clinically, there are white, irregular, multiple patches that may be seen anywhere on the mucosa. The papular lesions represent the organisms growing in colonies and the necrotic epithelium that they are invading. Characteristically, these white areas can be wiped off, which is an aid in diagnosis (Fig. 6.81 and 6.82). The underlying and adjacent mucosa is usually red, after removal of white patches. At times candidiasis may resemble the lesions of lichen planus, another white lesion distinguishable because the white lesions cannot be wiped off. Besides being white, candidiasis may be red and white or just red, as in denture sore mouth. As mentioned in Chapter 4, candidiasis is a causative factor in central papillary atrophy of the tongue.

Candidiasis is treated with antifungal agents such as nystatin or gentian violet. Soothing mouthwashes and sometimes anesthetics may be required for pain and to aid eating.

Other fungal infections of the oral cavity are more rare than candidiasis. They usu-

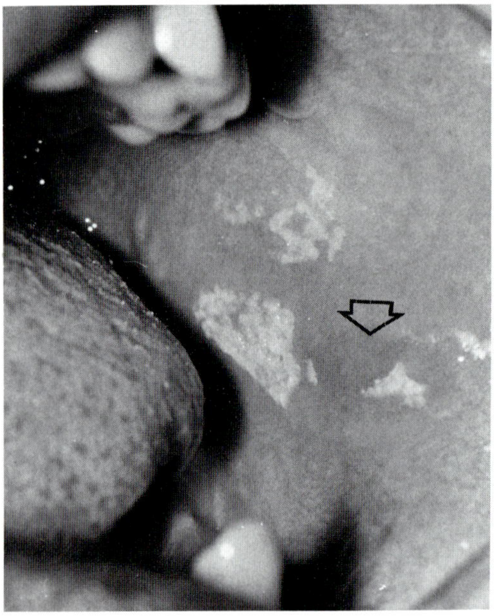

Figure 6.81. Candidiasis, buccal mucosa, in an adult female. The white lesions could be scraped away (*arrow*) and a smear was positive for fungal organisms.

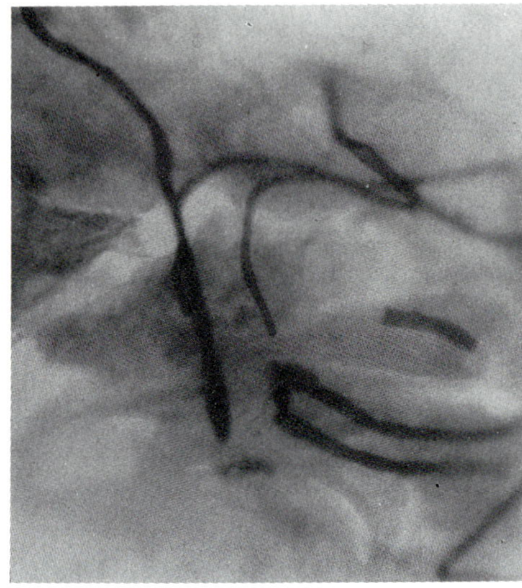

Figure 6.82. Oral cytology of a *Candida* infection showing multiple hyphae stained with PAS reaction.

ally are the deep fungal infections. They generally present as nonhealing ulcers suspicious for cancer and are diagnosed by biopsy and other studies, not by clinical appearance.

White Lesions

White lesions constitute that group of diseases and entities that clinically are characterized by being white or having some component that is white. The several possibilities of white lesions are listed along with pertinent features in Table 6.2. White lesions are visibly striking because they

Table 6.2.
White lesions

Lesion			
Simple hyperkeratosis Hyperkeratosis with dyspnea (premalignant) Carcinoma (malignant)	Leukoplakia; clinically not distinguishable	Keratototic lesions	Do not wipe off
Nicotinic stomatitis		Keratototic lesions	Do not wipe off
Lichen planus			Do not wipe off
White hairy tongue			Do not wipe off
Geographic tongue			Do not wipe off
White sponge nevus Leukoedema Fordyce's granules	Spongiosis	Bilateral	Do not wipe off
Gingival cysts of the newborn			Do not wipe off
Desquamative gingivitis			Wipe or rub off
Burns, ulcers, bullae (necrotic pseudomembranes)—most common			Wipe or rub off
Candidiasis			Wipe or rub off

stand out against the normal pink-red mucosa. Moreover, they are important because a white lesion may be premalignant or malignant.

The main subgroup of lesions commonly considered when a white lesion is seen or mentioned is that of the keratotic lesions. Among these are leukoplakia, nicotinic stomatitis, and lichen planus. Whereas the latter two clinically can be diagnosed easily because of their characteristic appearances, leukoplakia poses a problem because it may represent one of three separate keratotic conditions.

Leukoplakia is a clinical term indicating the presence of an abnormal white patch that is firmly adherent to the mucosa. It must be defined carefully, because it has been used to indicate only premalignancy. In this chapter, it is used as a clinical term only and refers to the lesions that present as white patches or areas. Accepting this, leukoplakia microscopically may be simple hyperkeratosis, hyperkeratosis with dysplasia, or actual carcinoma. Of oral carcinomas, 60 percent present as a white, keratotic lesion or are associated with such lesions. Consequently, white plaques are to be respected and held suspicious until a final diagnosis can be achieved. Further information on oral cancer is given in Chapter 7.

The white plaques of simple hyperkeratosis and hyperkeratosis with dysplasia are clinically indistinguishable. They appear as white, raised lesions that vary in size, shape, form, and consistency. They may be thin, almost transparent or thick, rough, and skinlike. Often they become stained by tobacco, coffee, tea, or other material. They cannot be scraped away or wiped off with a wooden tongue blade or spatula.

Histologically simple hyperkeratosis is an increase in the surface (corneal) layers accounting for the rough texture and white appearance. Depending on the lesion, the keratin layer may be a few layers in thickness or several—to the extent that the keratin or parakeratin layer is thicker than all the other layers of epithelium. By contrast hyperkeratosis with dysplasia contains other cellular changes. Besides a hyperkeratosis, there are the cellular changes of cancer within the epithelium. The only criterion that is lacking to call it cancer is that of invasion into the connective tissue. Because of these changes, hyperkeratosis with dysplasia is considered premalignant. Some dysplasia is irreversible so that at some future time the lesion will become a cancer. The length of time for this ultimate change to take place is not known. However, statistically, a significantly high percentage of dysplastic lesions do become cancerous if left untreated. Thus, this is a very important lesion to diagnose.

These keratotic lesions occur usually in males with a ratio of two males to one female. Usually the patients are about 40 years of age or older. However, depending on the cause, this is not a rigid fact. Generally there are no symptoms and the lesions are found on examination.

There are several causes and factors responsible for hyperkeratosis with and without dysplasia. The most common cause is some local irritation to the mucosa. These include the same factors responsible for trauma to the tissue. Some of these are biting habits, sharp objects such as denture teeth, clasp arms, worn facings on crowns, decayed teeth with sharp enamel edges, and unusual oral habits (Figs. 6.83 and 6.84). These irritate the mucosa, which builds a protection of keratin or parakeratin against the irritation. Another irritant is smoking, which has a drying effect on the mucosa. Cigars and pipes specifically affect the mouth. Cigars may cause a diffuse leukoplakia (Fig. 6.85). The pipe causes discrete lesions on the lower lip where the stem rests and on the soft palate where the smoke emits from the stem (Figs. 6.86 and 6.87). Cigarettes have their main effect on the lung system. The cilia of the bronchial tree become lost, and tars and chemicals build up in the lung. The individual becomes prone to serious diseases such as pneumonia, emphysema, bronchi-

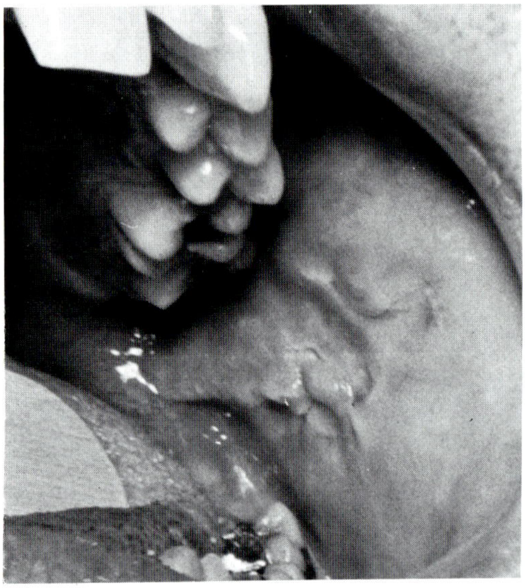

Figure 6.83. Cheek biting. Note many small nodular lesions and areas of leukoplakia.

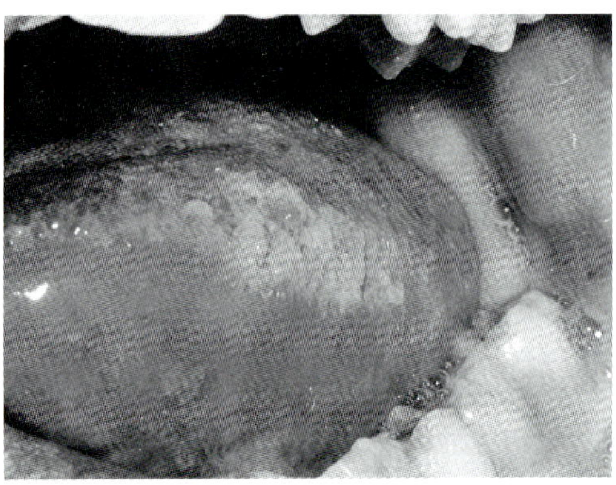

Figure 6.84. Diffuse hyperkeratosis of lateral border of tongue due to habit of biting and chewing on the tongue. (This pattern resembles hairy leukoplakia of AIDS.)

tis, and lung cancer. In addition, the oral mucosa is dried. The drying stimulates a growth of keratin for protection. Holding snuff against the mucosa can also cause similar changes. Nicotinic stomatitis is a clinically distinctive white lesion with simple hyperkeratosis that is specifically related to smoking. Some systemic diseases

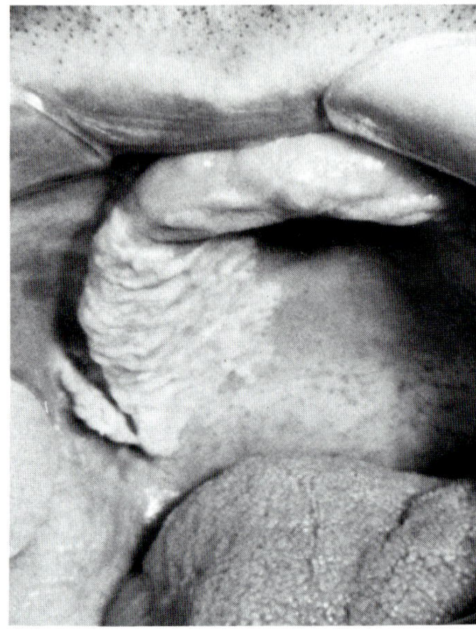

Figure 6.85. Diffuse leukoplakia in 45-year-old male who smokes 15 cigars per day. Biopsies have shown dysplasia.

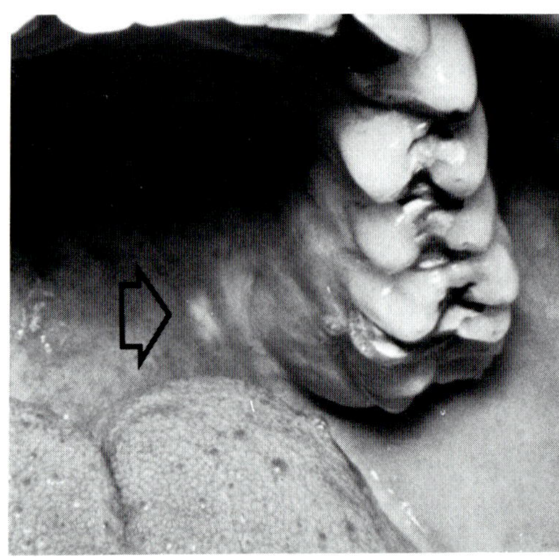

Figure 6.86. Leukoplakia, small discrete area of palate (*arrow*) in a pipe smoker, resulting from smoke and heat emitted at this area.

have oral manifestations that allow the mucosa to be sensitive to irritants. Syphilis (atrophic glossitis) and the anemias may result in a smooth bald tongue devoid of the

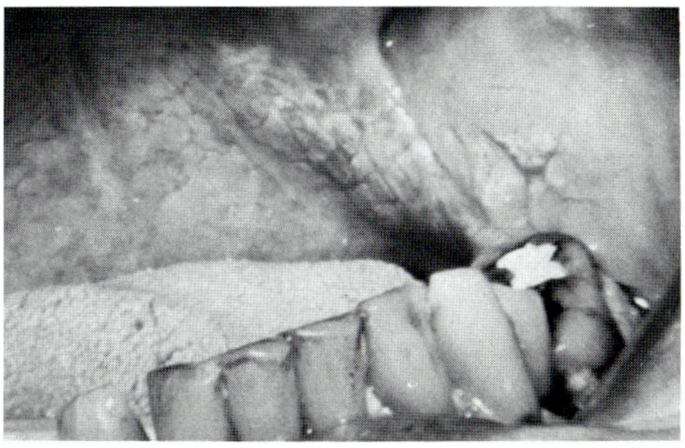

Figure 6.87. Diffuse leukoplakia, soft palate, buccal mucosa in a pipe smoker. Biopsy revealed changes of hyperkeratosis.

papillae that normally protect the dorsal surface. Frequently leukoplakia can be seen on these tongues, presumably a response to irritants.

Hairy leukoplakia is a white lesion, usually on the lateral border of the tongue, that does not rub off and has characteristic histologic features of hyperkeratosis, vacuolated (viral-induced) cells and a lack of inflammatory cells. It may occur bilaterally and can resemble fungal disease but does not respond to fungal therapy. It can respond to antiviral therapy and may regress spontaneously. It is consistently associated with HIV infection, is predictive of AIDS, and serves as a marker for AIDS. The Epstein-Barr virus appears to be etiologic.

The second most common cause of hyperkeratosis is idiopathic, because often no responsible irritant or sustaining factor can be found. Other factors may also play a role in the development of the simple or nonmalignant and premalignant hyperkeratosis. In women, hormonal disturbances may play a role. At menopause with a decrease in estrogen, some women develop areas of leukoplakia. A nutritional deficiency of vitamin A may cause white lesions in rare instances. Heredity probably plays a supporting role, since many of the factors mentioned may not cause changes in some individuals as they do in others who may be predisposed by a hereditary pattern.

The treatment for leukoplakia depends on the final microscopic diagnosis. A diligent effort should be made to find a source of irritation since that is the most common cause. If one can be found, the cause should be removed. Simple hyperkeratosis disappears usually on removal of the cause (Fig. 6.88 and 6.89). If a cause cannot be found or the lesion still persists 2 weeks after an attempt to remove it, a biopsy, either excisional or incisional, should be

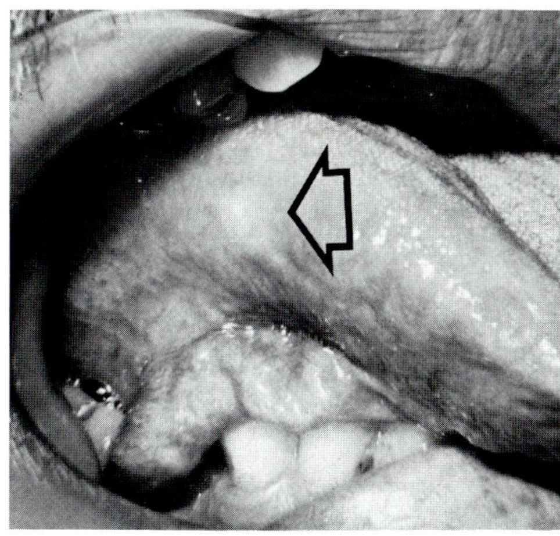

Figure 6.88. Leukoplakia, middle, lateral border of tongue (*arrow*). Patient rubbed tongue on sharp surfaces on lingual aspect of lower teeth.

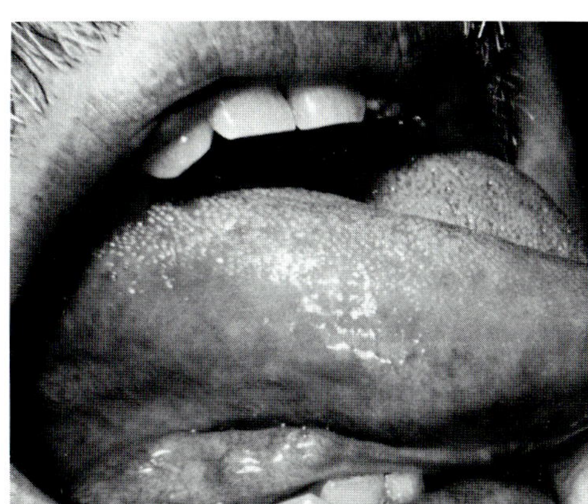

Figure 6.89. Same patient as in Figure 6.88, 1 week after the rough teeth were smoothed. The area of leukoplakia has disappeared.

done. If the microscopic diagnosis is simple hyperkeratosis, continue to search for a cause and remove it. The lesion should disappear. For hyperkeratosis with dysplasia, the lesion should be removed surgically with adequate margins. Any persistent white lesions should be followed and biopsied to determine the microscopic type. Approximately 10 percent of the leukoplakias excluding carcinomas are dysplastic, and 90 percent are simple lesions. However, clinically, they can look alike.

Nicotinic stomatitis is a white, hyperkeratotic lesion related, as the name implies, to the use of tobacco (Fig. 6.90). It is usually seen on the palate in smokers as numerous papules that are white with a central pink, slightly depressed dot. These red areas represent the opening of inflamed and plugged mucous ducts. The white areas represent the hyperkeratosis. These lesions may have a diffuse white background or may be associated with red areas. The palate may have an overall wrinkled effect (Fig. 6.91). A similar response may be seen in snuff holders, usually on the inner aspect of the lower lip or buccal vestibule (Fig. 6.92). In these cases there may be no papules, but the inflamed ductal openings stand out against the whitened background. The treatment includes removal of the smoking or snuff. The lesions are watched carefully to observe their disappearance. If any white lesions persist, a biopsy is necessary to rule out or to confirm premalignancy or malignancy.

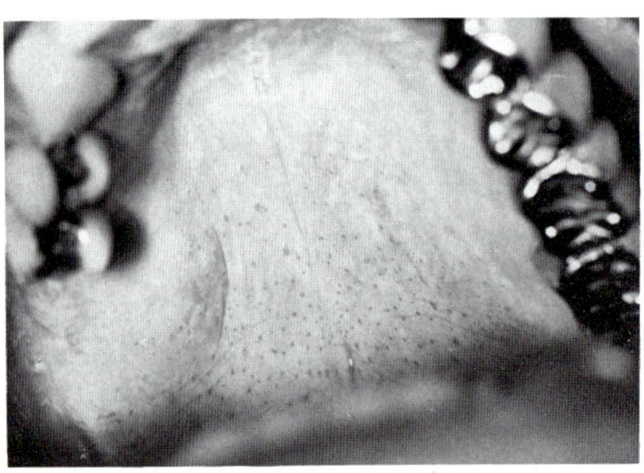

Figure 6.90. Nicotinic stomatitis, hard palate in a cigarette smoker. Note diffuse white background and multiple small areas corresponding to openings at inflamed mucous ducts.

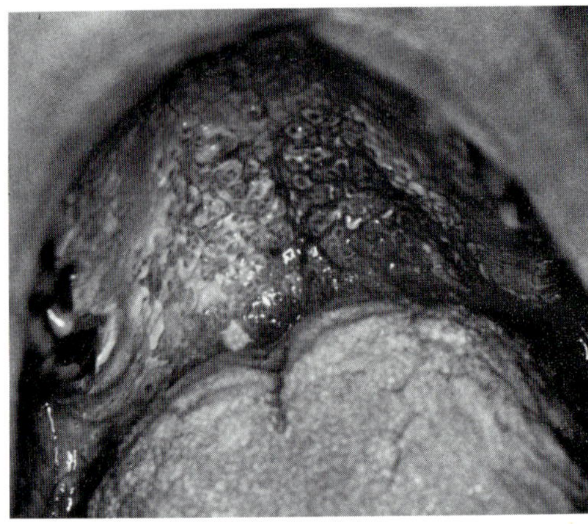

Figure 6.91. Nicotinic stomatitis, hard palate, severe involvement with red and white areas. Several biopsies revealed dysplastic changes.

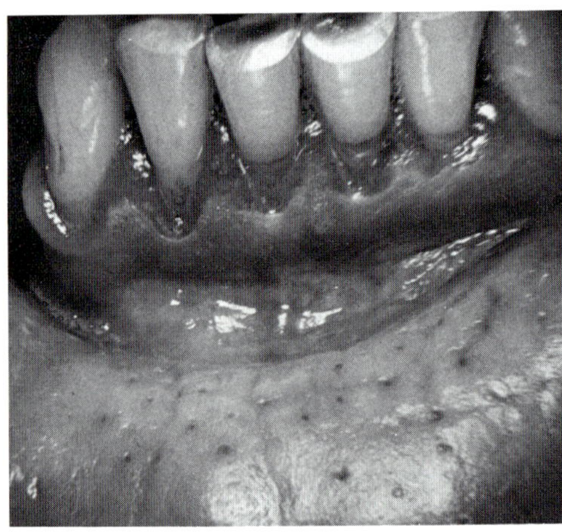

Figure 6.92. Nicotinic stomatitis, lower lip, in a snuff holder. Note leukoplakia and openings of inflamed mucous ducts.

Lichen Planus

Lichen planus is the other keratotic lesion that usually has a characteristic clinical appearance so that it can be diagnosed usually without biopsy. Lichen planus is a relatively common disease that affects the oral mucosa as well as the skin and is therefore considered a dermatologic disease. However, more often, there are oral manifestations without any skin lesions. The oral lesions consist of numerous tiny, white papules arranged in characteristic patterns. The lacelike pattern is most common and usually appears on the buccal mucosa, frequently on both sides (Fig. 6.93). The tongue, palate, gingiva (Fig. 6.94), and any other area may be affected. Other patterns are the circular, which on the tongue may mimic geographic tongue, and the plaque-like, which mimics leukoplakia and must be distinguished by biopsy (Fig. 6.95). The oral lesions usually are asymptomatic and are detected on routine oral examination. However, there is an erosive form of lichen planus that may cause discomfort. In these instances, characteristic lesions are usually seen at the edge of the erosive areas. The diagnosis is usually made by the clinical appearance. The coexistence of purple-violet papules on the flexor surfaces of the skin, chest, or genitalia may also be helpful in reaching a diagnosis. In those cases in which the clinical appearance is not characteristic and the lesions appear as a leukoplakia, biopsy is very helpful because lichen planus has a specific histologic appearance. Besides the hyperkeratotic surface, there is degeneration at the basement membrane area and a characteristic lymphocytic infiltrate congregated immediately adjacent to the epithelium. This pattern allows the pathologist to distinguish the disease as lichen planus.

Lichen planus is probably a psychosomatic disease, because there is usually some specific emotional event relating to the start of or the exacerbation of the disease. The actual cause is unknown. An immune disturbance is suspected. The disease is notable among diabetics. The treatment in most cases consists merely of diagnosis. The lesions may last for weeks, usually months, or even years. They eventually disappear with or without medication. Topical corticosteroids are very effective. Symptomatic treatment is required in erosive disease. Lichen planus is an innocuous

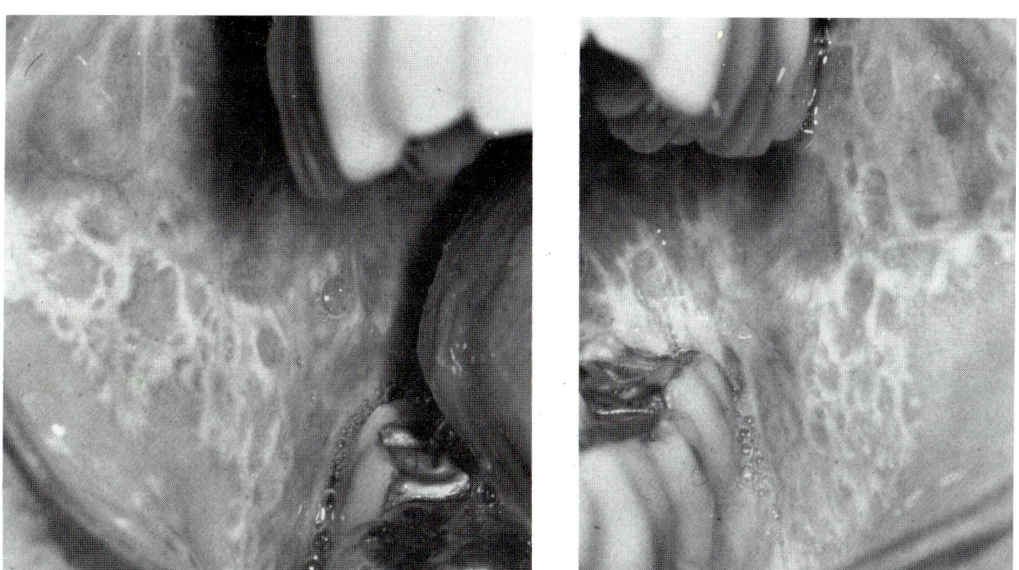

Figure 6.93. Lichen planus, white, keratotic, nonremovable lacelike lesions on both buccal mucosae. Two views of same patient, *A*, right side, and *B*, left side.

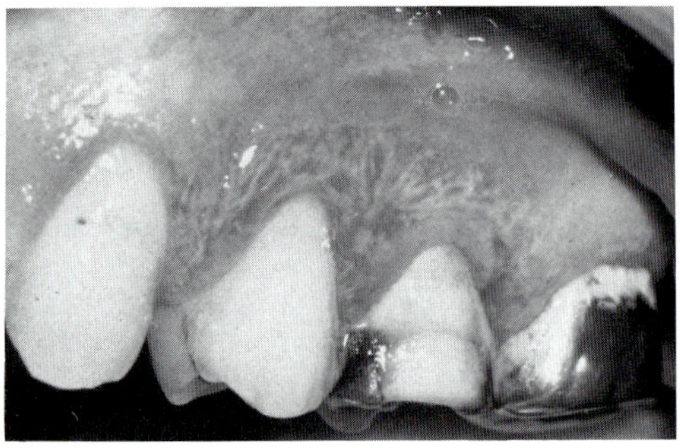

Figure 6.94. Lichen planus of attached gingivae. Note fine, lacelike pattern and red erosive background.

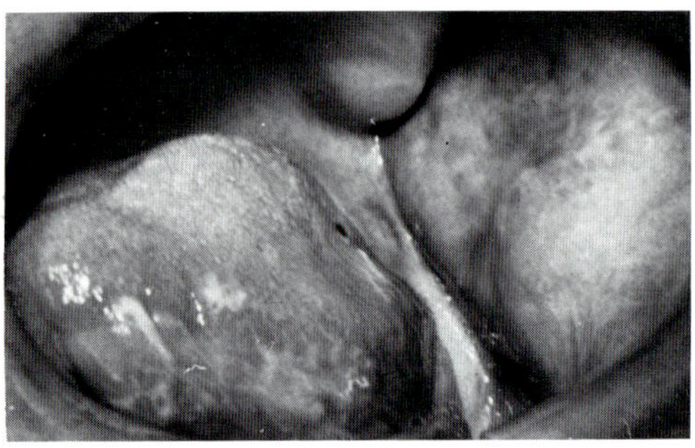

Figure 6.95. Lichen planus, buccal mucosa and tongue. Areas of leukoplakia occur along with a lacelike, linear pattern.

disease. Patients can be reassured that it is not cancer and is not serious.

Other White Lesions

White hairy tongue is a harmless condition in which the filiform papillae fail to shed normally and become elongated. The causes vary and include heavy smoking, antibiotic therapy, poor hygiene, emotional tension, and idiopathic factors. The mid-posterior dorsal surface is most often affected; however, the lateral borders may be involved. The "hairs" may pick up stains from bacteria, smoking, tea, coffee, or candies. Brushing the tongue aids in promoting removal.

Geographic tongue has white lesions at the periphery of the atrophic reddened areas. These desquamative and hyperkeratotic areas often assume circular patterns similar to lichen planus and traumatic glossitis from denture irritation. However, characteristically the atrophic areas heal in one area and appear in others—helping to distinguish this harmless condition from other white lesions.

White sponge nevus is a hereditary condition that presents as white, soft folds of tissue bilaterally mainly on the buccal mucosa, but also on the tongue and floor of the mouth. The white appearance is due to the spongiosis or fluid in the cells. It is usually diagnosed clinically on the basis of being bilateral and with the aid of a familial pattern. Biopsy would confirm the spongiosis and rule out hyperkeratosis.

Leukoedema also appears bilaterally on the buccal mucosa. There is a spongiosis of the spinous cells that yields a silvery, shiny white lesion with some wrinkles (Fig. 6.96). The linea alba is usually accentuated. Hyperkeratosis can be ruled out clinically by stretching the mucosa. When this is done the white lesion "disappears" (Fig. 6.97). Leukoedema is commonly seen in black patients. The cause is unknown. Some correlation exists between the severity of leukoedema and poorer oral hygiene. Leukoedema is essentially a normal condition and must be differentiated from the more serious white lesions.

Fordyce's granules (see Fig. 1.11, 1.16, and 4.15) are usually seen bilaterally on the buccal mucosa and on the lips. They may be noted as white or yellow-white submucosal clusters that appear more prominent when the tissue is stretched taut. They are normal sebaceous glands without hair follicles and occur so frequently they are considered normal. Sometimes a large cluster on the buccal mucosa concerns a cancerophobic patient. The patient should be reassured the granules are not cancerous. There is no treatment.

Gingival cysts of the newborn, commonly called Epstein's pearls, are mentioned here only because they are white lesions. They appear on the gingival pads

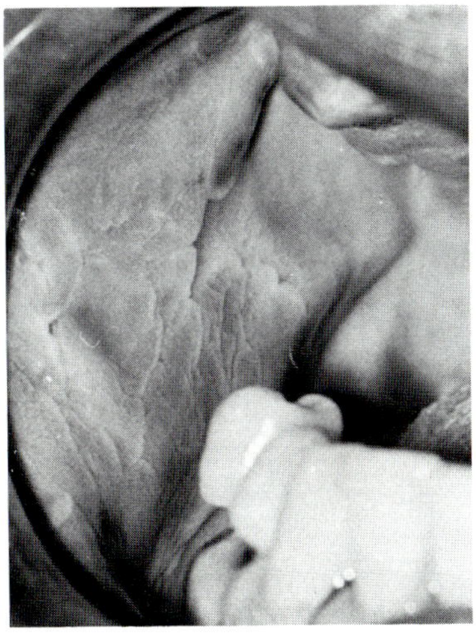

Figure 6.96. Leukoedema, buccal mucosa. Note folded, white spongy appearance.

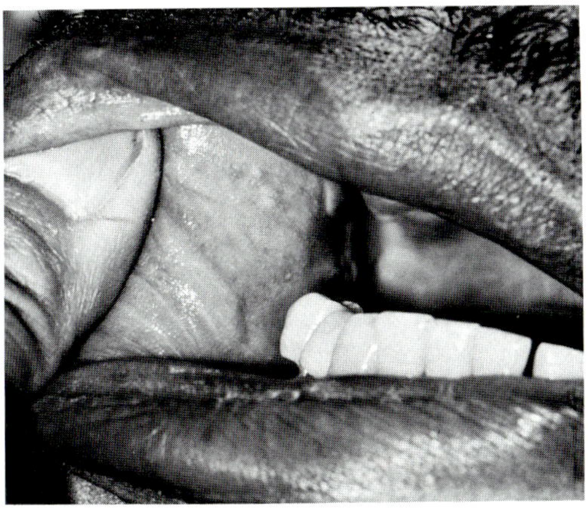

Figure 6.97. Leukoedema, same as in Figure 6.96. When tissue is stretched, the white disappears.

in infants, not adults (Fig. 6.98). These keratin cysts disappear spontaneously. Sometimes they mimic an erupting tooth.

The following group of white lesions can be distinguished readily from the keratotic variety because they can be wiped away with a wooden tongue blade or metal spatula.

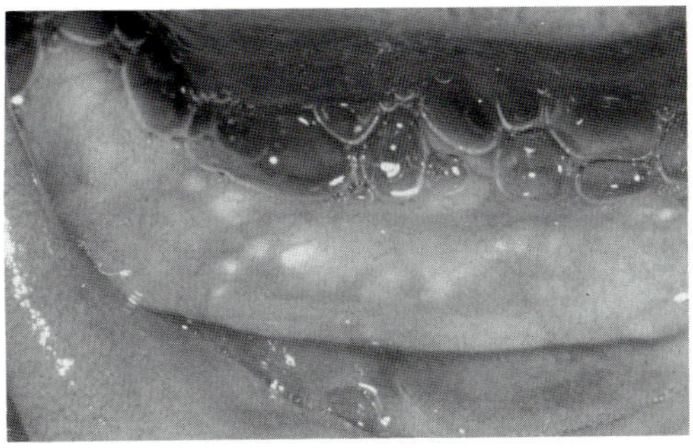

Figure 6.98. Gingival cysts of the newborn (Epstein's pearls) on gum pad of a 6-week-old boy.

Desquamative gingivitis is a condition seen primarily in women about the age of menopause. It may present as a burning sensation affecting the gingiva. There are erosive or red areas associated with white areas representing the desquamating epithelium that can be wiped away exposing more reddened areas. Desquamative gingivitis is actually a clinical term, because the condition can be seen in other diseases such as allergies and dermatologic-oral diseases.

Three diseases that can present with desquamative gingivitis are erosive lichen planus, mucous membrane pemphigoid, and pemphigus.

Pemphigus, like lichen planus, is a dermatologic disease with oral manifestations, but unlike lichen planus, it is quite serious because it is fatal if left untreated. Moreover, the oral lesions are often present before the skin lesions and afford the observer an opportunity to refer the patient for early diagnosis and treatment. It affects older patients of Jewish or Mediterranean origin. Pemphigus is an autoimmune disease affecting spinous cells. Large vesicles can form anywhere in the mouth and soon rupture. The necrotic epithelium is white and accounts for the white lesion against a red background (Fig. 6.99). The lesions may be seen on routine examination or are reported to have been present for some

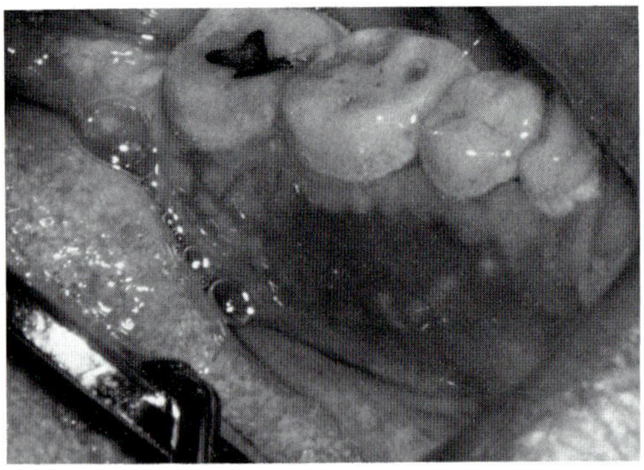

Figure 6.99. Pemphigus vulgaris, presenting as a desquamative gingivitis. Biopsy, smear, and other tests were positive.

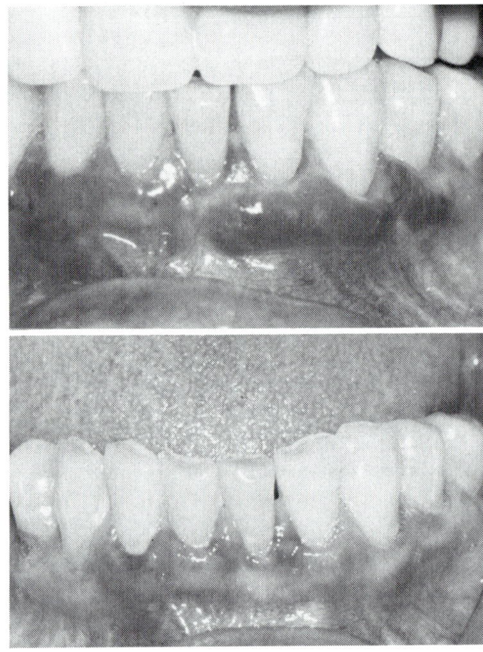

Figure 6.100. Mucous membrane pemphigoid. *A*, a desquamative gingivitis with blood-filled blisters in an older female. *B*, same patient showing improvement after treatment with topical corticosteroids.

time. As nonhealing ulcers and erosions, they should be suspicious. Biopsy is important, because pemphigus has a specific microscopic picture. Besides intense chronic inflammation, there is an intraepithelial vesiculation and acantholysis. This can be contrasted with other bullous and erosive diseases that have subepithelial vesicles. Pemphigus can be debilitating and fatal, because the lesions on the skin ulcerate and expose a large surface area, with loss of fluids similar to third degree burns. It can be effectively treated by immunotherapy.

Mucous membrane pemphigoid affects older women with blisters primarily on the gingivae and other areas such as the palate (Fig. 6.100). An autoimmune disease, it shows subepithelial blistering with antigen–antibody complexes in the basement membrane zone. The skin may be involved as well as the conjunctiva, in which case scarring may lead to blindness. Thus, corticosteroid therapy is required.

Another dermatologic-oral disease with sloughing white blisters is erythema multiforme. An acute condition, it is characterized by lip lesions that crust on the skin side. Within the mouth, the lesions are white from necrotic epithelium and red. On the skin, there may be a rash in many forms (multiforme), including a lesion with concentric rings (target lesion) (Fig. 6.101). The genitalia may be involved. When the

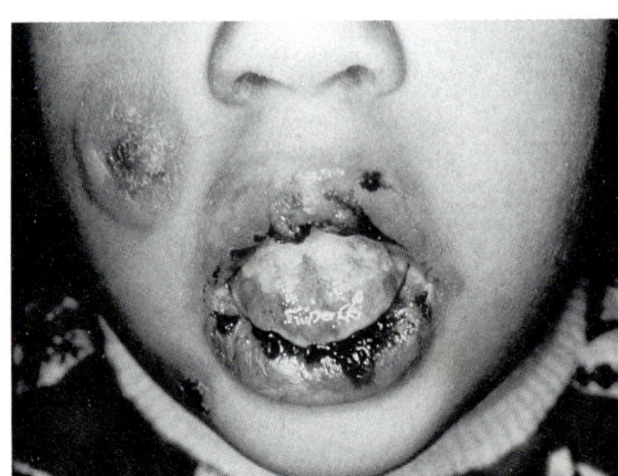

Figure 6.101. Erythema multiforme. Target lesion on skin of face; crusting bullous lesions on lips and blisters on a hairy tongue. The patient was allergic to aspirin and had multiple episodes.

disease is severe and the conjunctiva are involved, it is called Stevens-Johnson syndrome. The cause is unknown, but usually there is an allergen or hypersensitivity state. If discovered, the allergen should be removed; otherwise there will be recurrences. The use of corticosteroids is effective even though the disease is self-limiting and spontaneously regresses with supportive therapy.

Burns, ulcers, and other lesions with a white, necrotic surface or pseudomembrane constitute the most common group of white lesions. The white part of the lesion wipes off and leaves a raw surface. This fact, plus additional history and clinical features, usually distinguish them from the keratotic lesions. On the other hand, there are serious diseases among this group. Oral cancer may present as an ulcer.

Chapter 7
BENIGN AND MALIGNANT CONDITIONS

Neoplasia

An introduction to neoplasia was presented in Chapter 2. This section offers further clarification and some details of a most complex aspect of pathology.

The term neoplasia refers to a new growth of tissue. If growth of tissue relating to developmental and inflammatory hyperplasia is excluded, there are essentially two categories of neoplasia—benign and malignant. Any tissue of the body that is capable of dividing is capable of developing a neoplasia, a basic tissue response to various stimuli, in which the growth control mechanism is defective. The resulting growth may show cellular changes with little, if any, variation in morphology or behavior from the normal. This is one extreme of a large spectrum of changes that may occur. At the other extreme, the cells may not resemble or behave like the cells of origin, in which case they are called poorly differentiated. Thus, new growth may be hyperplastic; if the cause is removed, the growth of normal tissue stops. The growth may be abnormal: With little variation from the normal, it is benign; with marked variation, it is malignant.

Benign growths are those that are not malignant or highly injurious. Their cells resemble those of the tissue of origin. They are usually slow growing, encroaching on normal tissue as they expand. With expansion, a connective tissue capsule develops around them and the growth remains localized. Usually the removal of them is straightforward, recovery is favorable, and they do not recur. However, as a growth they create a mass that must be distinguished from a malignant growth (Fig. 7.1).

Malignant growths, by contrast, are highly injurious. Their cells are atypical and deviate markedly from the cells of origin. The nuclei are usually enlarged and occupy more of the cell than normal. The cell size is often enlarged, and there may be giant cell formation. The cells may lose all resemblance to the normal cells and cannot be recognized (anaplasia). Numerous mitotic figures account for the rapid growth. Some of these mitoses may be abnormal. The cells lose contact with one another, and the arrangement of cells is disorderly. They

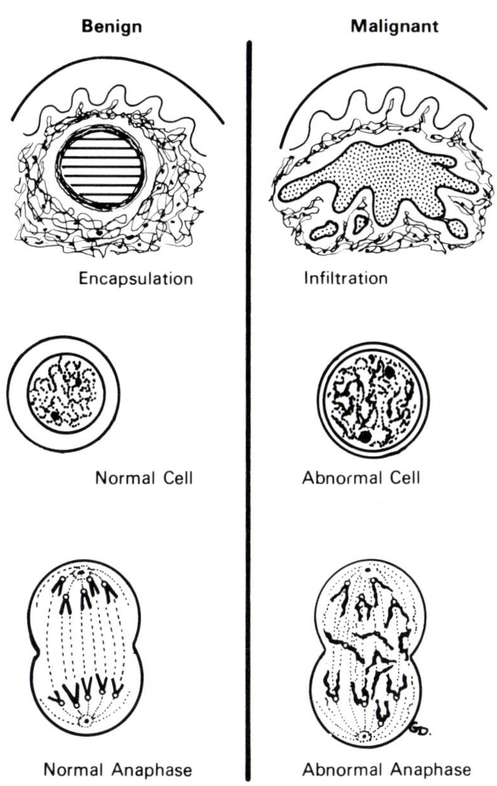

Figure 7.1. Diagram comparing features of benign and malignant tumors

grow by infiltration and invasion into the surrounding normal tissue. No capsule is formed; there is no localization. The hallmark of a malignant growth is its capacity to spread, i.e., metastasize. The growth may spread directly by extension, by sending cells into the lymphatic or vascular channels. The cells may grow at a distant site but generally do so at sites of preference, usually related to a rich blood supply. Thus, the lung is a frequent site for metastasis. Breast and prostatic malignancies metastasize to bones. Consequently, a radiolucency in the jaw can be due to a metastasis. Because of metastasis, the treatment of a malignancy is not straightforward and recovery is not always favorable. The prognosis depends upon the extent of size and spread of tumor (staging) at the time of discovery. The greater the spread, the worse the prognosis. Recurrences are not unusual. A patient with one malignancy is likely to develop another. Consequently, malignancies are followed closely and are measured in terms of 5- or 10-year cure rates. Some of the features distinguishing benign from malignant growths are given in Table 7.1.

The naming of neoplasms is generally done by utilizing the name of the tissue of origin. Table 7.2 offers a classification of some of the benign and malignant neoplasms. Most benign neoplasms are designated by adding the suffix "-oma" after the name of the tissue of origin. For example, a benign neoplasm composed of fibrous connective tissue is called a fibroma. If two or more tissues constitute the neoplasm, the terms are combined and the tissue of greater prominence appears last, as in neurofibroma. However, although the suffix "-oma" connotes a tumor or neoplasm, exceptions do exist. A granuloma is not a neoplasm, although it may present as a swelling or tumor. A lymphoma is not a benign neoplasm or lymphocytes but is, in fact, malignant. *Cancer* is the general term used for a malignant neoplasm. Cancers of epithelial origin are called *carcinomas*; cancers of mesodermal or connective tissue origin are called *sarcomas*. Exceptions are the lymphoma and the melanoma, for which the prefix malignant offers no confusion. The leukemias are malignancies of the blood-forming cells.

The effect of the neoplasia on the patient depends on the site or location, on the type of neoplasm, and on the individual patient. Benign growths create masses that are usually investigated to determine the presence of a malignancy. They usually are not fatal but can be if they expand and cause pressure on vital parts. Some benign tumors of glandular origin may produce secretions or hormones that can severely affect the patient. An adenoma of the parathyroid gland can cause an excess of hormone so that calcium is mobilized from bones and osteolytic and radiolucent lesions are seen in bones. These may appear in the jaws as a manifestation of the systemic disease called von Recklinghausen's disease of bone. The

Table 7.1.
Distinguishing features between types of a neoplastic mass

Neoplasia	Benign	Malignant
Clinical	Mass	Mass
	Capsule (localized)	No capsule (infiltrating)
	Slow growth	Rapid growth
	No metastases	Metastases
	Usually not fatal	Fatal if untreated
Microscopic	Cells, typical; normal	Cells, atypical; abnormal size, shapes
	Regular arrangement	Loss of regular arrangement
	Few mitoses	Many mitoses, often abnormal
	Normal nucleus	Large nucleus

Table 7.2.
Classifications of neoplasms

Cell or Tissue of Origin	Benign	Malignant (Cancer)
1. *Epithelium*		*Carcinoma*
Surface		
Squamous	Papilloma	Squamous cell carcinoma Verrucous carcinoma Basal cell carcinoma
Respiratory	Papilloma Inverted papilloma	Nasopharyngeal carcinoma
Glandular	Adenoma	Adenocarcinoma
Salivary duct	Pleomorphic adenoma	Malignant pleomorphic adenoma
Pigment cells	Pigmented nevus	Melanoma (malignant melanoma
Tooth	Ameloblastoma	Malignant ameloblastoma
2. *Connective tissue*		*Sarcoma*
Fibrous	Fibroma	Fibrosarcoma
Adipose	Lipoma	Liposarcoma
Cartilage	Chondroma	Chondrosarcoma
Bone	Osteoma	Osteosarcoma
Neural nerve	Neuroma	Neurosarcoma
Schwann cell combined	Schwannoma (Neurilemoma) Neurofibroma	Malignant schwannoma Malignant neurilemoma Neurofibrosarcoma
Vascular	Angioma	Angiosarcoma
Blood vessels	Hemangioma	Hemangiosarcoma
Lymph vessels	Lymphangioma Cystic hygroma	Lymphangiosarcoma
Pericytes	Hemangiopericytoma	Malignant hemangio-pericytoma
Granular cells	Granular cell tumor	Alveolar soft part sarcoma
Blood forming		Lymphoma, leukemia, myeloma
Tooth	Odontogenic fibroma	
Muscle		
Smooth	Leiomyoma	Leiomyosarcoma
Skeletal	Rhabdomyoma	Rhabdomyosarcoma
Histiocyte	Fibrous histiocytoma	Malignant fibrous histiocytoma
3. *Mixed*—epithelial and connective tissue		
Tooth	Odontoma Ameloblastic fibroma	Ameloblastic fibrosarcoma

removal of the parathyroid adenoma cures the bone lesions. Other effects of benign growths may arise from complications such as hemorrhage or infections that can arise because of their presence.

Similar effects can arise from malignant growths. Cancer and benign growths may present in many ways. On body surfaces that can be readily examined, the growth may be a "lump" or a sore that fails to heal. On internal organs, it may present as pain. However, cancer is usually painless until its later stages. There may be bleeding or some other sign, depending on the organ affected. An example is hoarseness in cancer of the larynx. The most important physiologic effect, though, is cachexia, a wasting resulting in weakness and weight loss. This may directly cause deaths, but the primary danger is that it predisposes the patient to infections. Prime causes of death in cancer patients are infection (pneumonia) and suicide. Another factor governing the effect of the growth is the state of the resistance of the individual patient. Resistance is a complex and poorly understood physiologic phenomenon. Contributing to it is immunity and its role in counteracting or containing malignancies.

The cause of cancer in humans is unknown. It appears that there are many factors that may act in concert with one another to produce an irreversible change in the nucleus of a cell so that, given a chance to proliferate, it grows uncontrollably. Some factors that are recognized as having a probable effect in the cause of cancer are viruses, chemicals, hormones, family susceptibility, physical agents, immunity, aging, diet, and gender.

Oncogenes are genes that have important roles in the day-to-day life of cells, in growth, and in cell division. Some suppress growth, whereas others accelerate it. If there is a malfunction, the cell can race out of control and give rise to a malignancy. If the oncogene is a negative regulator of growth and it is inactivated or lost, either by exposure to harmful chemicals or other carcinogens, then a malignant growth is unleashed. If the oncogene accelerates growth, then, when it is abnormally activated by cancer-causing agents in the environment or chemicals, or if the chromosomes are damaged, the oncogenes may produce too much of their normal chemical signals and cause the cells they are in to become malignant.

There are recognized viruses that cause cancer in animals. In humans, a strain of herpes virus, Epstein-Barr, is responsible for the Burkitt's lymphoma, a malignancy of the maxilla affecting children in certain parts of Africa.

Chemicals that can cause cancer are called carcinogens. Polycyclic hydrocarbons painted on or implanted in animals produce cancer. Similar compounds have been associated with cancer in humans. Smoke from cigarettes contains many carcinogens. The tars and chemicals adhere to the lung tissue. With a decreased resistance, familial tendency toward cancer, and the carcinogens, a lung cancer or bronchiogenic carcinoma may develop. Cigarette smoking is directly related to the incidence of lung cancer.

An imbalance of hormones can be related to cancer. An excess of hormones may lead to hyperplasia of cells at the target organ. Such a stimulation could eventually result in neoplasia. Cancer of the breast has been related to the hormone estrogen as well as to a familial susceptibility toward the disease. Certain families are more prone to certain types of cancer. Given a predisposing set of factors for cancer, individuals in these families can react in a similar pattern, resulting in neoplastic disease.

Immunity plays a significant role. If the immune response is decreased, there is a greater chance of inducing neoplasia, and existing neoplasia is enhanced. Interestingly, immunity decreases with age. With age there is a greater susceptibility to cancer. With some exceptions, cancer is a disease of older age. One can ponder that those individuals dying of lung cancer related to smoking at age 55 probably would have died of the same disease at age 75. The smoking and other factors may have altered the immune response so that the development of the neoplasia occurred years earlier.

Various physical agents are related to cancer production. Ionizing radiation such as roentgenograms, in chronic exposures, can cause cancer. Diagnostic radiation may affect the unborn fetus, who later in life may get leukemia. Radiation from the sun can be a factor in skin cancer. This is particularly true of light-skinned individuals who are exposed either by occupation or by choice to sunlight. Likewise, chronic mechanical trauma or irritation can contribute to neoplasia. Irritation constantly applied to an area coupled with other factors can produce a neoplastic growth.

Nine out of ten cancers diagnosed have *behavior* of the patient as a factor in their development. Smoking alone accounts for one-third of cancer deaths. Exposing the skin to sunlight accounts for 500,000 or more cancers of the skin. Exposure to industrial pollutants accounts for at least 5 percent of cancer deaths.

In the development of a neoplasia, a neoplastic change is imposed on a cell in the mitotic phase. If a differentiated cell is the target, a benign tumor results. If an undifferentiated or stem cell is the target, a malignant tumor results. Three steps are recognized: initiation, promotion, and progression. In initiation there is the exposure to the mitotic cell by a carcinogen. A single exposure is enough. But other factors, promoting agents such as chemicals (esters) and irritation, are required to promote the changed cell to proliferate. Other factors, not defined, allow the progression of this group of cells to the development of a malignancy. In the epithelium, there is a recognizable premalignant phase called epithelial dysplasia. Dysplasia may progress to include all of the epithelium, called carcinoma in situ. The cells have all of the attributes of cancer cells, but there is no invasion into the underlying tissue. Once the cells invade and permeate the connective tissue, the growth of changed cells is called a carcinoma. Then the cancer cells can spread. Epithelial cancers generally spread first to lymph nodes and secondly to the bloodstream. Sarcomas tend to spread by blood vessel; the multistep process of metastasis may follow. If the cells survive they are transported to a distant organ, arrest in, and penetrate the capillary. Again exposed to further body defenses, the cells may survive and proliferate, setting up a cancer in the secondary site (metastasis) (Fig. 7.2).

The treatment for neoplasia varies. Benign neoplasms are cured usually by simple surgical removal. They generally do not recur. Malignant neoplasms are treated by surgery, radiation, chemotherapy, or a combination of these. Some malignancies behave like benign growths and are easily cured. Others are not easily cured and may offer a grave prognosis depending on the type of cellular characteristics. Because

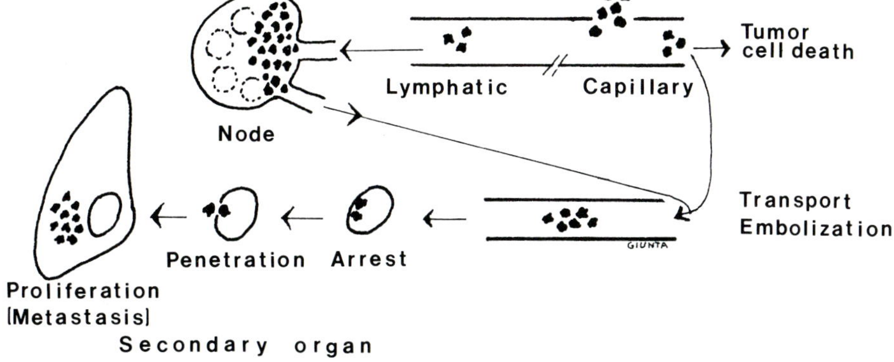

Figure 7.2. The development of a squamous cell carcinoma and a metastasis. Features are: invasion; spread via lymph and blood vessels; and steps progressing to a secondary neoplasm (metastasis).

there is a spectrum of cellular changes in cancers, these can be graded by the pathologist. Generally a low-grade malignancy (the cells of which tend to resemble the tissue of origin) has a better prognosis than a high-grade malignancy. Some cancers may be inoperable and incurable, in which case palliative and supportive therapy is used to relieve pain and discomfort. Even when an apparent cure is accomplished, patients with cancer must be watched closely because of the possibility of metastases being present and not discernible, because recurrences are frequent and because they are prone to more than one primary cancer.

Cancer is indeed a malicious disease. It is the second leading cause of death in the United States. Because of this impact, extensive efforts continue both clinically and at the research level to unravel the secrets of neoplasia, a common response of the body to the various stimuli about it, sometimes resulting in hundreds of diseases (cancers).

Benign Tumors of the Oral Cavity

Of the neoplasms, the benign tumors are much more common than the malignant tumors and compose a large percentage of the most common oral lesions observed and biopsied in dental practices. They can arise from any tissue of the oral cavity, including that within the bone. Usually they present as a swelling or nodular mass projecting outward from the mucosa. They may be attached to the mucosa by a narrow stalk or pedicle, in which case they are called pedunculated. If the base of the lesion is broad or wide the attachment is called sessile. In many instances the diagnosis is strongly suspected clinically, and because the treatment is usually surgical removal, the tissue is submitted for confirmation by microscopic analysis. In other circumstances the diagnosis is not definite, and an incisional or excisional biopsy is done for definitive diagnosis. Any nodular mass or swelling of tissue should be suspected as being a neoplasm, inflammatory hyperplasia, or developmental hyperplasia, and should be followed up until adequate diagnosis and care are instituted.

Fibroma (Irritation Fibroma)

The fibroma is a nodular mass composed of dense fibrous connective tissue. It is one of the most common lesions of the oral cavity and may occur in any location, although the buccal mucosa, tongue, lower lip, and gingiva are sites most affected. The fibroma appears as a pale pink to white, raised, smooth-surfaced, firm mass that may be pedunculated or sessile and can vary in size from a few millimeters to centimeters (Fig. 7.3). Because it is associated with some irritation or trauma, it is often referred to as an irritation fibroma, inferring that it is not a true benign tumor. Rather, it may reflect the end stage of a chronic inflammatory response, but the dense bundles of collagen, of which it is composed, are indistinguishable from those of a true fibroma. In addition, some inflammatory cells are invariably present. Cheek biting may lead to a fibroma on the buccal mucosa. Other habits such as rubbing a rough area with the tongue may likewise result in a lesion called a fibroma. Fibromas are readily diagnosed clinically. Treatment is simple surgical excision and microscopic examination. Fibromas may recur if the irritant is not removed.

Other lesions are composed of the same dense, firm tissue as the fibroma. Several of these affect the gingivae or the mucosa of the alveolar ridge. Because the area affected is diffuse, the term fibromatosis is used to indicate that the large mass of tissue resembles the fibroma. Fibromatosis of the gingivae has been referred to under developmental lesions (see Chapter 4). In this familial disease the gingivae are enlarged and tumorlike, but microscopically they are composed of dense fibrous connective tissue. Dilantin hyperplasia of the gingivae is a similar condition, but the cause is the administration of the drug dilantin for epilepsy. In some patients receiving the drug, the gingivae enlarge with a fibromatosis (Fig. 7.4). Transplant organ recipients

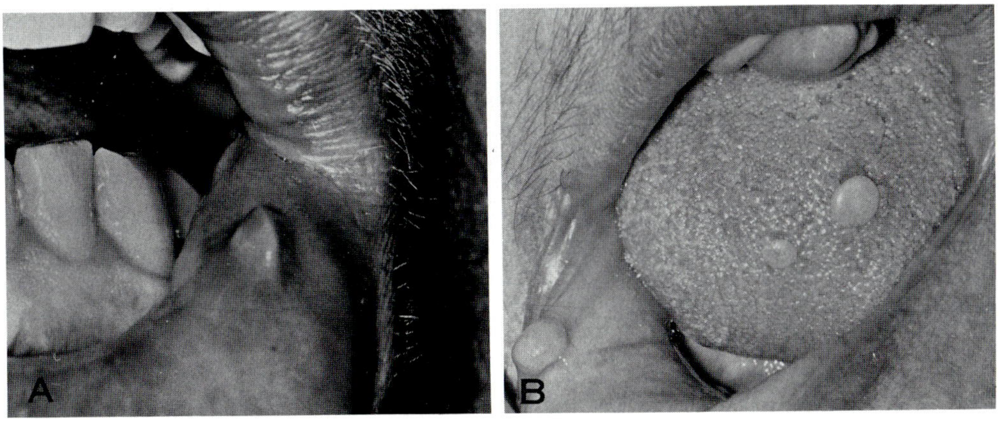

Figure 7.3. *A*, fibroma, sessile base, lower lip. Patient had habit of biting lip at this site. *B*, multiple fibromas, tongue and buccal mucosa.

receiving immunosuppressants may get a similar fibrotic reaction of the gingivae. Removal of the drug or gingivectomy is the treatment. Fibromatosis unrelated to a familial tendency or to dilantin is frequently seen in some patients in the maxillary tuberosity areas. These area may be so enlarged that they favor periodontal disease or, in edentulous patients, they interfere with fabrication of dentures. Surgery is the treatment. A fibroma on the gingiva may be large or small and, because of its location at the interdental papilla, may be termed a fibroid epulis. They are like fibromas elsewhere but must be distinguished from the peripheral giant cell granuloma, the pyogenic granuloma, and the hemangioma.

Angiomas are benign tumors composed of vascular channels. If the channels contain red blood cells, the tumor is called a hemangioma. If the vascular spaces are filled with lymph fluid, the tumor is a lymphangioma. The hemangioma is the most common benign tumor of the oral mucosa. Because of its cellular nature, it is often diagnosed but is not removed with such frequency as the fibroma. Moreover, the hemangioma, unrelated to irritation, is considered a true tumor. Some pathologists refer to it as a hamartoma, meaning that there was an overabundance of normal tissue formed, in this case, blood-filled channels.

Hemangiomas are often congenital and may be present at birth or appear in childhood. They tend to enlarge slowly and often regress in size at puberty. The hemangioma appears as a red, blue-red, or purplish lesion that may be flat or raised and can vary widely in size (Fig. 7.5). The color may blanch on pressure, and a pulsing often can be felt in the smaller lesions. Hemangiomas occur in all sites of the oral cavity—the tongue, buccal mucosa, and lips being common sites. Sometimes the lesions may be extensive. Half or all of the tongue may be involved and create a macroglossia (Fig. 7.6). In lymphangiomas of the tongue there are usually small projections with clear fluid yielding a pebbly appearance rather

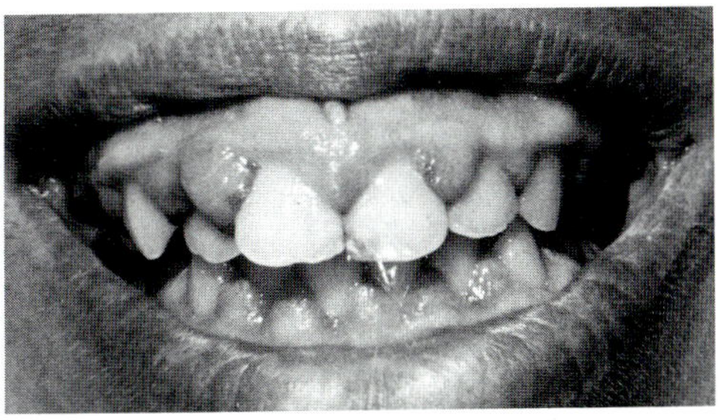

Figure 7.4. Dilantin hyperplasia of gingivae.

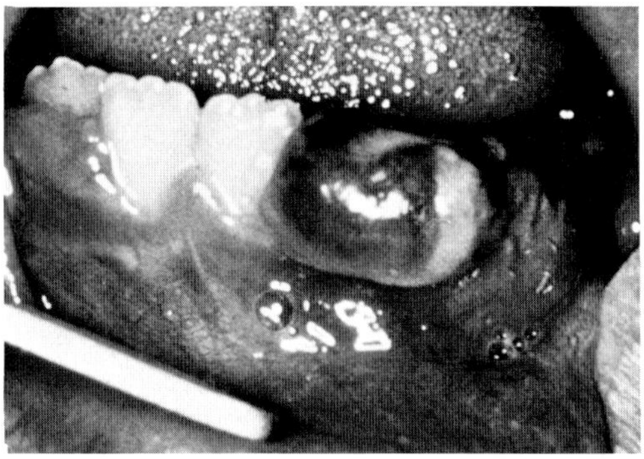

Figure 7.5. Hemangioma of gingiva (epulis) in a 6-month-old male. Lesion has been traumatized and has necrotic areas (*white*) on surface.

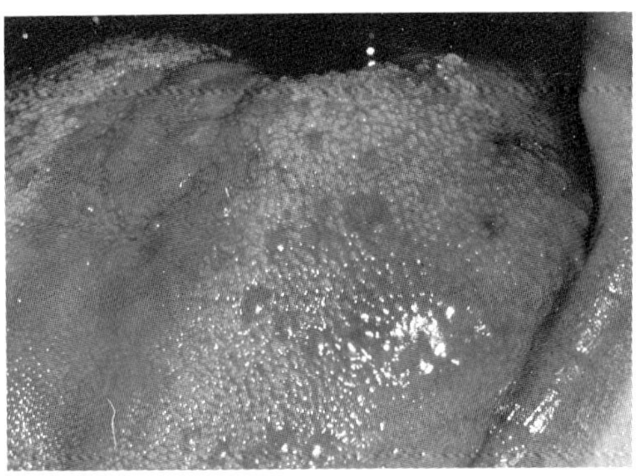

Figure 7.6. Hemangioma, left side of tongue, in a 9-year-old who also has central papillary atrophy (median rhomboid glossitis).

than a smooth surface. The treatment for hemangiomas varies with the individual circumstances. They may be left alone and observed. Precautionary measures should be taken against irritating or injurious factors. They may regress at puberty. Small lesions may be excised easily. Others may be injected with sclerosing solutions that promote scarring.

Hemangiomas are seen on the face and neck. Flat, large, red-purple areas, usually present from birth, are called port-wine hemangiomas or stains. These cause cosmetic difficulties but may be successfully covered since surgery and radiation are contraindicated.

There are other vascular lesions to be considered that are not tumors. A *hematoma* is a blood blister. It is a collection of blood beneath the mucosa. Usually deep purple, the lesion may be flat or raised. Secondary to trauma, the buccal mucosa and lower lip are common sites (Fig. 7.7). Patients on anticoagulants such as dicumarol are prone to bruising and may develop large hematomas (Fig. 7.8). The

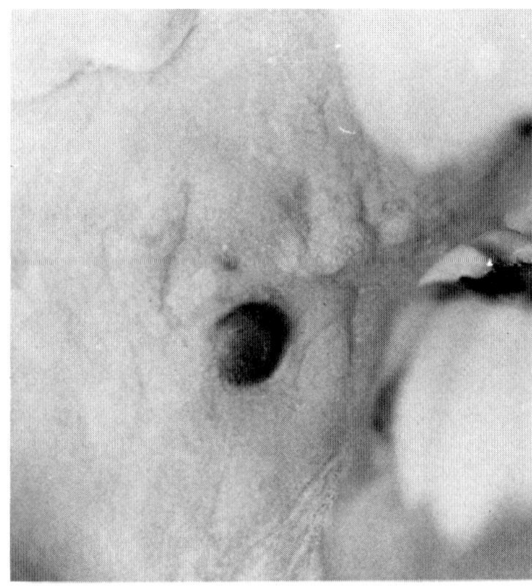

Figure 7.7. Hematoma or blood blister, buccal mucosa, caused by cheek bite.

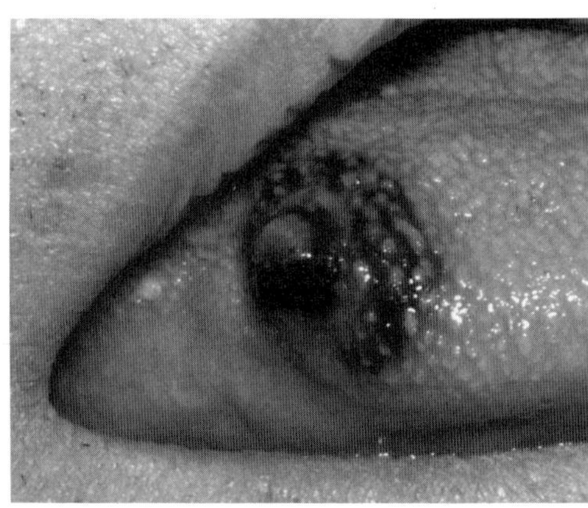

Figure 7.8. Hematoma, lateral tongue in male patient on Coumadin because of kidney dialysis treatment. Patient bit tongue and caused this bruise.

collection of blood cells is gradually resorbed, and the lesions disappear without intervention.

Vascular channels can dilate and become tortuous. This phenomenon of varicosities is common in aging individuals. It is seen most frequently on the ventral surface of the tongue and on the posterolateral surface near the lateral lingual tonsils and the lips (Fig. 7.9). They appear as prominent, deep purple or blue-black lesions. No treatment is required.

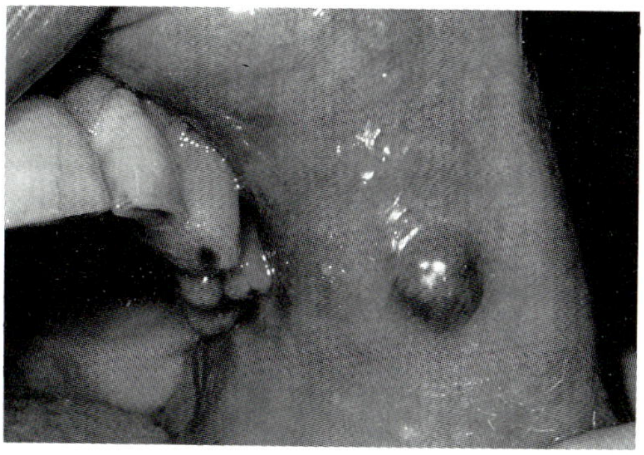

Figure 7.9. Varicosity or aneurysm of vein in the lip of an older person. This deep blue-purple swelling could also be a hemangioma or a Kaposi's sarcoma of AIDS.

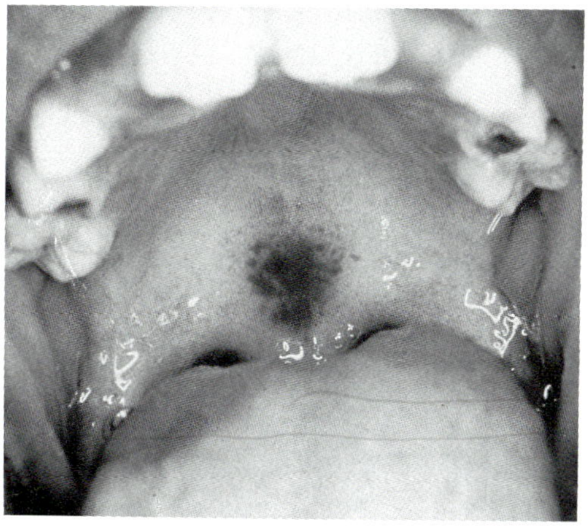

Figure 7.10. Multiple reddish, blue-purple petechiae coalescing to form an ecchymosis on soft palate. This may be due to trauma or may be a sign of a bleeding problem. It resembles the macular stage of a Kaposi's sarcoma in AIDS.

Capillary hemorrhage may cause red or purple macules called petechiae to appear on the mucosa. The soft palate is a common site (Fig. 7.10). Causes vary from the common cold or other viral diseases to trauma or bleeding disorders. The spots turn blue or yellow prior to their disappearance.

Telangiectasias are small, red macules or papules formed by dilated capillaries. They may be round or have spiderlike appearances (Fig. 7.11). They are common on the face, particularly the lips and nose. The causes vary, and there is a hereditary form. As with other vascular lesions, precautions against trauma and irritation should be taken.

The lymphangioma is a rare tumor of the oral cavity. It may occur singularly or be a component of a hemangioma. It is usually congenital and may cause severe enlargement of the affected part. The tongue is a usual site, and it may present as a macroglossia in an infant. Treatment is similar to that of the hemangioma.

Neuromas are rare lesions of the oral cavity. Because of the functioning nerve tissue, these nodular masses are usually painful. Some trauma is generally associated with their occurrence. Treatment is surgical removal.

A more common lesion is the neurofibroma, a benign tumor of combined origin

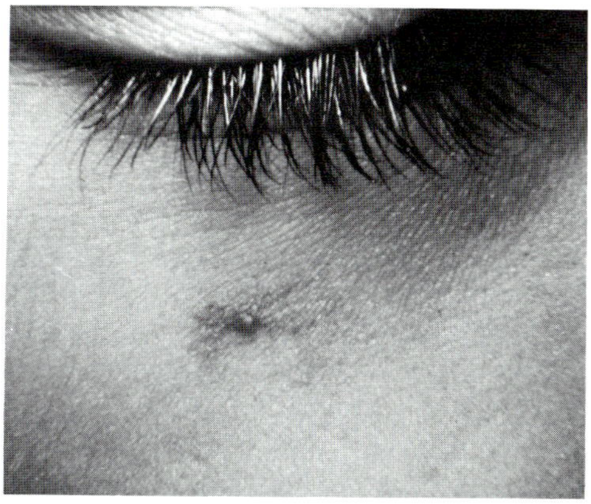

Figure 7.11. Spider nevus or telangiectasia on face below eye. This red lesion blanches upon pressure.

in which the basic fibroma has nerve elements. Neurofibroma produces nodular masses that may be large and softer in consistency than the firmer fibromas (Fig. 7.12). Like the fibroma, it may be multiple. However, when neurofibromas occur, they may be part of a systemic disease called multiple hereditary neurofibromatosis (von Recklinghausen's disease). Affected individuals have numerous neurofibromas on the face, the body, in the mouth, and in internal organs. In addition, they have pigmented, raised nodular lesions and several large brown macules called café-au-lait spots, like birthmarks, scattered over the body. It is important to diagnose and to watch these people, because some of the neurofibromas may become sarcomas later in life.

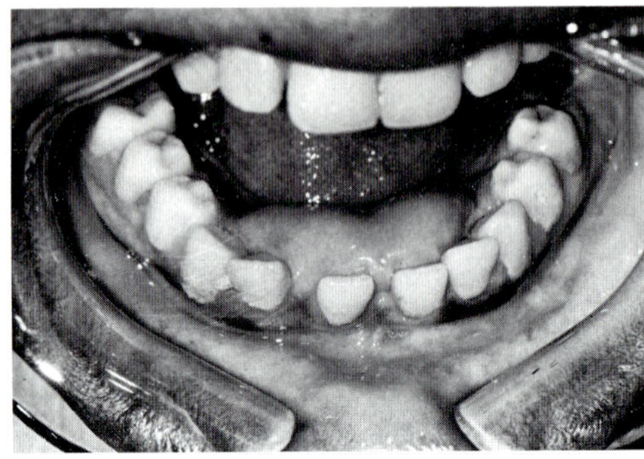

Figure 7.12. Neurofibroma, lingual gingiva. Note separation of teeth owing to pressure of tumor.

Lipoma

The lipoma is a rare benign tumor derived from adipose tissue or fat wherever it occurs in the oral cavity. The buccal mucosa and retromolar areas are common sites. The lesions appear as nodular masses that may be yellowish in color because of the fat. They tend to be soft in consistency. They are composed of normal fat cells. Treatment is simple excision.

Papilloma

The papilloma is a common tumor derived from squamous epithelium. It is a white lesion because of the keratotic surface. Nodular, it is usually characterized by a rough surface with a pebbly texture or with numerous small, slender, thick hairlike projections emanating from a pedunculated or sessile-based mass (Fig. 7.13). The size is generally confined, ranging from millimeters to about 1 centimeter. The papilloma can occur anywhere and is seen on the gingiva, tongue, uvula, floor of mouth, and lips. Similar-appearing lesions are seen on the skin of the face and fingers. They are called verrucae or warts because some are caused by the human wart virus (papovavirus). Some appear as a result of irritation. Papillomas are benign; however, large lesions may resemble a verrucous carcinoma. The treatment is complete surgical removal.

Pleomorphic Adenoma (Benign Mixed Tumor of Salivary Glands)

The pleomorphic adenoma is a benign tumor of salivary gland origin. It is derived from ductal epithelial cells and has a varied

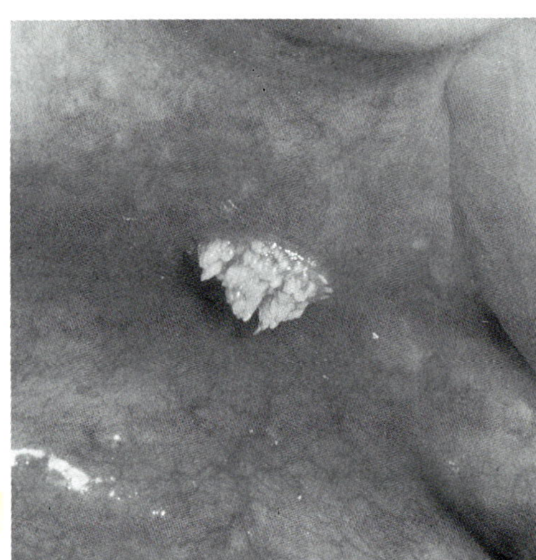

Figure 7.13. Papilloma, soft palate. Note white, keratotic, fingerlike projections and a flat (sessile) base. This is wartlike.

pattern (pleomorphic). These lesions are not common. Most of them occur as swelling emanating from the parotid gland where they comprise 75 percent of all the tumors at that site. Thus, a swelling at the angle of the mandible near the ear in a middle-aged person is probably a pleomorphic adenoma (Fig. 7.14). However, it cannot be distinguished from a malignant lesion or other tumors that can arise from the parotid. It is a swelling that must be investigated. The pleomorphic adenoma is also the most common intraoral salivary gland tumor. Its usual location is the palate, where it presents as a smooth-surfaced swelling resembling a fibroma (Fig. 7.15). The upper lip is the next most common site. Treatment is wide surgical removal, since they tend to recur.

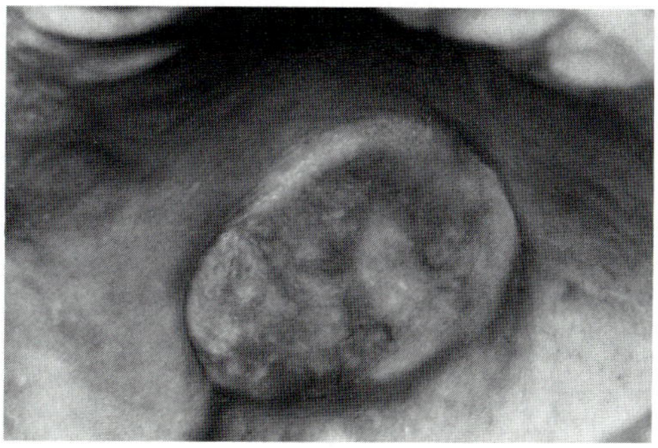

Figure 7.15. Salivary gland neoplasm, pleomorphic adenoma, hard and soft palate. This swelling was covered by a denture.

Osteoma

An osteoma is a rare benign tumor composed of bone, resembling normal dense or spicular bone. It usually occurs within the jaws, where it appears as a radiopaque circumscribed area not necessarily associated with teeth. There may or may not be expansion of the jaw, and it is usually asymptomatic. It also occurs rarely in the soft tissues and has been described in the tongue, mimicking a lingual thyroid. The treatment is for diagnosis and consists of surgical removal. It may occur as part of the syndrome in Gardner's syndrome of multiple polyposis of the colon and may be the first indication of the syndrome.

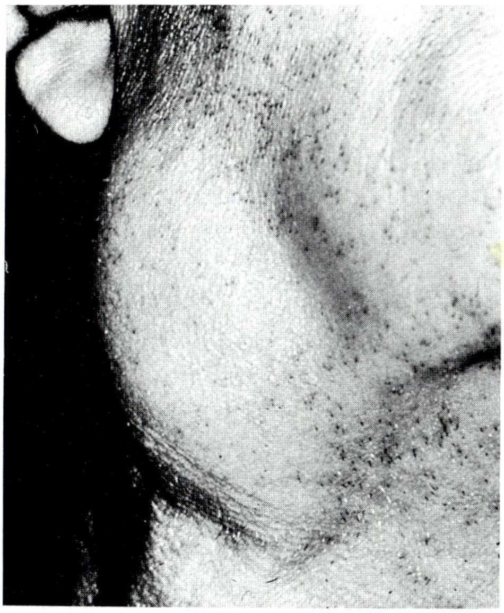

Figure 7.14. Pleomorphic adenoma, parotid. Large swelling at angle of mandible had been present and increasing in size over many years.

Odontogenic Tumors

Odontogenic tumors are those derived from cells that normally would form a tooth or part of a tooth. Most are benign. Very rarely, one is malignant.

Odontoma. The odontoma is the most common odontogenic tumor, occurring usually before the age of 20. It is generally noted on radiographic examination. There is usually a circumscribed area with a central radiopaque mass composed of numerous toothlike objects or dense irregular masses and spicules surrounded by a narrow radiolucent zone (Fig. 7.16). It occupies the space of a missing tooth or represents a developmental defect of a supernumerary tooth. Sometimes the jaw may be expanded or teeth may be separated. The odontoma may interfere with the eruption of a tooth. The radiographic picture is characteristic.

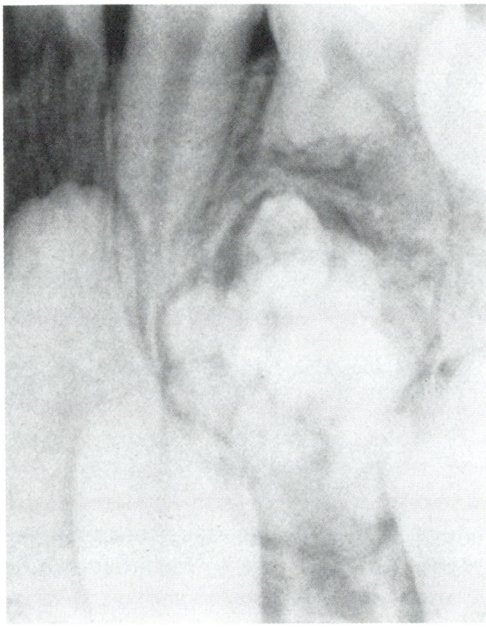

Figure 7.16. Composite odontoma, mandible, in 8-year-old. Multiple radiopaque toothlike masses with surrounding radiolucency. This was interfering with eruption of the premolar.

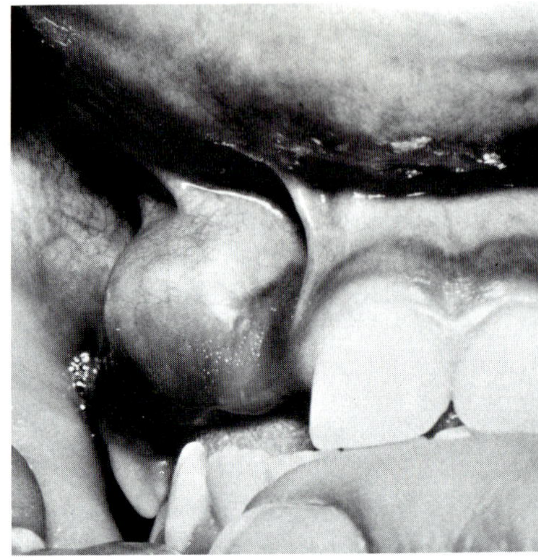

Figure 7.17. Odontoma, 11-year-old female. Presents as a hard swelling alveolar mucosa. Note missing teeth.

Conservative surgical removal is the treatment. The mass is composed of all the elements that form a tooth—pulp, dentin, cementum, and enamel—and is, therefore, mixed in origin. They may be either regularly arranged, like small teeth, or irregularly arranged (Figs. 7.17 to 7.19).

An odontogenic fibroma or pulpoma is derived from the connective tissue part of the tooth-forming organ. It probably represents the aborted development of a tooth in its early stages and is characterized by the proliferation of pulplike or fibrous tissue. Radiographically, there would be a radiolucent lesion.

Ameloblastoma. The ameloblastoma is a benign tumor derived from dental lamina, enamel organ cells, or cyst epithelium, and composed of epithelial cells resembling those of the enamel-forming organ of a tooth. It is histologically benign but can be locally aggressive, invading and destroying bone. It usually occurs at age 30 or older but can appear at any age. Its common location is the posterior part of the mandible. As it slowly increases in size, the jaw enlarges causing disfigurement (Fig. 7.20). Radiographically, there is a radiolucent cystlike appearance. It may mimic a solitary cyst but usually has a multicystic or

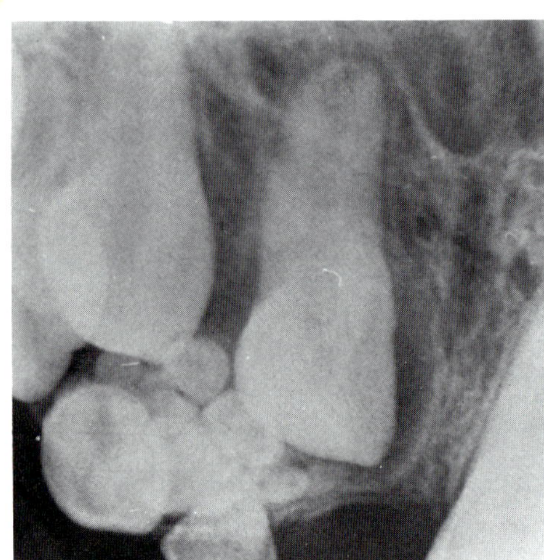

Figure 7.18. Radiograph of odontoma, multiple small radiopaque objects. Also note unerupted permanent teeth.

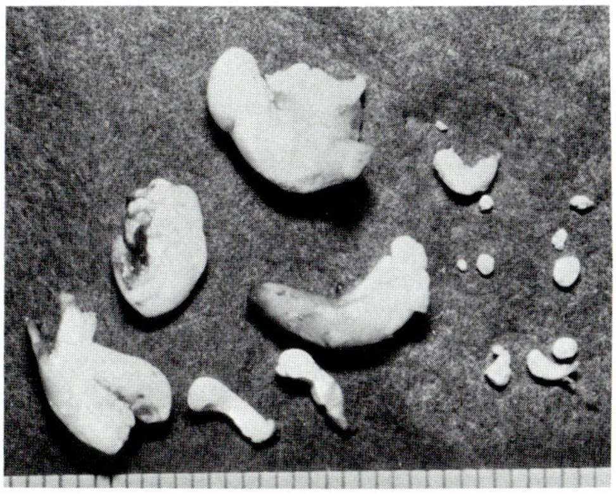

Figure 7.19. Multiple irregularly shaped, tooth-like objects removed on surgery.

compartmentalized appearance as if several soap bubbles were joined together (Fig. 7.21). There can be extensive destruction of the bone. Nonencapsulated islands of ameloblastic cells and stellate reticulum infiltrate and permeate the marrow spaces of the bone. Consequently, treatment consists of wide excision and, depending on the case, may involve removing a segment of or half of the jaw. They may also arise from the wall of a dentigerous cyst, usually associated with an impacted lower third molar (Fig. 7.22), in which case they behave less aggressively.

Two other odontogenic tumors may manifest as dentigerous cysts radiographically overlying an impacted tooth. Both occur in younger people than the ameloblastoma does, usually in the first or second decades. The adenomatoid odontogenic tumor is a nonaggressive encapsulated lesion of ameloblastic cells with duct formations. Usually occurring in females about a maxillary, impacted canine, it is easily removed and does not recur. The other tumor, derived from both ameloblastic cells and dental papilla tissues (a mixed tumor), is the ameloblastic fibroma. Frequently seen in youngsters in the posterior mandible, this tumor is encapsulated and removes easily from the bone but may recur.

Cementoma. The true cementoma (cementoblastoma) is a rare odontogenic tumor composed of cementum with an active and aggressive growth pattern. Usually it is noted on a radiograph as a dense, opaque mass surrounding and attached to the cementum of the root end of the tooth. In its early stages it could resemble hypercementosis. It may occur in the absence of a tooth, in which case it resembles enostoses or other opaque bone lesions. Because of progressive growth and intimate attachment, the tooth and tumor usually are surgically removed together.

Nontumor Bone Lesions. Periapical

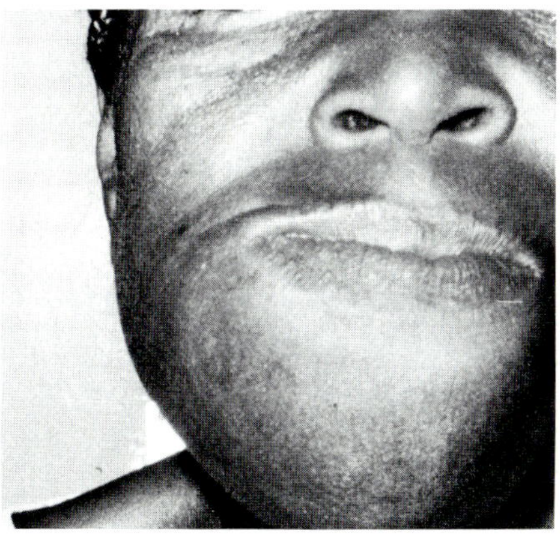

Figure 7.20. Ameloblastoma, mandible. Note disfigurement and enlargement of jaw.

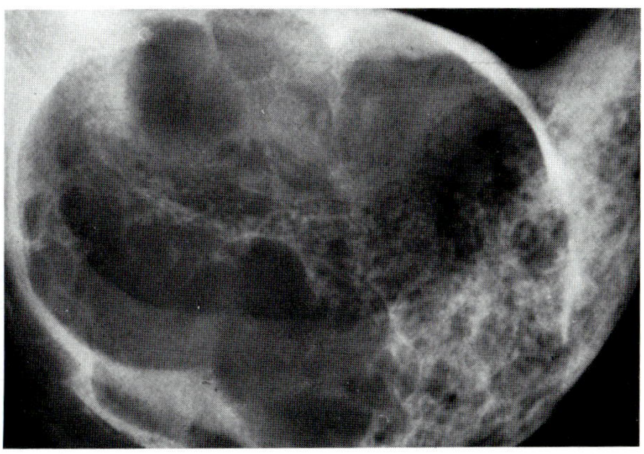

Figure 7.21. Ameloblastoma, multiocular or soap-bubble radiolucencies and thin radiopaque trabeculations.

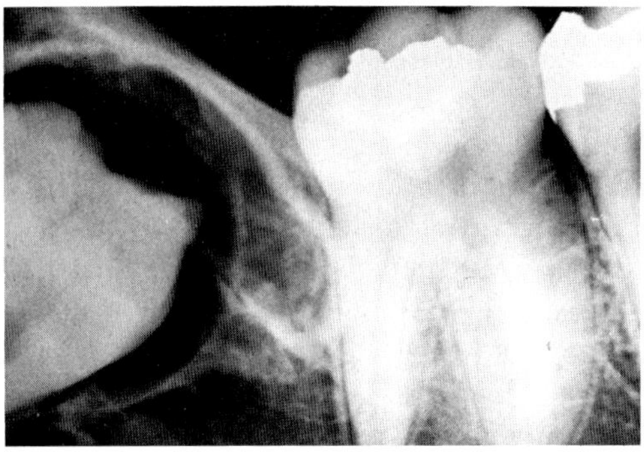

Figure 7.22. Ameloblastoma arising in dentigerous cyst.

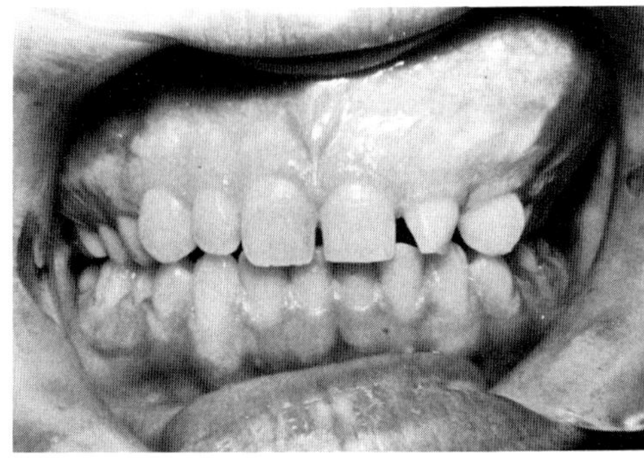

Figure 7.23. Fibrous dysplasia of maxilla in a 20-year-old male. Note enlarged left maxilla and separated teeth. This was a firm mass.

cemental dysplasia, commonly called cementoma, is not a tumor of odontogenic origin composed of cementum. As partly described in Chapter 5, it is a condition of unknown etiology, occurring in tooth-bearing bone that, in its early stage, may resemble periapical inflammatory disease. There are three stages that can be recognized in the development of this condition, the radiographic appearance reflecting what is happening microscopically within the bone. The earliest stage is a radiolucent lesion; fibrous tissue replaces the bone. With time, calcified masses form within the fibrous tissue giving a combined radiolucent and radiopaque (ground glass) lesion. The final stage is one in which there is more bone or cementum than fibrous tissue, resulting in a mostly radiopaque or cotton-wool appearance. The mandibular anterior region is most often affected. The teeth test vital. There is no jaw enlargement, and the cementoma requires follow-up by radiographs and biopsy only to rule out other entities.

Fibrous dysplasia of bone is a disease of young people and is of unknown cause. There is a replacement of bone with fibrous tissue containing varying amounts of abnormal bone. These can affect long bones and those of the skull and jaws. The jaws may be enlarged, and teeth may migrate or separate (Fig. 7.23). The radiographic appearance and histologic stages are similar to cemental dysplasia (Fig. 7.24). However, the sites vary, with the maxilla and posterior mandible being preferred sites. The bone lesions are diffuse and not well defined. The treatment consists of diagnosis, and possible surgery for cosmetic reasons only.

Condensing osteitis, previously mentioned in Chapter 5, may resemble end-stage cemental dysplasia. A sequela or sign of a chronic pulpitis, the radiopaque lesion is most often noted surrounding the root or roots of a lower molar tooth that usually

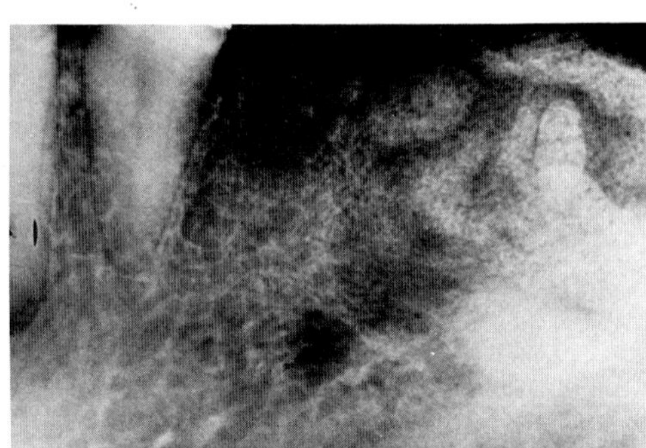

Figure 7.24. Radiograph showing changes in a confirmed case of fibrous dysplasia. There is a combination of radiolucent and radiopaque areas including a ground glass and cotton-wool appearance.

has a large restoration or decay (Fig. 7.25). Biopsies show some chronic inflammation about dense bone spicules.

Eosinophilic granuloma is a bone disease that can mimic a tumor, a cyst, periodontal disease, or an oral infection. Probably of immunologic origin, it is characterized by proliferation and accumulation of macrophages (histiocytes) plus eosinophils. The unifocal variant of an entity called histiocytosis X, eosinophilic granuloma is characterized by a punched-out, cystic radiolucency or a radiolucency about the roots of teeth looking like advanced periodontal disease or infection (Fig. 7.26). The teeth may be mobile, an unusual sign because eosinophilic granuloma occurs in young people. Biopsy is needed to prove the diagnosis. Treatment is surgical excision or low-dose radiation. The disease may recur and act aggressively.

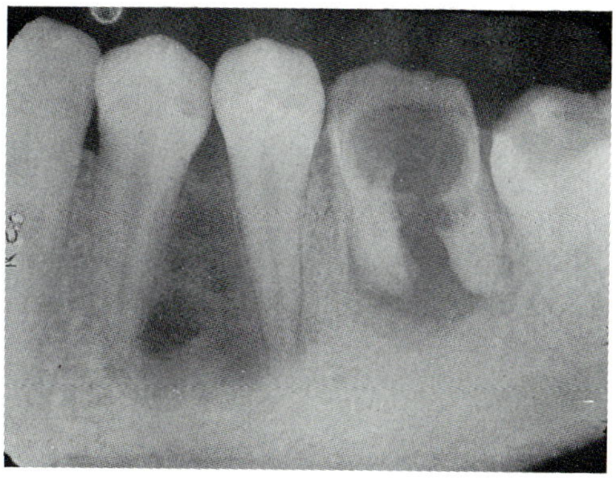

Figure 7.26. Eosinophilic granuloma, radiolucency on the left, mimicking local periodontal disease, among other bony lesions, in a 13-year-old male. The severely carious tooth has furcation involvement with a periapical granuloma.

Oral Cancer

Oral cancer is the most important disease to detect in the oral cavity, because it is a killer and because it occurs with relatively high frequency. It comprises approximately 5 percent of all malignancies. About 15,000 to 20,000 cases are detected in 1 year. However, only 7,000 to 10,000 of people with cases detected are cured and living in 5 years. The cure rate for intraoral cancer is worse than that for cancer of the uterus. This comparison is made because the oral cavity is more accessible for visible examination than the uterus. Oral cancer is detectable in its early stages, so it can be found and cured. Greater efforts at early detection, patient awareness, and motivation would change the present bleak statistics.

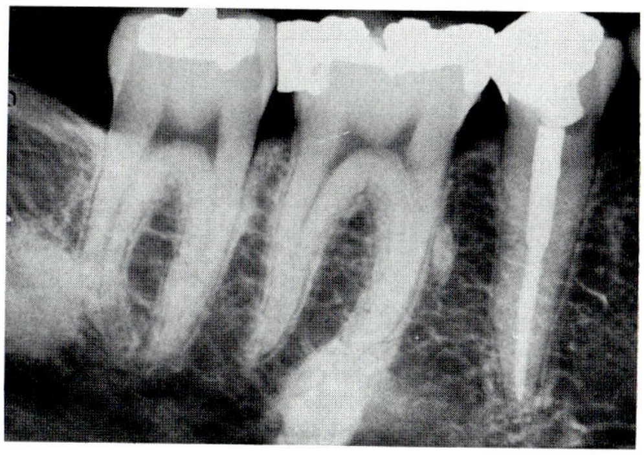

Figure 7.25. Radiograph with multiple lesions. Opacity near mesial root of first molar at middle third is consistent with a retained primary root tip. Opacity at apical end of mesial root is consistent with condensing osteitis. Opacity distal to second molar is consistent with periapical fibrous dysplasia or enostosis. Also note overhanging margin of restoration of first molar on distal and calculus on mesial.

The etiology of oral cancer is unknown. However, there are several factors associated with an increased incidence of oral cancer.

Tobacco use is a prime factor. In the mouth it has a drying effect that causes irritation and promotes the buildup of keratin. Cigars, pipes, and smokeless tobacco are particularly harsh on the oral mucosa. Cigarettes also have an effect but primarily involve the lungs. Tobacco also contains carcinogens that may act locally in susceptible individuals. Oral cancer occurs in significantly more smokers than nonsmokers.

Alcoholic consumption on a regular, habitual basis is another factor. Few cases of oral cancer appear in individuals who do not drink alcoholic beverages. Often smoking and drinking are combined habits.

Chronic irritation is another prominent factor. Oral cancer is associated with keratotic lesions in about 60 percent of the cases. This implicates chronic irritation. Sources of irritation are ill-fitting dentures, sharp edges on partial dentures, jagged restorations or rotten teeth, and any oral habit that inflicts damage.

Other factors that are responsible for predisposition to irritating factors are syphilis and anemias. Atrophic glossitis of tertiary syphilis and certain anemias result in a bald tongue that is prone to irritation and leukoplakia. A percentage of such patients get cancer of the tongue.

Poor oral hygiene is a condition associated with oral cancer. Frequently, a typical oral cancer patient is one who smokes heavily, drinks heavily, and disregards oral hygiene. Such patients are not motivated to visit the offices of dentists or physicians. Therein lies the challenge for early detection. On the other hand, oral cancer does occur in mouths of those who do not drink or smoke and who are motivated toward good health habits.

Oral cancer affects males more than females in a ratio of 4:1. This statistic may change, because the female is smoking as much as the male now. The age of occurrence is 40 or older; however, younger individuals are not immune.

Of all oral cancer, 95 percent is squamous cell or epidermoid carcinoma derived from the epithelium of oral mucosa (Fig. 7.27). Because they are mucosal, changes can be seen. The high-risk areas in order of frequency are the lower lip, lateral border of tongue, floor of mouth, buccal mucosa, palate, tonsils, and gingiva. Oral cancer can be separated into lip cancer and intraoral cancer because of the differences in prognosis.

Lip cancer occurs primarily in males past 50 years of age. It affects the lower lip, usually in the lateral aspects (Fig. 7.28). The lesions are usually painless, small keratotic or white areas with erosion and ulceration. There may be crusting at the skin surface. They may feel hard. With time they grow into large masses and present as ulcerative swellings of the lip. These are usually well-differentiated, low-grade lesions that generally do not metastasize. They offer a good prognosis, with 5-year survival rates of 90 to 95 percent. Tobacco and actinic radiation are associated factors. Actinic radiation from the sun affects

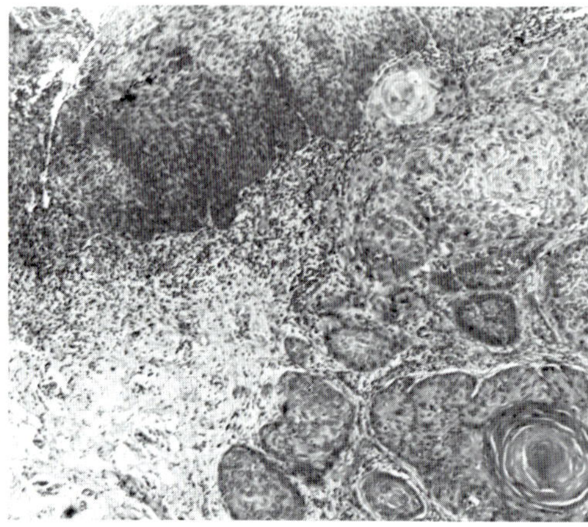

Figure 7.27. Squamous cell (epidermoid) carcinoma invading connective tissue (*right*). Adjacent surface epithelium (*left*) is dysplastic. Tumor is forming keratin (*lower right corner*).

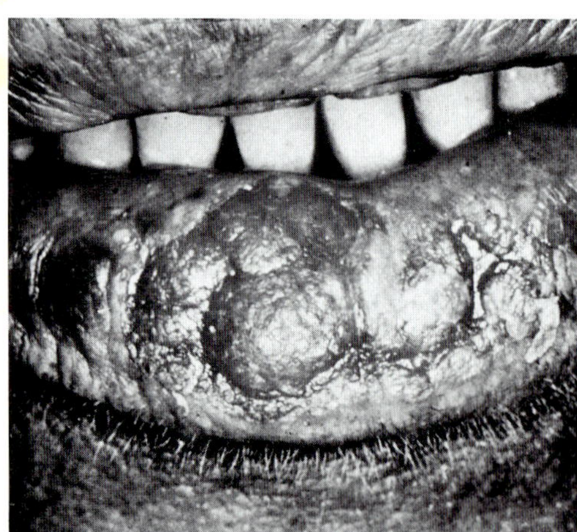

Figure 7.28. Epidermoid carcinoma, lower lip, diffuse involvement.

light-complexioned individuals who work out-of-doors and produces changes in the skin and lower lip. The skin appears flushed and burned with prominent telangiectasis over the cheeks, nose, and lower face. The lower lip appears blanched and dry, smooth and swollen, and often has small white plaques. This is called solar cheilosis and is considered to predispose to a small number of lip cancers. Treatment usually consists of a stripping of the vermilion border or wedge resections and plastic surgery for favorable esthetic and functional results.

Intraoral cancer comprises all areas other than the lip. The tongue is the most common site. The areas of the tongue of high risk are the posterolateral surfaces and the ventral surface, not in the dorsum or midline (Fig. 7.29). Intraoral cancer is painless until late stages are reached. A patient may be unaware of even a large lesion. The early changes to be searched for are ulcers, white areas, smooth or rough areas, red and white pebbly areas, red velvety areas, a swelling, or a papillary mass (Figs. 7.30 and 7.31). The late changes may be firm ulcers, masses, pain, bleeding, difficulty in swallowing, lymphadenopathy (metastases), weakness, and weight loss. There is no specific description of oral cancer. It is detected by a systematic routine of careful and deliberate oral examination and by having a high index of suspicion. A nonhealing ulcer or red pebbly lesion, particularly a red and white lesion, that persists beyond 2 weeks should be considered cancer until proven otherwise. Keratotic lesions must be biopsied to rule out premalignancy and malignancy, since a large percentage of oral cancer is associated with white lesions. Erythroplakia, a red plaque not considered part of a known disease, must be biopsied, since most are dysplastic or cancerous. Only a constant awareness of the possibility that any lesion not otherwise accounted for may be cancer

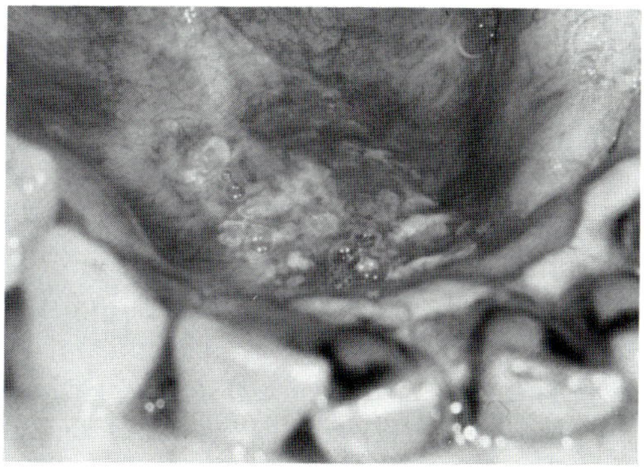

Figure 7.30. Epidermoid carcinoma, floor of mouth and lingual ridge. This was a speckled red and white slightly raised painless lesion.

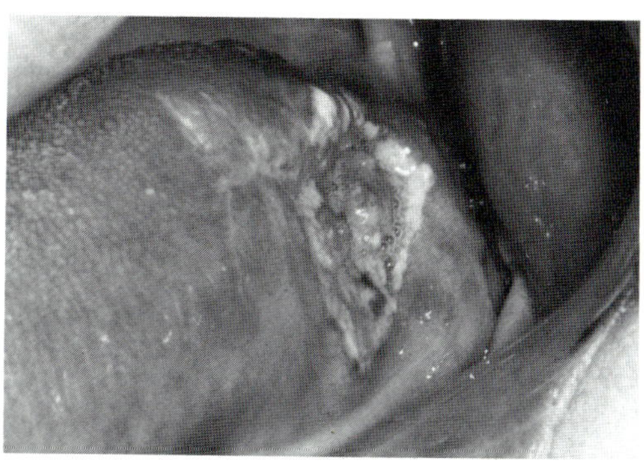

Figure 7.29. Epidermoid carcinoma, posterolateral border of tongue in a 60-year-old smoker and drinker. There is a large ulcer as well as adjacent red and white lesion.

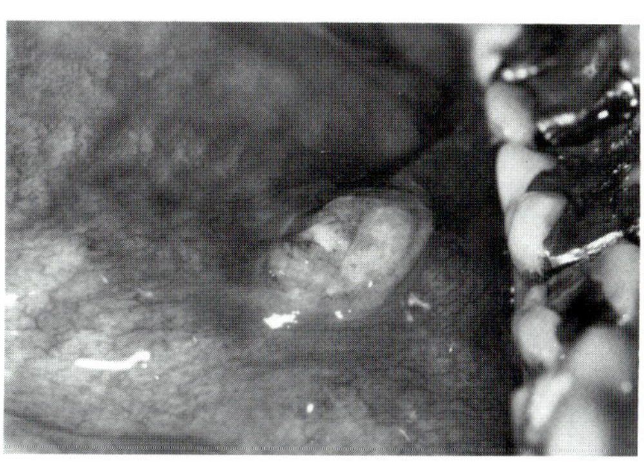

Figure 7.31. Epidermoid carcinoma, floor of mouth, in a 43-year-old female smoker and exdrinker. This small size and early discovery means a better prognosis.

will ensure that early cancer will be detected.

Oral cancer is diagnosed by biopsy. The oral biopsy is accurate in diagnosing oral cancer on the first biopsy in nearly 100 percent of the cases. Oral cytology may be valuable and can detect cells from the mouth. However, it is accurate in only 85 percent of the cases and should not be used instead of the biopsy. Any patient with a suspicious lesion should be referred to a dentist or physician for biopsy and follow-up.

Intraoral cancer contrasts with lip cancer. The type of cancer tends to be of a higher grade and tends more to metastasize to the lymph nodes of the neck. The more posterior the tumor, the more the tumor has spread at time of diagnosis, and the worse the prognosis (Fig. 7.32). The prognosis is only fair, because there is a 5-year survival rate of 50 percent. The survival rates reflect treatment of these patients. This rate increases markedly, though, if the original lesions are less than 1 cm and if there are no metastases, stressing again the importance of early detection. The treatment consists of surgery, radiation therapy, a combination of the two, or chemotherapy when only palliative therapy is useful. Precautions must be taken when radiotherapy is used in the head and neck. Since it induces xerostomia, the teeth should get treatments to prevent radiation caries (Fig. 7.33). Treatment is usually directed by a team of cancer specialists. If the lesion is small, limited surgery or radiation alone can effect a cure with limited disfigurement. In larger lesions and those with metastases, extensive, mutilating surgery may be required. Plastic surgery and prosthetic appliances may be required to ameliorate the resulting defects. All oral cancer patients are followed closely, because they may have a second primary tumor or a recurrence.

Intraoral malignancies other than the squamous cell carcinoma are rare. Making up only 5 percent of all oral malignancies, there are many separate tumors of diverse origin, making any one of them alone very rare. However, many of them are lethal, they affect younger as well as older individuals, and they are to be respected and understood. The most common is that of salivary gland origin. Intraorally, about half of the salivary gland tumors are malignant. The most common site is the palate, where either an adenocystic carcinoma (cylindroma) or a mucoepidermoid carcinoma can occur as a swelling mimicking an abscess, a fibroma, or a torus. The mass is usually firm and painless with either a slow or a fast growth pattern. In the palate it can invade bone, and treatment includes a maxillectomy. The prognosis can be poor, particularly for the cylindroma.

Next in frequency are the metastatic malignancies from other sites in the body to the jawbones. The most common malignancies to metastasize to the jaws are primary from the breast, prostate, thyroid, lung, and colon. They present as radiolucencies of the bone, usually the posterior mandible. There may be loosening of the teeth, pain or no pain, or a paresthesia (tingling or numbness) of the lower lip and face. The histopathology is the same as the primary tumor. Sometimes the metastasis is the first sign of the malignancy. Because of the metastasis, the prognosis is poor.

Other malignancies are those of connective tissue origin. These sarcomas, like fibrosarcomas and osteosarcomas are very rare, rapidly growing nodular masses of the soft tissue that may be ulcerated or of the bone that may be expanded. They may occur in younger individuals. If the tumor presses against the inferior alveolar nerve, there may be paresthesia. Surgery is the usual treatment and offers a chance for cure and reconstruction. Also occurring rarely are melanomas, malignant tumors of nevus cells that produce melanin. They normally are seen on the skin, particularly the face, but they may occur intraorally where the site is likely to be the palate or the gingiva. The macular or nodular black-brown area is biopsied to distinguish the melanoma from normal pigment or a benign nevus. Treatment may be chemo-

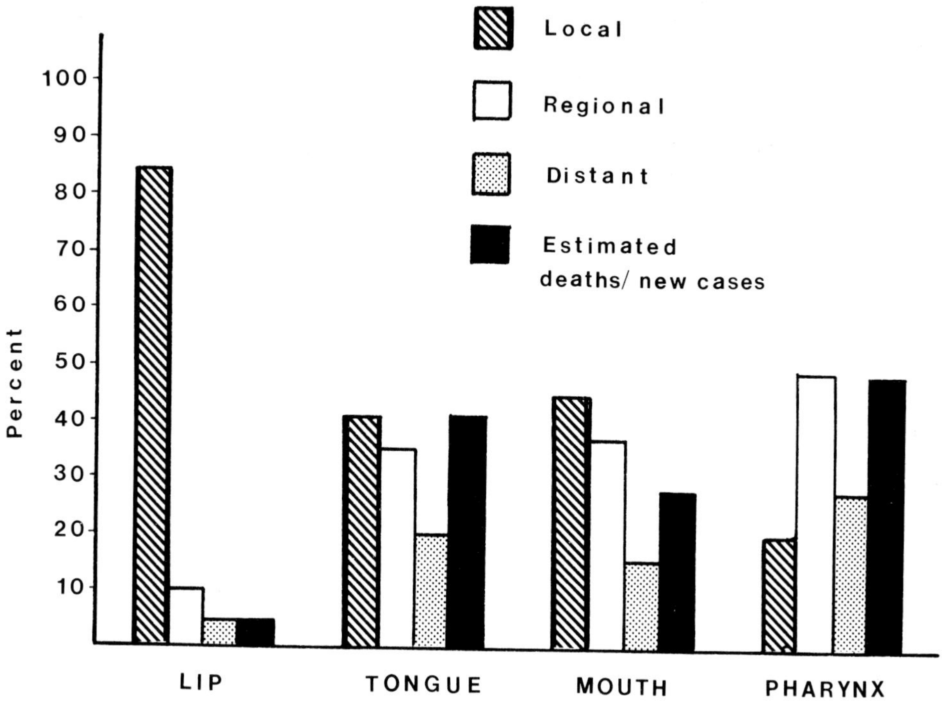

Figure 7.32. Bar graph comparing the extent of spread with estimated deaths (prognosis) for cancers of the lip, tongue, mouth, and pharynx. As the cancer is more posterior, the spread at initial discovery is greater, and the prognosis is worse.

therapy with or without further surgery. The prognosis is guarded and is usually poor.

Regarding lesions in the bone, either primary or secondary, there are significant symptoms. If a patient complains of a tingling (paresthesia) of the lip or any numbness, pain, or swelling and it is not associated with a dental origin, a malignancy of bone should be suspected and further investigation is required.

Extraoral cancers of the face and neck are usually visible on examination (see Figs. 1.3 and 1.4). The most common cancer of skin is the basal cell carcinoma, commonly seen on the upper face and neck. It is a tumor rising from and composed of the basal cells of the epithelium of the skin. It is found in older, generally fair-skinned individuals who are exposed to the sun. The lesions occur anywhere—upper lip, nose, ear, and neck. Usually they are small, rounded, raised or only slightly raised, red or scaly lesions often with a central depressed area of ulceration. It is a "sore" that fails to heal. Characteristically, it is slow growing and localized, it spreads by local

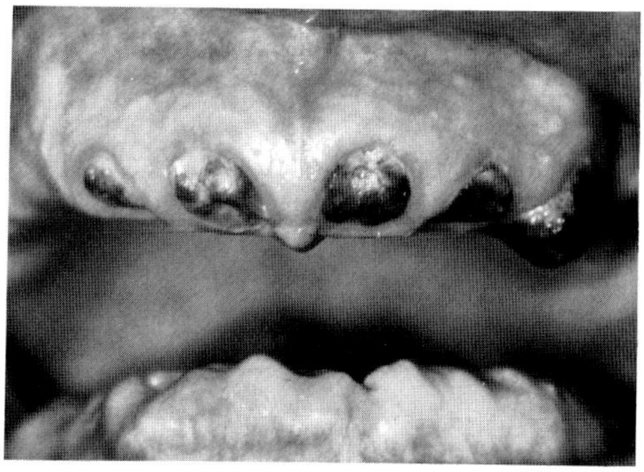

Figure 7.33. Radiation caries secondary to xerostomia in an oral cancer patient treated with radiation only. Unfortunately, poor hygiene and lack of fluoride therapy resulted in this preventable loss.

extension, and it rarely if ever metastasizes. It is easy to cure with conservative surgery or radiation. If left untreated, or if discovered as a large lesion, extensive infiltration and destruction can occur, and the treatment is more radical and less likely to achieve a cure. When diagnosed and treated early, there is usually a 95 percent cure rate.

Pigmentations

Pigmentations are of two types, endogenous and exogenous. Those pigments produced by the body are endogenous. Those introduced from the environment are exogenous. Some of the pigmentations seen in the oral cavity are listed in Table 7.3, which separates them into categories of diffuse and focal. Diffuse or spread-out pigmentation usually signifies that there is a systemic problem elsewhere in the body. Such a manifestation of systemic disease is seen in Peutz-Jeghers syndrome. The oral signs are numerous brown macules or spots of melanin about the lips and perhaps in the mouth. The systemic problem is inherited multiple polyps or growths in the intestine. These have the potential of causing obstruction and rarely become malignant. Patients with diffuse pigmentation should be suspected of having a systemic problem and should be referred to a physician.

Certain occupations and some medical therapy can introduce heavy metals into the body. These settle out in many organs, one of which can be the mouth, particularly along the marginal gingiva. In some countries it is fashionable to tattoo the maxillary attached gingivae for beauty. This appears as a diffuse blue-black or gray color spread from canine to canine.

The more common pigmented lesions of the oral cavity are those that are focal or localized, not diffuse. Normal melanin pigment is seen frequently, particularly on the attached gingivae (Fig. 7.34). Usually physiologic melanin is symmetrical, but a single patch may occur. History may help differentiate it from a melanotic macule. There is no clinical significance to physiologic melanin except to recognize it as normal. Hemosiderin and bilirubin are pigments of blood breakdown. The hematoma is a collection of blood that presents as a blue-black round lesion, usually on the buccal mucosa. Petechiae are macules of hemorrhage that are blue-black at first and then change to a yellowish color as the blood products are broken down and disappear. Bleeding into the dentinal tubules leaves red blood cells that break down and cause a staining so

Table 7.3.
Pigmentations

Distribution	Endogenous	Exogenous
Diffuse—spread out	Metabolic—systemic disease	Industrial
	Melanin spots	
	Peutz-Jeghers syndrome	Lead, silver, etc.
	Adrenal insufficiency	Tattoo (self-applied)
	Bilirubin	
	Jaundice—black teeth	
Focal—localized	Normal melanin	Amalgam tattoo—common
	Hemosiderin	Foreign bodies
	Blood product	(pencils, etc.)
	Black teeth	
	Melanotic macule	
		Tetracycline—yellow-brown
	Nevus—rare in mouth	
	Melanoma	

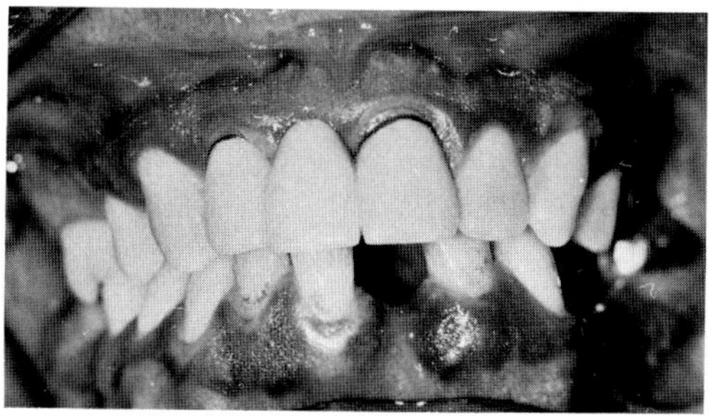

Figure 7.34. Normal melanin pigmentation, gingivae.

episode of jaundice. Causes of stains and discolorations of teeth are listed in Table 7.4.

Other focal lesions are associated with melanin but are rare to the oral cavity. A melanotic macule (freckle) is a brown spot caused by melanin in the basal cell layer (Fig. 7.37). A nevus is a flat or slightly raised benign tumor mass with nevus cells and melanin in the connective tissue. A melanoma is a malignant nevus, appears black, and occurs rarely in the mouth, its

that the tooth appears darkened (Fig. 7.35). This is commonly seen in anterior teeth that have been traumatized. A dark tooth should be investigated for pulpal or periapical pathology. Black or gray-black teeth may be due to medications and a systemic condition causing a breakdown of blood into bilirubin pigment causing jaundice. The pigment remains in the dentinal tubules and stains the teeth black (Fig. 7.36). This has been seen in children born of mothers with an Rh incompatibility with the baby (erythroblastosis fetalis). The newborn can be transfused with blood and saved; however, black or gray-black primary teeth remain as a reminder of the

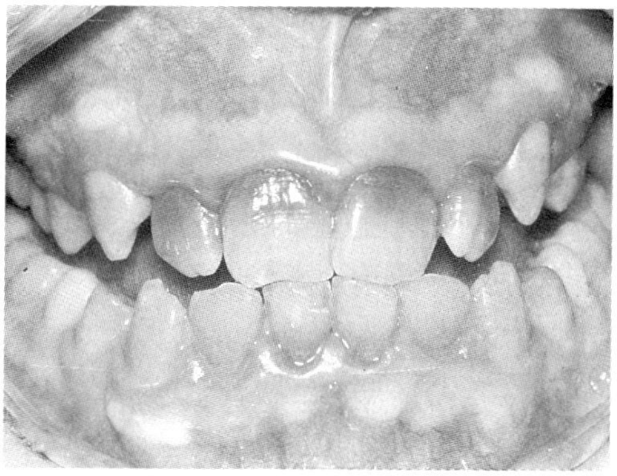

Figure 7.36. Staining of teeth due to excess bilirubin. This resembles tetracycline staining and dentinogenesis imperfecta.

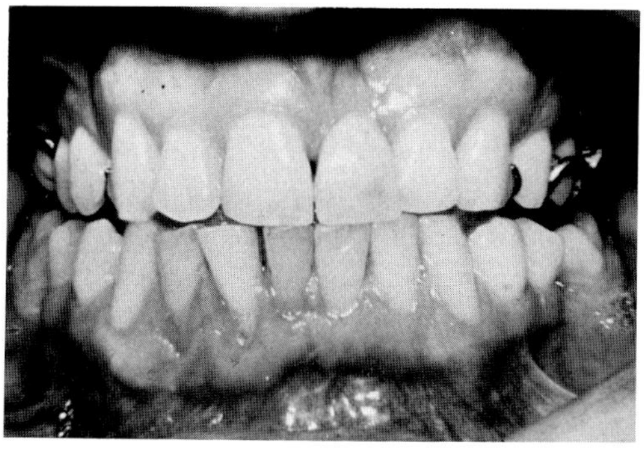

Figure 7.35. Intrinsic staining, lower incisor. Gray color due to bleeding into dentinal tubules. Patient had history of being hit by a baseball bat. Also note the supernumerary lower incisor (five incisors).

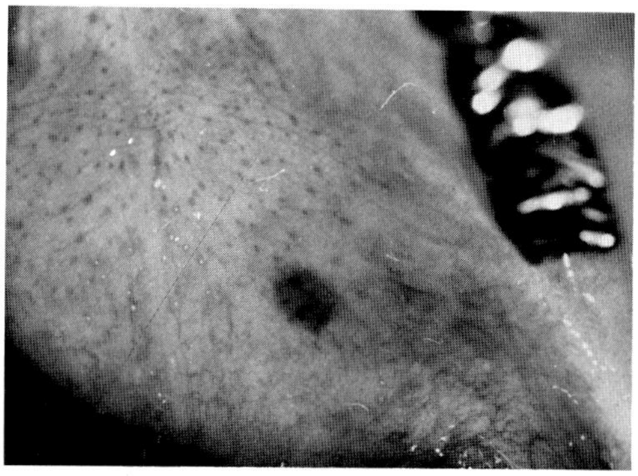

Figure 7.37. A melanotic macule on the soft palate. This could be simple melanin pigmentation, a nevus, or a melanoma; also note the nicotinic stomatitis.

Table 7.4.
Causes of stains and discolorations of teeth

Extrinsic
- Chromogenic bacteria in plaque—green, black, brown; poor hygiene; arrested dental caries—brown, black
- Discoloring agents
  - Foodstuffs—coffee, tea, berries; color of food item
  - Tobacco and by-products; brown, black
  - Restorative materials—e.g., amalgam; gray, black
  - Medicaments
    - Iron sulfide—black
    - Stannous fluoride on caries—brown
    - Chlorhexidine—gray, black
  - Industrial dusts; proprietary health aids

Intrinsic
- Blood-borne pigments
  - Congenital erythropoietic porphyria; red, brown
  - Bile duct defects—bile pigment; green
  - Hepatitis—bilirubin; black, gray
  - Hemolytic anemias—hemosiderin
    - Rh incompatability (erythroblastosis fetalis)—only primary teeth; gray
    - Thalassemia and sickle cell anemia—either primary or permanent teeth; gray
    - Iron deficiency anemia—gray, black
  - Trauma to tooth—hemosiderin
    - Transient—flush, red
    - Permanent—maybe pulpal necrosis; gray, black
    - Hemorrhage; incomplete root canal therapy; gray, black
  - Transfusion reaction hemolysis—hemosiderin; gray
- Drug administration
    - Tetracycline—primary or permanent teeth; yellow; gray
    - Sulfur (Sul-spansion)—bilirubin; black
    - Fluorides; white and/or brown spots
    - Liquid iron supplement—gray, black
- Other—hypoplastic and hypocalcified disease states
    - Hereditary—both primary and permanent teeth
      - Amelogenesis imperfecta; yellow, brown
      - Dentinogenesis imperfecta; blue, gray, black
    - Dental fluorosis—white, yellow, brown, black
    - Dental caries—yellow, brown, black
    - Abrasion, attrition, erosion—yellow of dentin

common site being the palate and alveolar mucosa.

The other focal pigmentations are exogenous. The most common is from the embedding of amalgam particles in the connective tissue of the mucosa. These "amalgam tattoos" appear as small, well-defined, blue-black lesions, occurring in association with the alveolar ridge. The particles of amalgam may show as radiopacities on a radiograph. They may result from the placement of retrograde root canal fillings, appearing in the mucobuccal fold (Fig. 7.38). They occur in older individuals who have usually had extensive dental treatment. Often they are noted on the alveolar ridge after extraction of teeth. In the floor of the mouth, they may resemble melanin pigmentations. Amalgam tattoos are so common that they should always be considered when a black lesion is noted. Other diagnostic considerations should include the mucocele, hemangioma, and melanin pigmentations.

Other foreign materials may cause pigmented lesions. Many individuals habit-

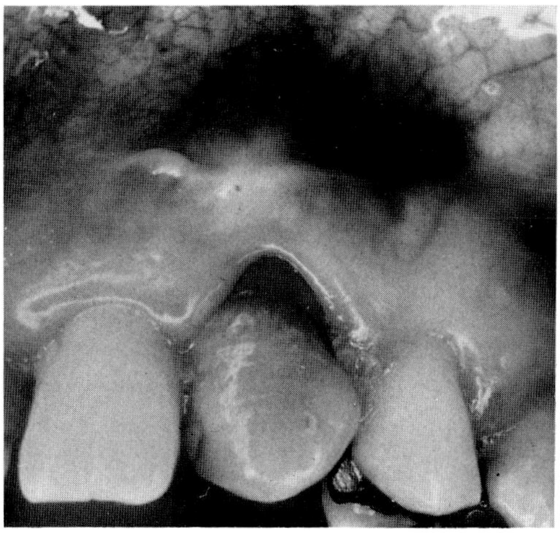

Figure 7.38. Amalgam tattoo, labial sulcus due to retrograde amalgam filling of cuspid that has a dead pulp and is stained due to hemosiderin in dentinal tubules.

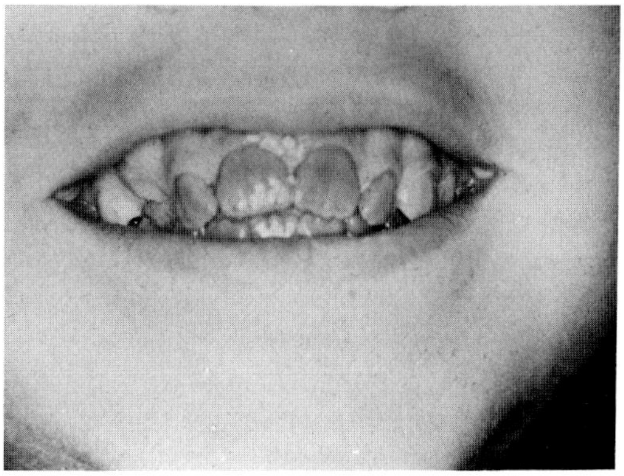

Figure 7.39. Tetracycline staining. This change is permanent, but bleaching or bonding may help eliminate the surface discoloration.

ually introduce lead pencils into the mouth. Graphite from the pencil can be forced into the mucosa and leave a dark, black circumscribed macule resembling the amalgam tattoo (see Fig. 6.13). A careful history aids the differentiation.

The antibiotic tetracycline may cause permanent intrinsic staining of either the primary or permanent teeth. If tetracycline is given over an extended period of time to the mother during pregnancy or to the infant, the teeth developing at that time become stained from a mild yellow to an unsightly yellow-brown or gray (Fig. 7.39). The change is permanent. The permanent teeth may need bleaching, bonding, or crowns to improve the esthetics.

Chapter 8
ORAL MANIFESTATIONS OF SYSTEMIC DISEASES

Numerous examples of oral manifestations of systemic diseases have been mentioned in other chapters. Viral diseases, tuberculosis, syphilis, lichen planus, pemphigus, and pigmentations are some examples. The oral cavity is commonly involved in many systemic diseases. Sometimes the resultant lesion is easily categorized and specific so that the disease entity is recognized, e.g., lichen planus. Other times the oral lesion is nonspecific. The lesion(s) may be common for several disease states that must be distinguished by means other than the clinical lesion itself. Thus, the oral manifestation may be gingivitis, glossitis, cheilosis, macroglossia, stomatitis, hemorrhage, infection, ulceration, pigmentation, changes in tooth eruption patterns, enlargement of bone, or other general disease states. One or more of these conditions may exist and, along with other body signs and symptoms, reflect a generalized, systemic disease rather than merely a localized, oral disease (Table 8.1). More examples are noted in this section.

Angular cheilosis refers to a fissuring or ulceration of the lips, specifically at the angles of the mouth. The condition may be

Table 8.1.
Differential diagnosis of general oral conditions of local or systemic etiology

Angular cheilosis	Gingivitis
Loss of vertical dimension	Imbalance of sex hormones (estrogens)
Excess salivation	Diabetes
Candidiasis	Vitamin C deficiency
Nutritional deficiency	Leukemia
Anemia	Bleeding disorder
Allergy	Eosinophilic granuloma
Smooth tongue (atrophic glossitis)	Local plaque
Nutritional deficiency	Primary herpes
Anemia	Allergy
Allergy	Macroglossia
Candidiasis	Congenital
Trauma	Hereditary—Down syndrome
Geographic tongue	Developmental—hemangioma
	Idiopathic—cause unknown
	Acquired
	Inflammatory edema—trauma, stomatitis, radiation
	Habit—biting, hypertrophy
	Tumor—neurofibromatosis
	Hormonal disturbance—acromegaly, hypothyroid
	Metabolism—amyloid deposits

painful, annoying, and long lasting. There are several causes. A common localized etiologic factor is the loss of vertical dimension of the occlusion in partially or totally edentulous individuals. Without the appropriate stops, the mandible overcloses toward the maxilla. The lips are forced against one another and appear grooved inward at the angle of the mouth (Fig. 8.1). Saliva leaks out and creates a moist environment that harbors microorganisms. Eventually the tissue breaks down and ulcerates. In this case, the vertical dimension can be restored by appropriate dental prosthetic appliances. Other causes of angular cheilosis are excessive salivation, with drooling and infection with *Candida albicans*, in which case the name of *perleche* is synonymous with cheilosis. Nutritional deficiencies, anemias, and allergy may also be etiologic factors in angular cheilosis.

True nutritional deficiencies are rare in the United States, although they may be found in deprived individuals or in those who practice "diet" fads. Vitamin B complex rather than an individual vitamin B deficiency may result in angular cheilosis as one of its signs (Fig. 8.2). Usually coupled with the cheilosis and generally regarded as the main oral sign is an atrophic or "bald" tongue (Fig. 8.3). There is atrophy and loss of the filiform and fungiform papillae. The tongue appears smooth; is prone to irritation; and often becomes red, swollen, and painful.

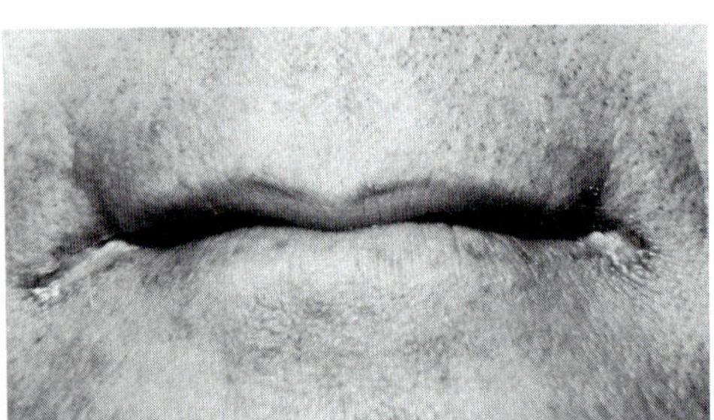

Figure 8.1. Angular cheilosis due to loss of vertical dimension in a full denture wearer.

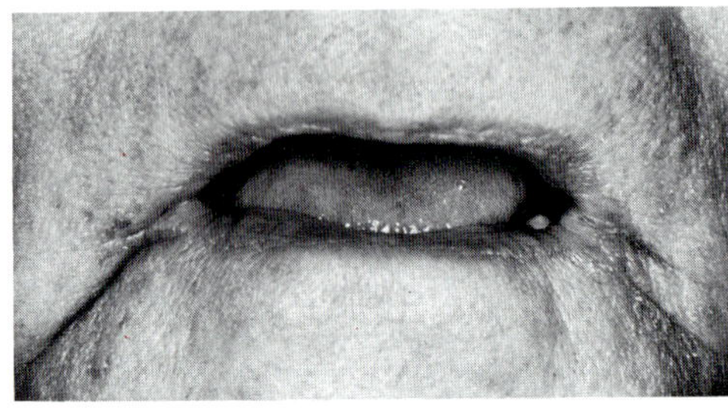

Figure 8.2. Angular cheilosis associated with vitamin B complex deficiency as well as loss of vertical dimension.

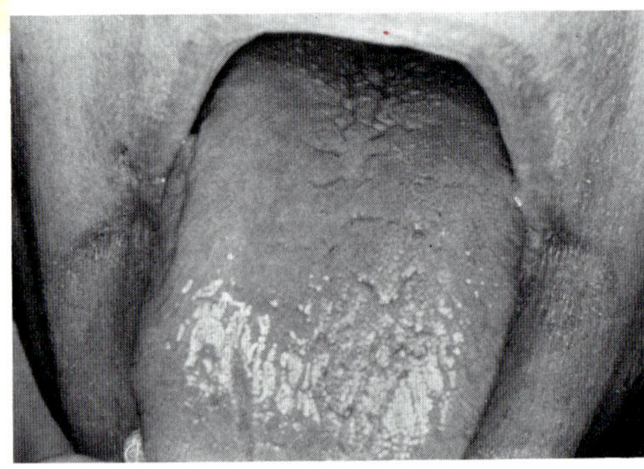

Figure 8.3. Smooth balding tongue and angular cheilosis associated with vitamin B complex deficiency. Same patient as in Figure 8.2.

Atrophic glossitis is also seen in anemic states. Anemia refers to an insufficient number of erythrocytes or hemoglobin, resulting in a decrease in the amount of oxygen to the tissues. There are many types of anemia including nutritional; pernicious; hemorrhagic (from a large loss of blood; hemolytic (from the premature rupturing of the red blood cells); those caused by parasites, toxins, antibodies, and heredity (thalassemia); aplastic anemia from the destruction of the red bone marrow from tumors, toxins, radiation, or some medications; and sickle cell anemia, a hereditary trait with abnormal hemoglobin leading to hemolysis of the red cells. The lack of oxygen results in the patient feeling fatigued, being intolerant to cold, and showing a paleness caused by lack of hemoglobin. The tongue is sensitive to such changes in its nutritional state and responds with a loss of papillae, resulting in a smooth tongue (Figs. 8.4 and 8.5). Blood tests must be done to diagnose the type of anemia accurately.

Pernicious anemia is a hereditary disease affecting middle-aged individuals. The patient lacks production in the stomach of intrinsic factor that is required to absorb vitamin B_{12}, the extrinsic factor, from the intestine. The B_{12} is necessary in the formation of hemoglobin. Some malabsorption conditions and treatment with tetracycline can cause a similar lack of vitamin B_{12} and a state of anemia.

After diagnosis and treatment with monthly injections of vitamin B_{12}, the mucosa returns to normal (Figs. 8.6 and 8.7). It should be recalled that the endarteritis of syphilis produces atrophic glossitis in the tertiary stage of the disease. The loss of papillae may occur gradually, leaving patchy areas that may mimic traumatic glossitis or geographic tongue. Tongues with atrophic glossitis are susceptible to the development of leukoplakia and therefore may also have white patches over the smooth red surface.

Another sign of anemia may be a burning tongue and paleness of the skin and

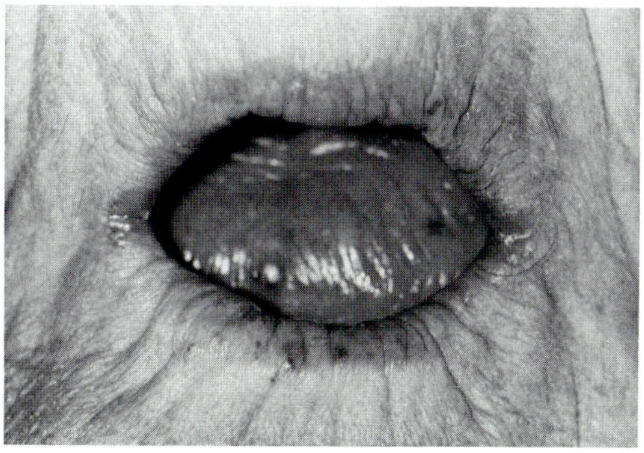

Figure 8.4. Angular cheilosis and pallor of the lips associated with iron deficiency anemia in a 76-year-old female with Plummer-Vinson syndrome.

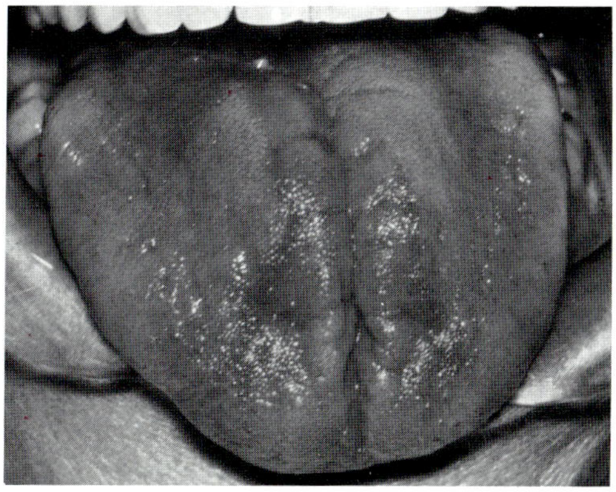

Figure 8.6. Smooth patchy red tongue due to vitamin B_{12} deficiency secondary to pernicious anemia.

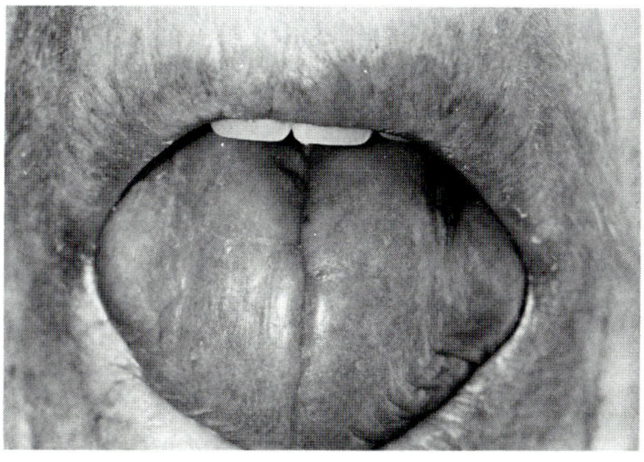

Figure 8.5. Smooth bald tongue associated with iron deficiency anemia. Same patient as in Figure 8.4.

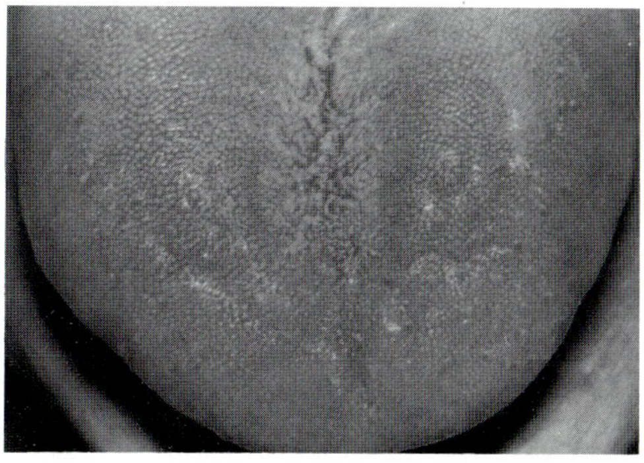

Figure 8.7. Normal-appearing tongue of patient in Figure 8.6 after treatment with injection of vitamin B_{12} showing regeneration of lingual papillae.

mucosa. The lips may be white with a bluish tint, in addition to the cheilosis and glossitis.

The opposite of anemia is polycythemia, an abnormal increase in the number of red blood cells. The hematocrit and blood pressure rise, and thrombosis from too many cells in the vessel ensues, along with hemorrhage. Because of the possibility of hemorrhage, surgery is contraindicated until the patient's hematocrit is lowered. The oral tissues appear very red and there may be gingivitis and spontaneous hemorrhage.

Gingivitis, with red, boggy, swollen, bleeding gingivae, may be a sign of systemic disease. Systemic disease may alter the response of the tissue to local factors or it may, in itself, cause a hyperplastic response. The resulting clinical picture is recognized only as a gingivitis. Generally, patients with gingivitis of local cause heal dramatically after a scaling and curettage. If after such treatment(s), a patient fails to heal or the lesions on the gingiva persist, some systemic disease or component should be considered. An imbalance of sex hormones at puberty, in pregnancy, during menstruation, or via oral contraceptive agents has been associated with gingival inflammation. Uncontrolled diabetic patients are prone to severe periodontal problems and an exaggerated gingivitis (Fig. 8.8). Eosinophilic granuloma (see Chapter 7), a bone disease mimicking a cyst or periodontal disease, may first manifest as a gingivitis along with mobile teeth in the first and second decades (Fig. 8.9). Bleeding and hyperplastic gingivae may be a sign of vitamin C deficiency (scurvy), although this would be very rare now except for poor dieting.

Leukemia may present as a gingival hyperplasia. Leukemia is a malignant disease of blood-forming tissues. Usually, in acute leukemia there is uncontrolled growth of immature leukocytes. In chronic leukemia there is an accumulation of mature leukocytes. The human T-cell leukemia-lymphoma virus (HTLV-1) is associated with leukemia. The crowding out of normal cells in the marrow creates anemia and bleeding problems from a decrease in platelets. Owing to the lack of normal leukocytes

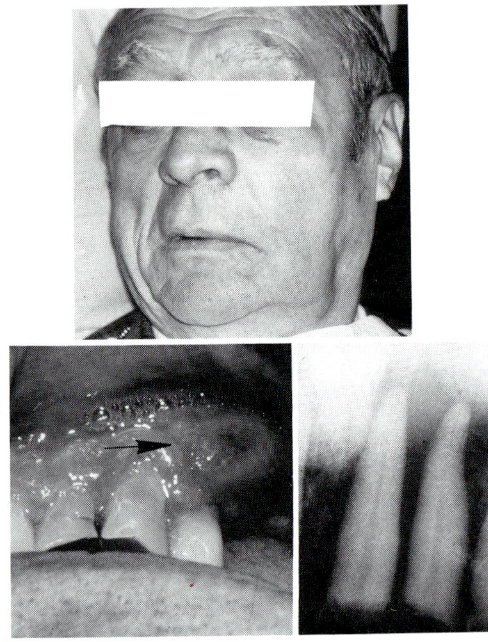

Figure 8.8. Uncontrolled diabetic patient with multiple episodes of acute apical and periodontal abscesses; infection spread to cause a cellulitis of left face up to the eye; there is a large fluctuant gum boil or periodontal abscess over the premolar, and the radiograph reveals severe loss of bone. Patient was medicated with antibiotics and teeth were extracted.

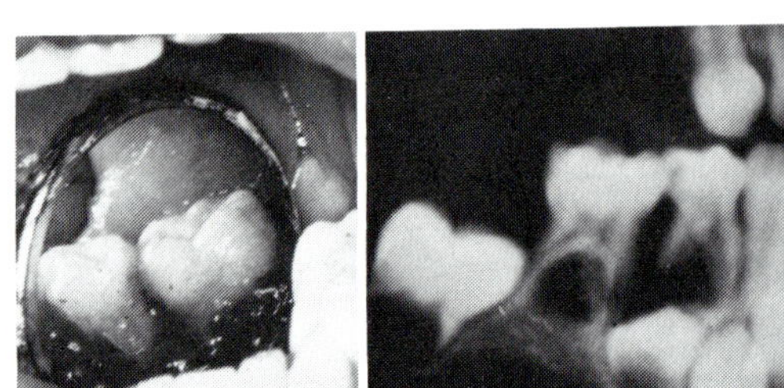

Figure 8.9. Eosinophilic granuloma in a 4-year-old; the deciduous teeth were prematurely loose with severe recession and gingivitis; radiographs show severe loss of bone mimicking periodontal disease, with teeth floating in the radiolucency.

to fight organisms, the patients are prone to infections. In the oral cavity the manifestations may be spontaneous bleeding, abnormal infections by organisms normally not in the oral cavity, ulcerations, candidiasis, and gingival hyperplasia. The hyperplasia may be the first sign and may be due to inflammation or an infiltration of the leukemic cells. Generally, acute or chronic monocytic leukemia manifests in the mouth (Fig. 8.10). In children, the gingival swelling may be present but is not the first sign of the disease.

Bleeding may occur from the gingivae or into the oral tissues as a result of a bleeding or hemorrhagic disorder. Petechiae and ecchymoses are often signs of platelet deficiency (thrombocytopenia). When the platelet count falls below 60,000 (normal = 200,000 to 400,000; see Appendix B), then capillary bleeding may be easily provoked or spontaneous, particularly below a count of 10,000. The oral signs are blue-purple macules either as tiny dots (petechiae) or as large areas (ecchymoses). Platelet deficiency may be caused by sundry conditions, including reaction to medications or organisms, radiation, cancers, and unknown causes (primary thrombocytopenic purpura).

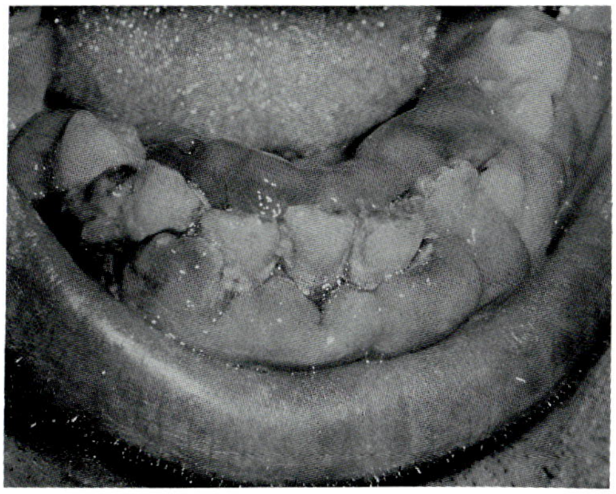

Figure 8.10. Acute monocytic leukemia; middle-aged male developed sudden growth of gingivae that bled spontaneously (note labial gingivae of canine and premolar); white blood count was 50,000; biopsy revealed abnormal macrophages.

The oral manifestation of a bleeding disorder is a hematoma, petechiae, or ecchymoses (see Fig. 9.10); spontaneous bleeding; or delayed bleeding after a surgical procedure. It may occur along with a gingivitis. Either fresh blood or clots, some of which may be very large, are noted. The cause becomes apparent after the appropriate tests are done for the factor(s) that may be deficient. In von Willebrandt's disease, there is a deficiency of clotting factor VIII. Other hemophilic factors, either combined or singularly deficient, show similar signs of bleeding. Because several clotting factors are manufactured in the liver, one should remember that liver disease, particularly cirrhosis, may be associated with bleeding problems. There are several diseases that are treated by thinning the blood or purposefully causing the bleeding time to be longer. For example, patients with severe kidney disease requiring dialysis are placed on dicumerol. This predisposes the patient to bleeding and bruising problems (see Fig. 7.8).

Neutropenia refers to a marked decrease or lack in the number of neutrophils. Without neutrophils the body cannot fight infections properly, and organisms get the upper hand. This results in tissue destruction. In the oral cavity there can be necrosis of the gingivae and a severe loss of alveolar bone resembling periodontal disease. The causes for neutropenia are many, including unknown or idiopathic, leukemia, radiation, drug or medication reaction, and a genetic enzyme deficiency.

Autoimmune Diseases

Lupus erythematosus is an autoimmune (collagen) disease with damage to small blood vessel walls resulting in inflammation. There is a chronic, low-grade disease that can affect the skin primarily and eventually heals. A more serious systemic form attacks young women in their reproductive years. They have antinuclear antibodies, and the vessel damage can affect major organs like the kidney and heart. Triggering factors are medications, exposure to excessive sunlight, stress, and infections. A skin rash may appear on the body, and when on the cheeks and bridge of the nose may resemble a "butterfly" (Figs. 8.11 and 8.12). In the oral cavity lupus lesions resemble lichen planus with erosive areas and white, keratotic, linear and oval lesions. Biopsy and several special tests are required for diagnosis. It is treated with corticosteroids.

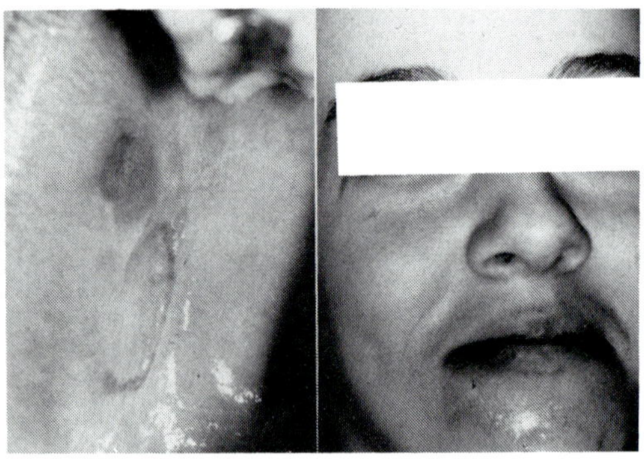

Figure 8.11. Oral and facial manifestations of systemic lupus erythematosus; oval erosive and reticular lesions on buccal mucosa resemble lichen planus; the patient has a mild rash over the cheeks and bridge of nose (butterfly rash); coincidentally, she has a hemangioma of the lower lip and chin.

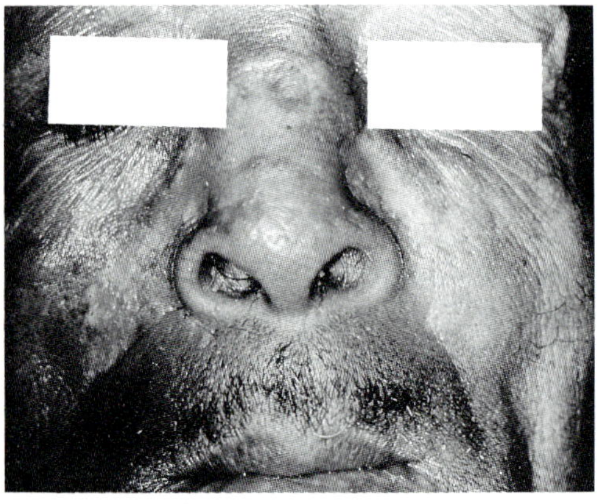

Figure 8.12. Healed (scarred) "butterfly" rash of chronic discoid erythematosus in a male. The disease occurred in his younger days.

Another autoimmune disease with oral consequences is scleroderma. Characterized by excessive deposition of collagen in the tissues, it causes the skin to become hardened, taut, and shiny. Correspondingly, the oral opening becomes restricted and collagen deposition is seen in the form of firm gingivae, sometimes with swellings, and in a general, bilateral widening of periodontal ligaments, particularly of the posterior teeth in a small percentage of patients. Occurring in all patients with scleroderma is Raynaud's phenomenon.

Raynaud's phenomenon refers to the spasm of end arterioles of the hands, primarily, and toes. Triggered by cold and emotions, the digits become pale for several minutes due to the ischemia. There is pain and burning and then the circulation returns. The phenomenon occurs with underlying diseases such as autoimmune diseases and may be occupational (jackhammer operators). When there is no underlying disease identified, the phenomenon is called Raynaud's disease. The oral cavity rarely may be affected with spasms of end arteries, as on the tongue (Fig. 8.13).

Rheumatoid arthritis is an autoimmune disease with antigen-antibody complexes arising against the patient's own tissues in the joints, resulting in inflammation, swelling, and pain in the joints. It is associated with many of the other autoimmune diseases and in particular with Sjögren's syndrome. Sjögren's syndrome is a clinical complex comprising rheumatoid arthritis (or other immune diseases), a dry mouth, and dry eyes (conjunctivitis). The clinical diagnosis may be made if any two of the three exist in the patient. The dry mouth is significant and can lead to severe dental caries despite good hygiene (Figs. 8.14 and 8.15). Therefore, the patient should be offered saliva substitutes along with remineralization treatments to prevent loss of the teeth. The lack of saliva is often reflected in changes in the salivary glands such that a biopsy shows lymphoproliferative changes and may manifest as an enlargement of the parotid gland(s). There is a chance that a lymphoma may arise in some patients.

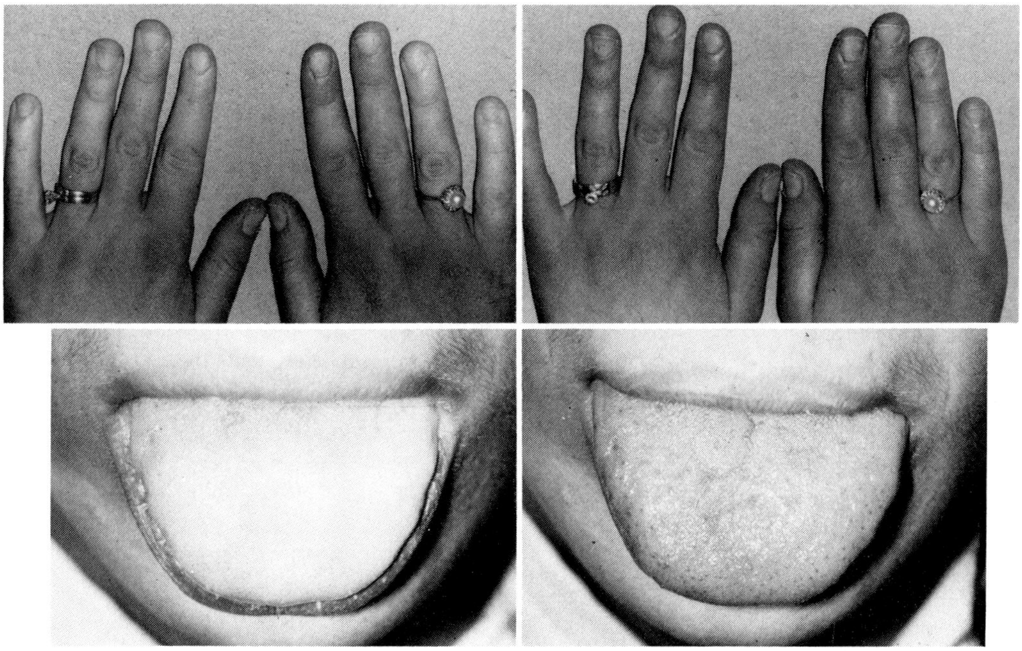

Figure 8.13. A 24-year-old female with Raynaud's disease of hands and mouth triggered by emotions and cold. On left, the tissues are blanched due to spasm of end arterioles, lasting for 15 minutes; on right, tissues returned to normal tone. Raynaud's phenomenon includes spasm of the fingers and some other underlying disease, usually autoimmune in nature.

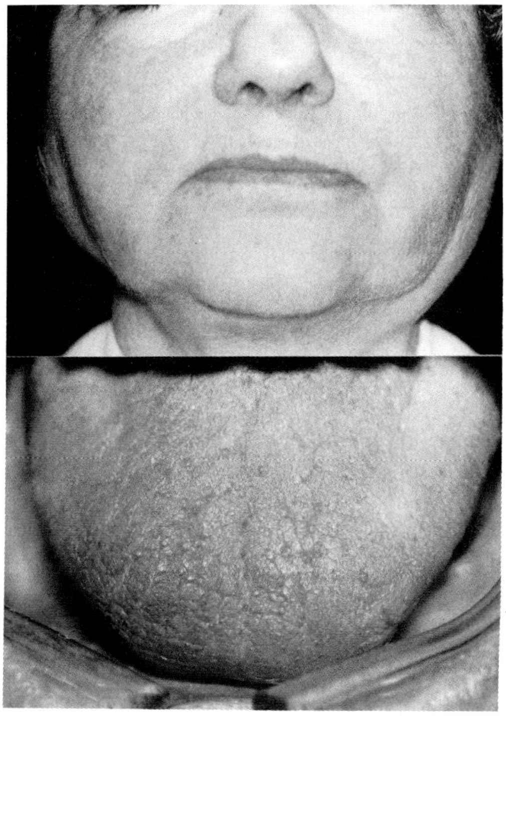

Figure 8.14. Sjögren's syndrome; older female has dry mouth and dry eyes and has developed bilateral enlargement of the parotid glands resembling mumps or tumor. The tongue is smooth and dry from lack of saliva.

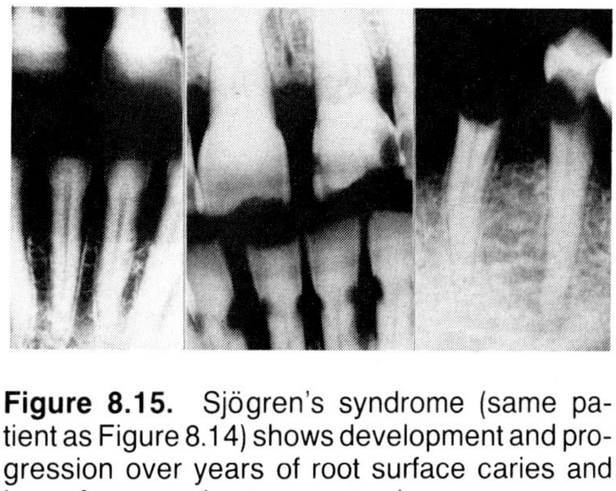

Figure 8.15. Sjögren's syndrome (same patient as Figure 8.14) shows development and progression over years of root surface caries and loss of crowns due to xerostomia.

Endocrine Disturbances

There are many hormonal disturbances or endocrinopathies, some of which manifest in the oral cavity. Acromegaly, though not common, is a condition that may be noted first by the dental team. Acromegaly is caused by an adenoma arising in the pituitary gland causing the sella turcica to enlarge. The adenoma produces several hormones that affect other areas of the body. An increase in growth hormone in an adult causes the distal, extreme (acro) parts to grow. The hands, feet, ear lobes, and mandible enlarge prominently over time (Fig. 8.16). Internally, the major organs such as the heart enlarge. The mandibular growth causes a change in occlusion and mandibular prognathism. This change may be the first indication of disease, because the enlargement of the hands and feet is slow enough not to impress the patient. In addition, macroglossia is a prominent feature, along with large edematous lips. The oral manifestations should lead the clinician to send the patient for diagnosis. Treatment consists of ablating the tumor with drugs, radiation, or surgery.

Hypothyroidism results from a hyposecretion of thyrotropic hormone. During growth, it results in cretinism with lack of

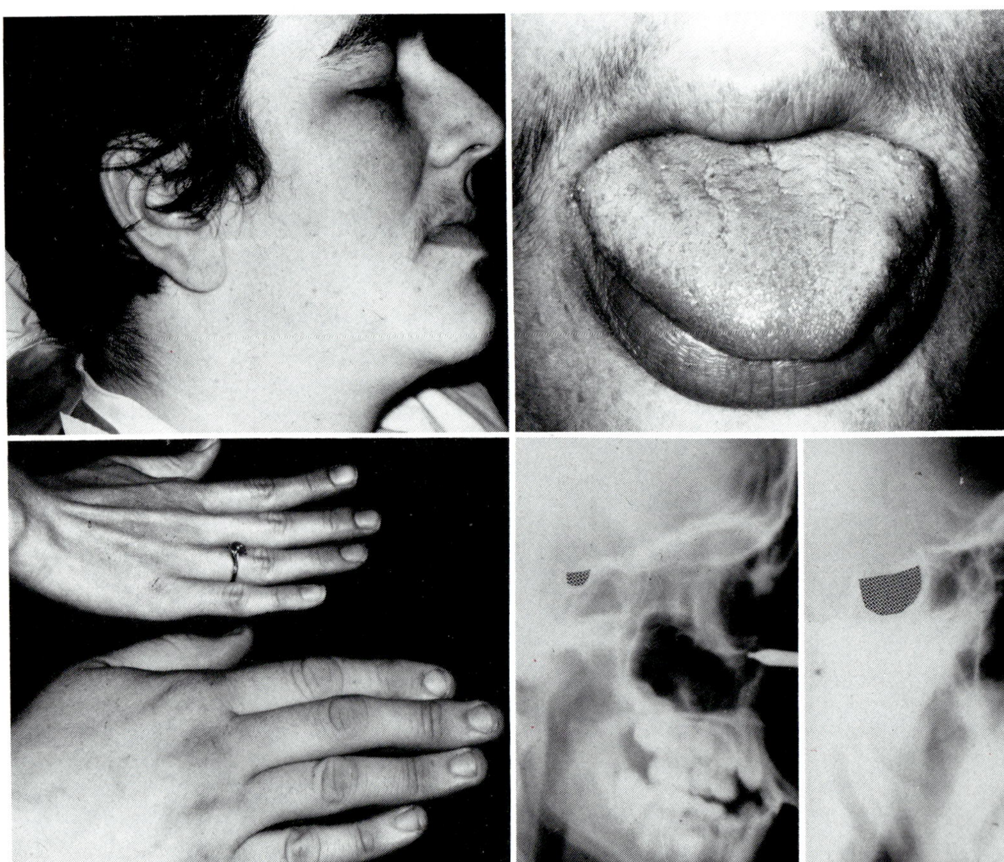

Figure 8.16. Acromegaly in a 31-year-old male; note prognathic mandible, large lower lip, and large ear lobe; large tongue (macroglossia); enlarged hand of patient compared to a size 8 hand (feet were also enlarged); enlarged sella turcica on right compared to a normal one on the left; the size of the sella is indicated by gray area.

skeletal growth and mental retardation. Fat pads accumulate, and the infants have large bellies and large protruding tongues. In adults, it results in myxedema with slow heart rate, lethargy, muscle weakness, and weight gain. Facial tissues become swollen and rounded. Intraorally, the edema causes the tongue to enlarge, with a scalloping caused by pressure against the teeth (see Fig. 4.3). A delay in the eruption of teeth may be one of the signs to raise the diagnosis of hypothyroidism.

Hypersecretion of thyroid hormones is hyperthyroidism. Generally, the thyroid enlarges and is called a goiter. There can be edema behind the eye, causing the eye to protrude (exophthalmos) and a high metabolic rate yielding high energy and weight loss. Orally, there may be increased salivation, premature eruption of teeth, and osteoporosis. A lower than average amount of iodine in the diet may also be a cause of goiter, since iodine is required for thyroxine production.

Parathyroid gland dysfunction may also have oral manifestations. The parathyroid glands regulate blood calcium levels, interacting with calcitonin from the thyroid, estrogens, and androgens, among others. They synthesize and release parathyroid hormone (PTH), which increases blood calcium by acting on the gut, the bone (through osteoclastic activity), and the kidney to increase phosphate excretion and to activate vitamin D. In hypoparathyroidism there is low blood calcium, resulting in tetany and convulsions. If the episode occurs during tooth development, then there is delayed eruption and hypoplasia of the enamel and dentin (Fig. 8.17) of the teeth affected during the tetany. In hyperparathyroidism there is an increase in blood calcium. With time there can be lethargy and a generalized osteoporosis (thinning of the endosteal plates of bone). Orally, the changes are noted radiographically in some patients. There may be a loss of the lamina dura and radiolucent cystic lesions, which have a giant-cell granuloma histology. After removal of the benign tumor or hyperplastic parathyroid tissue causing the condition, the serum calcium returns to normal and the bone lesions heal.

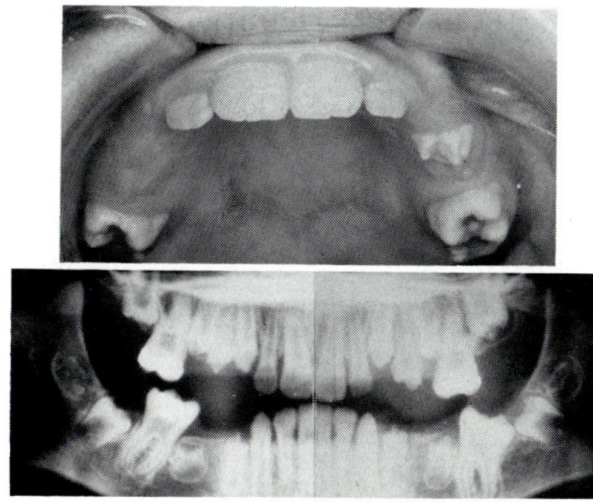

Figure 8.17. Hypoplasia of teeth secondary to an episode of hypoparathyroid disease. Erupting premolar shows lack of tooth structure. Radiograph shows bilateral involvement of premolars and second molars, which were forming at the time of the convulsions owing to the lowered serum calcium.

Adrenal glands produce many hormones. If there is a hyposecretion of the glucocorticoids, then Addison's disease (primary adrenal insufficiency) results. There may be lethargy, weight loss, hypoglycemia, low blood pressure, and weakness. The low corticoid level triggers the homeostatic mechanism to produce ACTH from the thalamus in an effort to get the adrenal to produce more steroids. The melanin-stimulating hormone is also triggered, and one of the signs on the skin and the mouth is an increase in melanin pigmentation. Diffuse melanotic macules may appear early or late in the disease. If early, they may lead to the diagnosis. Treatment is with corticosteroids.

Cushing's syndrome results from a hypersecretion of adrenal glucocorticoids, particularly cortisone. Fat is redistributed, resulting in a "moon face," "buffalo hump" on the back, and a plump abdomen. Facial skin is flushed. Oral manifestations of steroid excess would be osteoporosis, perhaps presenting as periodontal disease or an exaggeration of it. In addition, there may be delayed healing and bruising, since steroids decrease proper collagen formation, yielding less scar tissue and weakened smaller blood vessels.

Diabetes is a class of diseases categorized by a deficiency of insulin or its activity. Insulin is produced by the beta cells of the islets of Langerhans' in the pancreas. In the controlled diabetic, it is questionable whether there are oral manifestations. In the uncontrolled diabetic there are recognized oral manifestations. There can be an exaggerated gingival hyperplasia with bleeding, a tendency toward multiple periodontal abscesses and multiple periapical abscesses. Also, a burning mouth or tongue may be a symptom of diabetes.

Estrogen, produced in excess by the ovaries, can result in oral manifestations. During puberty there is an imbalance of many hormones including estrogen. Pubertal gingivitis, an exaggerated response to plaque, is a recognized entity. A similar condition may occur during pregnancy and may occur with a pyogenic granuloma (pregnancy tumor) (see Chapter 6). A similar gingival reaction may be noted during menstruation. Also, there can be a desquamative gingivitis related to menopause. Birth control pills, particularly those high in estrogen, may cause small focal opaque dots on the radiographs of the mandible beneath the anterior teeth (Fig. 8.18), due to the fact that estrogen stimulates endosteal bone formation by turning off parathyroid hormone.

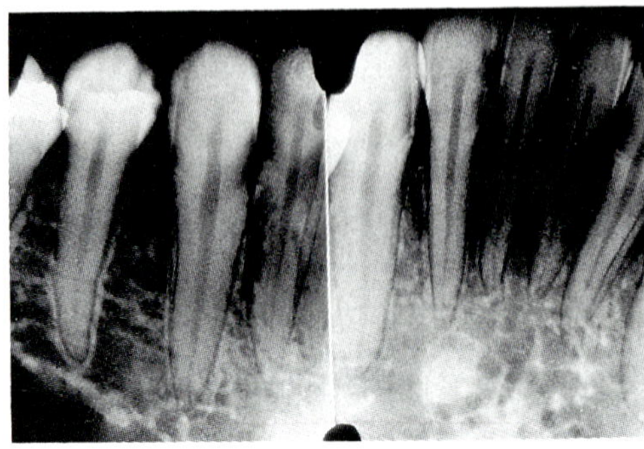

Figure 8.18. Osteosclerotic, white spots in basal bone below teeth due to increased size of endosteal bony plates in a female in her twenties; caused by use of birth control pills and the effect of estrogen on endosteal bone.

Allergy

Allergic or hypersensitivity reactions occur in the oral cavity and are a manifestation of an overactive immune response. The reaction may be immediate, as in an anaphylactic reaction or a reaction to a commonly used drug. For instance, a reaction to penicillin or sulfa drug can occur at any time that the drug is reintroduced to the body. There may be a very serious reaction that affects breathing, or there may be a skin reaction in the form of hives or welts. The drug must be stopped and Benadryl or other medication should be given. Because allergic reactions are part of the immune response, they are manifestations of systemic disease. However, the reactions may appear in many ways so that they are difficult to categorize. The oral manifestations may be blisters, ulcers, an erythema or rash, a white, necrotic lesion with a pseudomembrane, a white keratotic lesion, an erosion, an area of atrophy, or even a hematoma. It may mimic several disease entities. Therefore, allergy should be a consideration in many situations when establishing a differential diagnosis.

Erythema multiforme is a symptom complex categorized by blisters and a rash on the skin. It usually is traced to some allergen when a careful history is taken. The oral manifestation is usually lip involvement with blisters and crusts. A target lesion on the skin is helpful in making the diagnosis. An example of erythema multiforme secondary to aspirin gum allergy is noted in Figure 8.19. An allergy to chewing gum, mint, or cinnamon, may manifest as angular cheilitis, fiery red gingivitis, and reddened stomatitis. Patients may be allergic to the liquid monomer used in making temporary crowns and bridges or to other

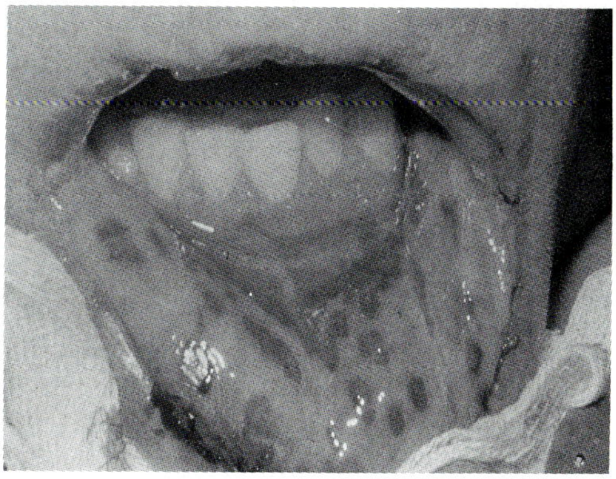

Figure 8.19. Erythema multiforme of lower lip, showing multiple coalescing blisters with white pseudomembrane and some crusting on skin side with no gingival involvement; caused by an allergy to aspirin chewing gum.

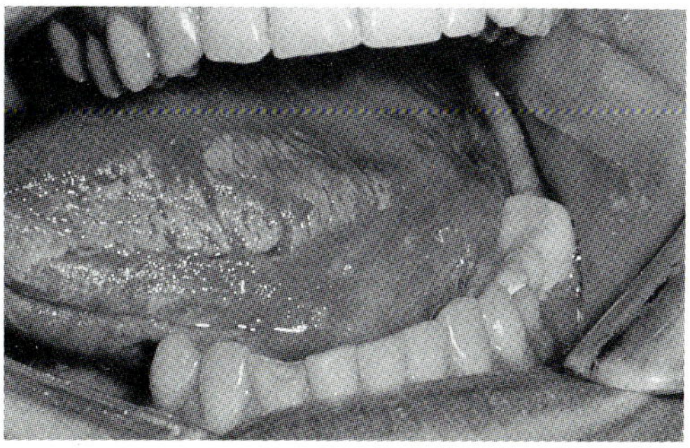

Figure 8.20. Allergy to acrylic liquid monomer in a hypersensitive female in her twenties. Note hyperkeratosis on lateral tongue and buccal mucosa, both having touched the temporary bridge, which had residual monomer. The reaction occurred 24 hours after placing the bridge and disappeared two days after bridge was removed. (This picture also resembles hairy leukoplakia of AIDS.)

dental materials. The reaction to monomer is a classic example of a delayed hypersensitivity reaction. In contrast to a direct chemical burn, in which there is an almost immediate reaction, the delayed reaction occurs after 24 hours. The patient complains of a burning sensation, and there may be a hyperkeratotic reaction or blistering with erosions (Fig. 8.20). The treatment is to recognize the offending agent and to remove it. The temporary restoration should be removed and then autoclaved to drive out the residual monomer. It may then be recemented or a crown of another material may replace it. The oral lesion resolves quickly after removal of the offending agent, and topical corticosteroids may help speed the healing. A more common allergen in the oral cavity is the medication benzocaine. It is used frequently in the many over-the-counter aids to alleviate oral and dental pain. The reaction is delayed and is characterized by blisters that leave the surface of the epithelium a necrotic white with areas of erythema (Fig. 8.21). The use of the medication should be stopped, and the pain and lesions may be treated. Commonly, the patient may have a history of being allergic to other agents.

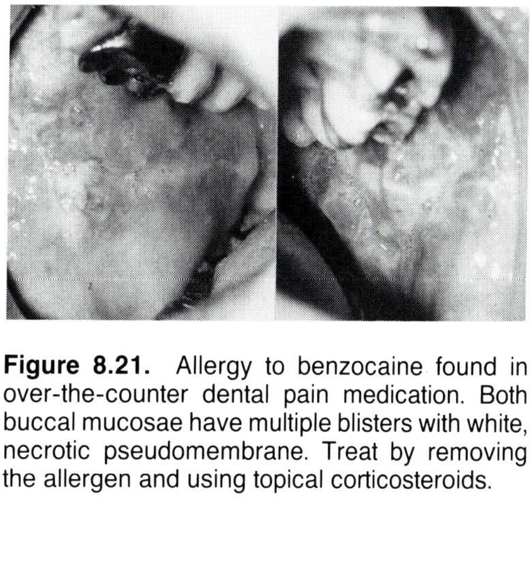

Figure 8.21. Allergy to benzocaine found in over-the-counter dental pain medication. Both buccal mucosae have multiple blisters with white, necrotic pseudomembrane. Treat by removing the allergen and using topical corticosteroids.

A special form of allergic response is seen in angioneurotic edema. The allergens can be anything but usually can be traced to foods, such as eggs, chicken, or shellfish, or to agents such as cosmetics. After a delay, the lips and sometimes the eyes swell greatly with fluid; the lips double or triple in size (Fig. 8.22), presenting as a pitting edema. The treatment is systemic Benadryl to counteract the histaminic reaction that

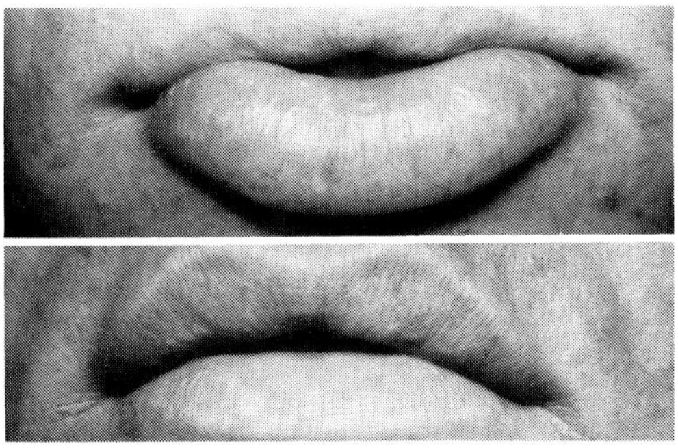

Figure 8.22. Angioneurotic edema of the lower lip in a 19-year-old male who by history was sensitive to shellfish in a meal the previous night. The swelling was sudden and had pitting edema. It resolved with Benadryl tablets and returned to normal (*bottom*).

has triggered the outpouring of fluid into the tissues.

Commonly used items may unexpectedly cause an allergic reaction. An example is toothpaste. The patient may be sensitive to the active ingredients or to the preservatives or binding agents. The exact agent is difficult to determine. There may be a sloughing of tissue with atrophy or erosions with a fiery erythema. Tissues touched by the material are affected. Thus, the gingivae, tongue, and buccal mucosae may be reddened with burning (Fig. 8.23). Withdrawal of the paste allows healing to ensue within a few days. To prove that the agent is the cause, it would have to be reintroduced to develop new lesions. This is not usually necessary. However, when an agent is unknown, it is suggested that the patient keep a careful diary so that the agent may be identified. If a food is suggested, then the patient must try an elimination diet, a tedious but sometimes rewarding experience.

AIDS

AIDS was discussed in the section on immunology. HIV infects the basic cells of the immune response, and without that response the patient is prone to many opportunistic infections. The oral cavity is very much involved in AIDS. Oral candidiasis may be the first sign of the disease. However, there are many oral manifestations:

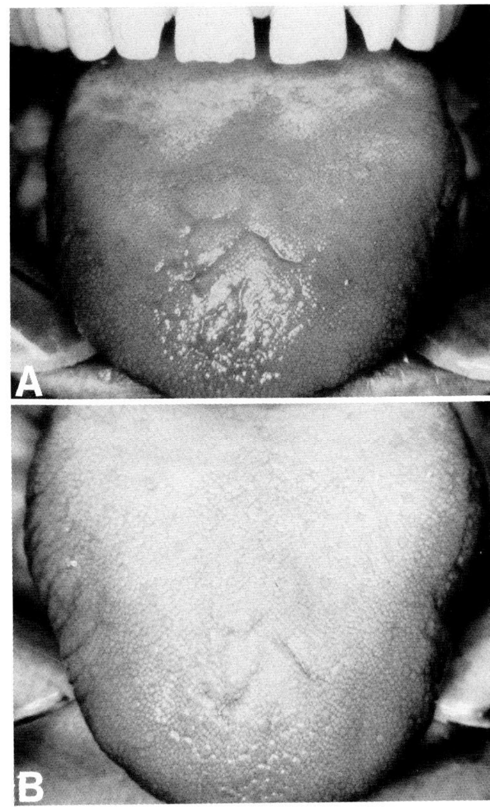

Figure 8.23. Allergy to toothpaste. *A*, atrophic, balding, red rash on tongue with burning. *B*, return of tongue to normal after removing offending toothpaste and replacing it.

- Cervical and postcervical lymphadenopathy—similar to infectious mononucleosis (see Fig. 1.10)
- Kaposi's sarcoma
- Hairy leukoplakia—a marker for HIV infection
- Candidiasis—the most common HIV-related infection
- Atypical periodontal disease—like severe ANUG
- Herpetic infections—primary and secondary
- Oral cancer—lymphoma and carcinoma at an early age

- Ulcers—like chronic aphthous stomatitis
- Other infections—like tuberculosis or any other unusual infection in the mouth

Of these, candidiasis, hairy leukoplakia, and Kaposi's sarcoma are key features. The candidiasis may appear in any of its forms, a white removable, a reddened atrophic, or even a keratotic lesion. What is important is to be suspicious if the patient fits into one of the high-risk categories. Hairy leukoplakia is a unique white lesion covering the lateral surface on one or both sides (Fig. 8.24). Classically it is slightly raised and corrugated with the appearance of "hairs," but it may resemble hyperkeratosis, candidiasis, lichen planus, and others. Again, one needs a high suspicion, and then a biopsy may be very useful because it has a very suggestive pattern. Hairy leukoplakia may be a first manifestation or may lead to a diagnosis of AIDS. Kaposi's sarcoma is a late-stage manifestation. A malignant tumor of blood vessels and fibroblasts, it is macular at first, like an ecchymosis, and then nodular like a hemangioma as it enlarges. Blue-purple because of its vascularity, it frequently appears in the mouth on the palate or gingiva, as well as on the face. But it may be just in the mouth at first and also may lead to a diagnosis of AIDS. The oral cavity is an important area in this disease with many oral manifestations.

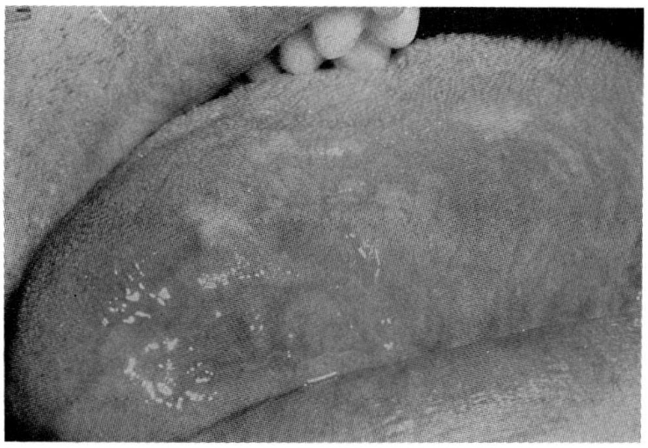

Figure 8.24. Hairy leukoplakia in a 38-year-old male homosexual. Slightly raised white lesions have a corrugated appearance and cover a large area on the lateral border of the tongue. This may be the first indication that the patient has AIDS and may serve as a marker for the disease. Note that this resembles lichen planus.

Macroglossia occurs in several conditions and has been referred to here many times. Because it is striking, its causes are interesting to review and they offer an overview of many catagories of disease. Essentially we are referring to a diffuse enlargement of the tongue, causes of which may be congenital, acquired, or idiopathic (Table 8.2).

Congenital macroglossia may be seen in patients with Down syndrome. This is a spontaneous or hereditary genetic defect with several manifestations, one being a large tongue. Down syndrome is the most

Table 8.2.
Macroglossia

Causes (Condition)	Category of Disease
Congenital	
Genetic—Down syndrome	Developmental
Developmental—hemangioma, lymphangioma	
Idiopathic	
Acquired	
Trauma—inflammatory edema, stomatitis	Inflammatory
Radiation therapy—edema	
Habit—hypertrophy	Hyperplastic
Tumor—neurofibroma	Neoplastic
Hormone disturbance—acromegaly, hypothyroidism (cretinism, myxedema)	Metabolic (systemic)
Metabolic disturbance—amyloid deposits	

common genetic disorder, characterized by having 47 chromosomes instead of the normal 46 (the extra chromosome being in the twenty-first pair, trisomy 21). The syndrome consists of mental retardation, short stature and stubby fingers, round head, slanting eyes, flat profile due to small maxilla, and a large tongue. The heart, ears, hands, and feet are malformed. In addition to the small maxilla and to macroglossia, these patients have excess saliva, a more alkaline saliva, and fewer dental caries. However, they have a marked tendency toward severe periodontal disease.

Hemangiomas and lymphangiomas are developmental benign tumors that may affect the entire tongue (angiomatosis) (Fig. 8.25). The hormonal disturbances of acromegaly and hypothyroidism are acquired, and one of the signs may be macroglossia. Amyloid deposition is another condition, usually systemic, in which protein metabolism is disturbed. The amyloid accumulates and infiltrates major organs. Amyloid may occur secondarily in association with malignant tumors. In the tongue it replaces the musculature and causes a macroglossia. Therefore, the dentist may be requested by the patient's physician to biopsy the tongue because it is much more accessible than the other organs that might be involved, to evaluate the possibility of amyloid deposition. The nervous habit of forcing the tongue against the teeth or dentures may result in a hypertrophy of the tissue with enlargement (Fig. 8.26). Many inflammatory situations, particularly in acute stomatitis, yield edema, scalloped tongue, and a large, full tongue. Acute herpetic stomatitis and erythema multiforme are examples. Similar edema may result during or following radiation therapy. Finally, there may be gross enlargement with a tumor. In von Recklinghausen's neurofibromatosis, multiple neurofibromas cause a pronounced macroglossia. There are many unknown causes listed as idiopathic. Thus, macroglossia, readily observed, may have many causes. The manifestation of a large tongue may be categorized according to the response of the body as developmental, inflammatory, hyperplastic, neoplastic, or metabolic (systemic) disease. If no observation is made, the pathology will be overlooked.

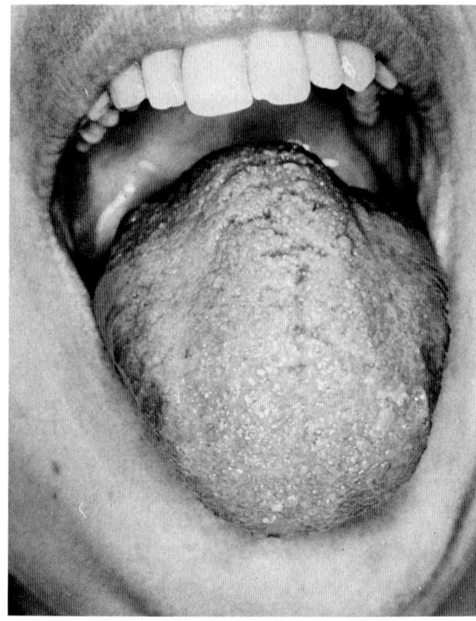

Figure 8.25. Macroglossia associated with angiomatosis of the tongue. The whole tongue was involved with a congenital hemangioma.

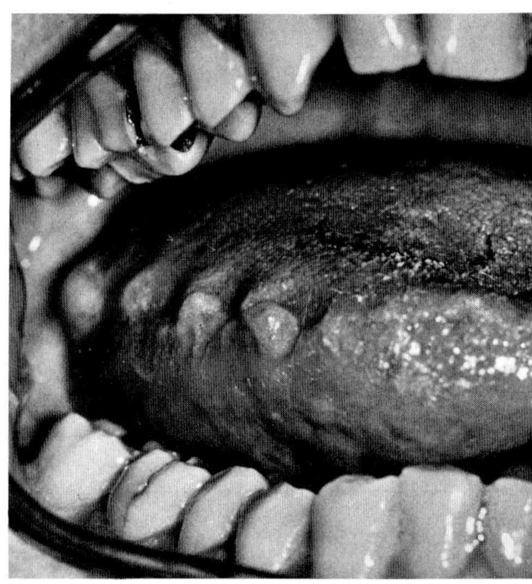

Figure 8.26. Macroglossia and scalloping of lateral border of tongue associated with nervous habit of tongue-thrusting.

Chapter 9
DIFFERENTIAL DIAGNOSIS

Differential diagnosis is defined as the determination of which one of two or more diseases or conditions is affecting a patient, by systematically comparing and contrasting their symptoms. For comprehensive coverage of differential diagnosis of oral lesions, refer to Wood and Goaz in the bibliography. This chapter presents an overview and an example of differential diagnosis.

The basis of the diagnosis is the history and physical examination of the patient followed by a radiologic study or some other imaging technique. The age, sex, and other identifying data are followed by a statement of chief complaint, such as, "I have had this lesion on my lip for several months or years." This is followed by the history of the present illness to find out more details about it, such as a history of pain or swelling or recurrences. Then the medical history is reviewed to include the family, social, occupational, and dental history. This would include questions on smoking and drinking, among many other things. Then a historical review of systems in completed. Following this, a physical examination is done (as described in Chapter 1), ending at the area of chief complaint. Inspection and palpation are the main means of accomplishing this. Should radiographs be required for further information, appropriate films are taken.

With the foregoing basic information, a differential diagnosis can be formulated. This entails arranging or listing in one's mind and recording the various possible diseases or entities the patient could have, listing the most probable first. Most often there can be a definite diagnosis. If it is not, then the number one possibility becomes the working or provisional diagnosis, and further information is sought to support or reject the working diagnosis. These additional studies may be medical laboratory studies such as a blood count, a blood sugar, hematocrit, hemoglobin, and platelet count; dental laboratory studies as in mounted models; a biopsy or removal of the whole lesion (excisional) or part of the lesion (incisional), either by knife or by needle, and receiving the report from a qualified pathologist; cytologic smear and the report, such as in herpetic or candidal infections; and the referral of the patient to a specialist or other doctor for another opinion. With this information, the clinician can hopefully render a final diagnosis, proven by the histories and several tests as required.

Based on the diagnosis, the patient is treated for that disease. Treatment may be rendered at the level of the provisional diagnosis, with modifications rendered after a final diagnosis is determined. Based on the diagnosis and response to treatment which includes follow-up, a prognosis can be made. Prognosis is a forecast of the outcome of the disease and the prospect of recovery based on the nature and symptoms of the case. The prognosis for recurrent aphthous stomatitis is fair to excellent depending on whether the patient gets the ulcers every week or every 2 years. For a carcinoma of the tongue, the prognosis depends on the size, histology, condition and age of the patient, metastases, and staging. It is guarded and spoken of in 5-year increments. A 5-year survival would be good, because half of these patients may die before 5 years have passed.

After a diagnosis is made it must be

communicated either to the record or to another person or practitioner. The language used to describe the lesion(s) is that presented in Chapter 6.

Case Study One

Following is an example of a case presentation for differential diagnosis, final diagnosis, treatment, and follow-up.

A 37-year-old sailor was in the dental office for a dental hygiene appointment. On examination, a white lesion—diffuse, slightly raised, and corrugated—was noted on the mucosal aspect of the left lower lip (Fig. 9.1). It was asymptomatic, and the patient did not known how long it had been present. On further examination, it was noted that the patient was edentulous on the left lower mandible behind the cuspid; that the lower anterior teeth had attrition; and that there was recession with brown staining of the labial surface of the cuspid. He had no replacement prosthesis. His history was significant in that he had used smokeless tobacco for more than 20 years and held it in the vestibule at the site of the lesion. He also smoked cigarettes occasionally and liked to drink beer, usually a six-pack. He was otherwise healthy and was not taking nor had he been taking any other drugs or medications. A petty officer in the Navy, he had spent much time at sea and was exposed to the sun frequently. Palpation of the stained area on the tooth revealed hard structure and no evidence of caries. Radiographs taken of the teeth in this area were within normal limits. The white lesion did not scrape away. The differential diagnosis was as follows:

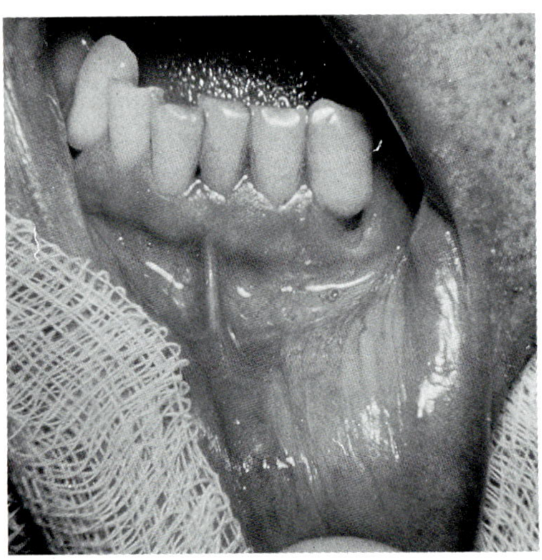

Figure 9.1. Asymptomatic leukoplakia in a 37-year-old male who used smokeless tobacco for more than 20 years.

1. Leukoplakia due to smokeless tobacco usage
   Benign hyperkeratosis
2. Leukoplakia with epithelial dysplasia
   Epithelial dysplasia with hyperkeratosis
3. Leukoplakia with carcinoma
   Epidermoid or squamous cell carcinoma with keratosis
4. Leukoplakia due to biting habit
   Benign hyperkeratosis
5. Lichen planus, keratotic, plaque type
6. Leukoedema, white sponge nevus
7. Candidiasis, keratotic type

Since the lip lesion was keratotic (it did not scrape away as in candidiasis or a pseudomembrane), the main clinical category to place it in is leukoplakia. Because it is impossible to know exactly what one is dealing with without the microscopic information, the various differential diagnoses encompass those possibilities of white keratotic lesions. Therefore, simple or benign hyperkeratosis would be the most probable, followed by the possibility of premalignancy (dysplasia) or malignancy (carcinoma may occur secondary to smokeless tobacco usage). Because trauma is responsible for most oral lesions, that possibility is listed and can be ruled in or out by careful history and observation of the patient. Lip biting can produce a leukoplakia. Lichen planus is listed because it may have a plaque variety. However, it usually occurs in females, and the most common location is the buccal mucosa, usually with a lace-like pattern. It would also have a distinctive microscopic pattern. Leukoedema is usually seen on the buccal mucosa and tends to disappear on stretching the tissue. That did not happen in this instance, but the white lesion does look shiny and wet like leukoedema, and it is listed low in the list of possibilities. It, too, would have specific microscopy. White sponge nevus is hereditary and would usually appear bilaterally and in other family members. Finally, candidiasis has many patterns clinically, the most common being whitened lesions on a reddened mucosa. Scraping away part of the lesion is helpful, and a smear can be done. In this instance, scraping led us away from candidiasis, but since this disease may have a keratotic variety, it was included and the organisms could be seen or stained for in a biopsy.

To find out more exactly what this can be, a biopsy is needed. Even the number one working diagnosis of leukoplakia due to smokeless tobacco would show changes microscopically that are indicative of the entity.

A letter of referral would be written to the dentist or specialist who will take the biopsy. For example:

Re: Mr. Seaman

Dear Dr. Good:

Mr. Seaman is a 37-year-old male who presented to this office for a regular cleaning and examination appointment. He has a white, keratotic, slightly raised and diffuse lesion on the mucosa of his lower lip opposite the incisor, lateral, and canine. The duration is unknown, but he has a history of holding smokeless tobacco in this area during the past 20 years. My provisional diagnosis is leukoplakia—benign hyperkeratosis secondary to the smokeless tobacco versus other types of leukoplakia. I would like the lesion to be biopsied, preferably incisional, to find out exactly what this represents.

Please perform an incisional biopsy of the lower lip lesion, send a copy of the biopsy report to this office, and return the patient here for follow-up care and treatment.

Sincerely,

The biopsy was performed, and the report indicated that there was simple hyperkeratosis with acanthosis, almost no inflammation, and atrophy with fibrosis of the mucous glands, all consistent with snuff-dipper's lesion. There was no evidence of premalignant or malignant changes.

Final diagnosis: Snuff-dipper's leukoplakia, benign hyperkeratosis.

The treatment would consist of speaking to and advising the patient of the effect of the smokeless tobacco on his tissues. If he can be convinced to stop the habit, the white lesion will disappear in 2 to 3 weeks.

Further discussion: The biopsy in this case was most helpful, because the microscopic pattern could rule out the other entities. Should the biopsy have been equivocal, other testing could have been ordered, depending on the value of the test. For example, special staining, immunohistochemistry, and elcctronmicroscopy may offer clues to the definitive diagnosis.

Case Study Two

The following case is presented to show the diversity of possibilities based on a single radiograph. Over the years, I have compiled cases that are like this, and therefore I offer them as a differential diagnosis. Because the radiograph immediately brings to mind a lateral periodontal cyst, this differential is for those lesions mimicking a lateral periodontal cyst.

A 21-year-old female presented to the dental office for routine care. A slight swelling of the buccal gingiva was noted on the mandibular left side between the canine and the first premolar. The lesion was asymptomatic, and the tooth was slightly mobile. A radiograph was taken and revealed a round to oval radiolucency in the superior portion of the alveolar bone between the canine and premolar (Fig. 9.2). The differential diagnosis was as follows:

1. Lateral periodontal cyst
2. Keratocyst (These can mimic many cysts.)
3. Gingival cyst (Causing pressure resorption of labial bone.)
4. Odontogenic tumor
   Squamous odontogenic (Can mimic a lateral perio cyst.)
   Adenomatoid odontogenic (Can appear other than maxilla and occurs in this age range.)
5. Normal
   Osteoporotic marrow defect of bone in anemic female
   Labial bone defect (Like Stafne's but on labial surface.)
6. Fibro-osseous—ossifying fibroma, fibrous dysplasia
7. Malignant tumor
   Fibrosarcoma (Rapid presentation of swollen gingiva causing pressure atrophy on bone or starting in bone.)
8. Central giant cell granuloma
9. Eosinophilic granuloma (Can present as loose tooth and punched-out lesion in bone.)
10. Central neurogenic tumor—neurilemmoma

Any of these conditions could be confirmed by biopsy to yield the final diagnosis. Treatment varies depending on the disease or condition. There are many examples of lesions listed like a differential diagnosis in several tables in this book. Appendix D is a listing of common oral lesions listed in a differential way. It is also a list of those entities commonly questioned on dental hygiene regional boards and may prove helpful to the student as a study guide. Other appendices offer information that may help in gathering data for a diagnosis and serve as references for some common baseline data.

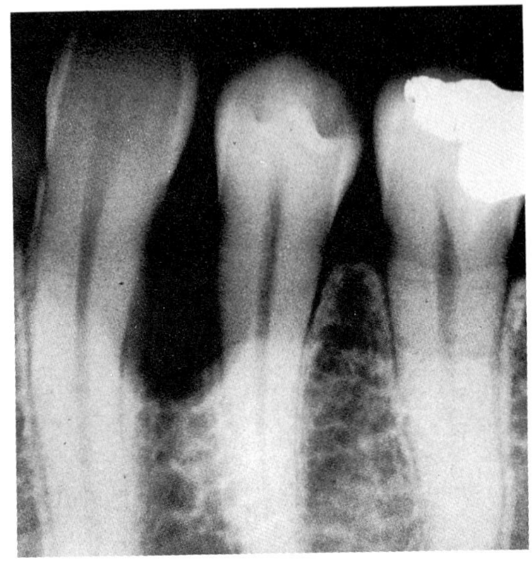

Figure 9.2. Asymptomatic radiolucency between the mandibular canine and first premolar in a 21-year-old female with a slight gingival swelling.

Bibliography

1. Bhaskar SN. Synopsis of oral pathology. 7th ed. St. Louis: CV Mosby, 1986.
2. Golden A, Powell D. Pathology—understanding human disease. 2nd ed. Baltimore: Williams & Wilkins, 1985.
3. Hill RB, LaVia MF. Principles of pathobiology. 3rd ed. New York: Oxford University Press, 1980.
4. Kerr DA, Ash M. Oral pathology: an introduction to general and oral pathology for hygienists. 5th ed. Philadelphia: Lea & Febiger, 1986.
5. Pindborg JJ. Pathology of the dental hard tissues. Philadelphia: WB Saunders, 1970.
6. Pindborg JJ. Atlas of diseases of the oral mucosa. 4th ed. Philadelphia: WB Saunders, 1986.
7. Robbins SL, Kumar V. Basic pathology. 4th ed. Philadelphia: WB Saunders, 1987.
8. Robinson HBG, Miller AS. Colby, Kerr and Robinson's color atlas of oral pathology. 4th ed. Philadelphia: JB Lippincott, 1983.
9. Shafer WG, Hine MK, Levy BM, Tomich CE. A textbook of oral pathology. 4th ed. Philadelphia: WB Saunders, 1983.
10. Shklar G. Oral cancer. The diagnosis, therapy, management and rehabilitation of the oral cancer patient. Philadelphia: WB Saunders, 1984.
11. Shklar G, McCarthy P. Oral manifestations of systemic disease. Boston: Butterworths, 1976.
12. Tortora GJ, Anagnostakos NP. Principles of anatomy and physiology. 5th ed. New York: Harper & Row, 1987.
13. Wilkins EM. Clinical practice of the dental hygienist. 6th ed. Philadelphia: Lea & Febiger, 1989.
14. Wood NK, Goaz PW. Differential diagnosis of oral lesions. 3rd ed. St. Louis: CV Mosby, 1985.
15. Young WG, Sedano HO. Atlas of oral pathology. Minneapolis: University of Minnesota Press, 1981.

Appendix A

Table A.1.
Chronology of permanent dentition listed in order of eruption

Teeth	1st Evidence Calcification	Enamel Completed	Eruption
1. First molar			
Mandibular	At birth	2¼-3 yr	6-7 yr
Maxillary	At birth	3-4 yr	6 yr
2. Mandibular incisors			
Central	3-4 mo	4-5 yr	6-7 yr
Lateral	3-4 mo	4-5 yr	7-8 yr
3. Maxillary incisor			
Central	3-4 mo	4-5 yr	7-8 yr
4. Maxillary incisor			
Lateral	1 yr	4-5 yr	8-9 yr
5. Mandibular canine	4-5 mo	6-7 yr	9-10 yr
6. First premolars			
Mandibular	1¼-2 yr	5-6 yr	10-12 yr
Maxillary	1½-1¾ yr	5-6 yr	10-11 yr
7. Second premolars			
Maxillary	2-2¼ yr	6-7 yr	10-12 yr
Mandibular	2¼-2½ yr	6-7 yr	11-12 yr
8. Maxillary canine	4-5 mo	6-7 yr	11-12 yr
9. Second molars			
Mandibular	2½-3 yr	7-8 yr	11-13 yr
Maxillary	2½-3 yr	7-8 yr	12-13 yr
10. Third molars			
Maxillary	7-9 yr	12-13 yr	17-21 yr
Mandibular	8-10 yr	12-16 yr	17-21 yr

The roots are completely formed generally 2 to 2½ years after eruption. The mandibular teeth generally precede the maxillary teeth in order of eruption.

Table A.2.
Chronology of deciduous teeth listed in order of eruption

Teeth	1st Evidence Calcification (In Utero)	Enamel Completed (After Birth)	Eruption
1. Central incisors			
Mandibular	14 wk	2½ mo	6½ mo
Maxillary	14 wk	1½ mo	7½ mo
2. Lateral incisors			
Mandibular	16 wk	3 mo	7 mo
Maxillary	16 wk	2½ mo	8 mo
3. First molars	15½ wk	5½-6 mo	14 mo
4. Canines	17 wk	9 mo	18 mo
5. Second molars	18-19 wk	10-11 mo	24 mo

The mandibular teeth generally erupt before the maxillary and girls' teeth generally erupt later than boys' teeth. By 7 years, there is a mixed deciduous and permanent dentition until age 12. The roots are completed generally 1 to 1½ years after eruption. The deciduous teeth begin their development at 4 to 5 weeks in utero.

Appendix B

Table B.1.
Normal Values for Selected Blood Tests

Test	Normal Value
Bleeding time	4-8 minutes
Blood urea nitrogen	8-23 mg/dl
Calcium (Ca++)	Adults: 4.3-5.3 mEq/L Children: 6 mEq/L
Cholesterol	
Total	150-250 mg/dl
HDL	29-77 mg/dl
LDL	62-185 mg/dl
VLDL	0-40 mg/dl
Clotting (coagulation) time	5-10 minutes
Glucose	70-110 mg/dl
Hemoglobin	Male: 14-16.5 g/100 ml Female: 12-15 g/100 ml Newborn: 14-20 g/100 ml
Hematocrit	Male: 40-54% Female: 38-47%
Iron, total	60-150 μg/dl
pH	Arterial: 7.35-7.45
Phosphorus	Adult: 1.8-4.1 mEq/L
Platelet count	250,000-400,000/mm
Prothrombin time	11-15 seconds
Red blood cell count, differential	
Neutrophils	60-70%
Lymphocytes	20-25%
Monocytes	3-8%
Eosinophils	2-4%
Basophils	0.5-1%
Total count	5,000-9,000/mm

After Tortora GJ, Anagnostakos NP. Principles of anatomy and physiology. 5th ed. New York: Harper & Row, 1987.

Appendix C

Table C.1.
Serodiagnostic tests for hepatitis B and their clinical significance

HBs Antigen	HBs Antibody	HBe Antigen	HBe Antibody	HBc Antibody	Clinical Status
−	−	−	−	−	No exposure to the virus
−	+	−	−	+	Previous exposure; patient immune to HBV
+	−	−	+ or −	+ or −	Chronic carrier, chronic hepatitis, cirrhosis, and/or liver cancer
+	−	+	−	+ or −	Highly infective carrier, acute severe hepatitis

Appendix D

This is a compilation of common oral lesions listed by differential diagnoses according to the predominant color or other clinical feature. These entities are commonly used in Dental Hygiene Regional Boards.

Structures mistaken for disease

- Tissue tags
- Fordyce granules
- Tonsils—accessory, lateral
- Circumvallate papillae
- Papilla of Stenson's duct
- Linea alba—bite line
- Varicosities
- Tori
- Retrocuspid papillae
- Fungiform papillae
- Edentulous floor of mouth

Developmental

- Cleft lip
- Cleft palate
- Torus, exostosis
- Macrognathia, micrognathia
- Malocclusion
  - Angle class 1, 2, 3
  - Anterior open bite
    - Mamelons
- Tooth related
  - Dilaceration
  - Dens in dente
  - Gemination
  - Fusion
  - Concrescence
  - Supernumerary

Tooth and tooth related

- Dental caries
- Periapical disease
  - Periapical granuloma
  - Periapical cyst
  - Periapical abscess
  - Condensing osteitis
  - Periapical cemental dysplasia
  - Acute dentoalveolar abscess
  - Chronic dentoalveolar abscess
- Discolorations and stains
  - Tetracycline
  - Fluorosis
  - Hemosiderin
  - Plaque
  - Hereditary
    - Dentinogenesis imperfecta
    - Amelogenesis imperfecta
  - Others (see Table 7.4)
- Malocclusion
  - Craniodental
  - Dentodental
  - Bruxism
  - TM dysfunction
  - Tongue thrusting
- Pulpitis
- Noncarious tooth destruction
  - Enamel hypoplasia
    - Systemic
    - Turner's
  - Attrition
  - Erosion
  - External root resorption
  - Internal root resorption
- Trauma
  - Tooth fracture
  - Jaw fracture
  - Jaw discoloration
  - Avulsed tooth

Periodontal (gingival)

- Gingivitis (see Table 8.1)
  - Localized
  - Systemic
- Hyperplastic gingivitis
  - Hormonal
  - Dilantin
  - Allergy (see Table 8.1)
- Epulides (gingival swelling) (inflammatory hyperplasias)
  - Pyogenic granuloma
  - Peripheral giant cell granuloma
  - Peripheral fibroma
  - Peripheral ossifying fibroma
  - Hemangioma
  - Parulis, gum boil
- Gingival infections
  - Primary herpetic gingivostomatitis
  - Recurrent herpes, intraoral, labial
  - Acute necrotizing gingivitis ANUG
- Periodontitis
  - Localized
  - Systemic
    - Periodontosis
    - Eosinophilic granuloma
    - Neoplastic
      - Benign odontogenic
      - Malignant
        - Localized
        - Metastatic
- Gingival cysts of newborn, Epstein's eruption

Mucosal lesions

- Ulcerations
  - Traumatic—mechanical, thermal, chemical, factitial, iatrogenic
  - Aphthous stomatitis
  - Herpetiform—herpes infections
  - carcinoma
  - Systemic—anemia, etc.
- Tongue
  - Fissured tongue
  - Geographic tongue
    - Stomatitis migrans
  - Median rhomboid glossitis
  - (Central papillary atrophy)
  - Macroglossia (see Table 8.1)
  - White, black hairy tongue
  - Ankyloglossia
- White lesions (see Table 6.2)
  - Leukoplakia—simple keratosis, dysplasia, carcinoma
  - Nicotinic stomatitis, snuff-dipper lesion
  - Lichen planus
  - Leukoedema
  - Pseudomembranous, desquamative
  - Candidiasis
  - Allergy
- Yellow lesions
  - Fordyce (ectopic sebaceous)
  - Bacterial plug
  - Pseudocyst of tonsil
  - Abscess
  - Buccal fat pad
  - Lipoma
- Benign tumors
  - Fibroma
  - Papilloma
  - Neurogenic, neuroma, neurofibroma
  - Lipoma
- Traumatic
  - Chemical (aspirin burn)
  - Denture-related
    - Epulis fissuratum
    - Inflammatory papillary hyperplasia
    - Atrophic glossitis
- Pigmented—blood-related
  - Hemangioma
  - Hematoma
  - Varicosity
  - Aneurysm
  - Telangiectasias
  - Eruption cyst
- Pigmented—nonblood-related (see Table 7.3)
  - Melanotic—macule, nevus, melanoma
  - Amalgam tattoo
  - Mucocele
- Red lesions
  - Trauma, iatrogenic
  - Allergy
  - Infections
  - Candidiasis
  - Erosive lichen planus
  - Systemic xerostomia, deficiency states
  - Neoplastic, carcinoma erythroplasia
- Blistering lesions
  - Herpetic infections
  - Allergy
  - Erythema multiforme
  - Mucous membrane pemphigoid
  - Pemphigus vulgaris
- Malignant tumors
  - Epidermoid carcinoma
  - Metastatic cancers
  - Salivary gland
  - Sarcomas
  - Melanomas
  - Basal cell carcinoma

Odontogenic cysts

- Periapical cyst
- Residual cyst
- Keratocyst
- Dentigerous
- Lateral periodontal

Nonodontogenic cysts

- Nasopalatine duct cyst
- Midline cyst
- Dermoid cyst
- Thyroglossal duct cyst
- Lymphoepithelial

Parotid swelling

- Mumps
- Recurrent parotitis
- Sjögren's syndrome
- Salivary tumor, pleomorphic adenoma
- Metastatic tumor
- Granulomatous disease (tuberculosis)

Odontogenic tumors

- Odontoma
- Ameloblastoma
- Ameloblastic fibroma
- Adenomatoid odontogenic
- Cementoma

Noncysts

- Stafne's defect
- Traumatic bone "cyst"
- Marrow defect
- Normal structure
- Eosinophilic granuloma

Neck mass or swelling

- Lateral or midline cyst
- Swollen lymph node(s)
  - Inflammatory
  - Neoplastic
    - Metastatic
    - Primary
- Lipoma
- Sebaceous cyst

Manifestations of systemic disease (see Table 8.1)

- Cheilitis
- Glossitis
- Gingivitis
- Macroglossia

Besides the foregoing, the regional boards frequently question the following:

Radiographic

- Nasal spine
- Incisive canal
- Floor of nose
- Hamulus
- Inferior border, mandible
- Calculus
- Tori, exostoses
- Missing bicuspids
- Artifacts
- Nasal septum
- Nutrient canal(s)
- Genial tubercle
- Maxillary tuberosity
- Double-rooted canine, premolar
- Impacted tooth
- Odontoma
- Defective margin
- Static electricity
- Median suture
- Maxillary sinus
- Coronoid process
- Mental foramen
- Age of patient, eruption pattern
- Hypercementosis
- Double exposure
- Type of restoration

Proper versus improper angulation for exposure

Other

- Proper versus improper position of periodontal probe
- Early loss of deciduous teeth
- Supereruption due to loss of opposing teeth
- Some laboratory values

Index

The letter f *following a page number indicates a figure; the letter* t *indicates a table.*